Humanitarian Reason

Humanitarian Reason

A Moral History of the Present

DIDIER FASSIN

Translated by Rachel Gomme

University of California Press

BERKELEY   LOS ANGELES   LONDON

University of California Press, one of the most distinguished
university presses in the United States, enriches lives around the world
by advancing scholarship in the humanities, social sciences, and natural
sciences. Its activities are supported by the UC Press Foundation and
by philanthropic contributions from individuals and institutions. For
more information, visit www.ucpress.edu.

University of California Press
Berkeley and Los Angeles, California

University of California Press, Ltd.
London, England

Originally published in French as *La Raison humanitaire. Une histoire
morale du temps présent*, Hautes Etudes–Gallimard–Seuil, 2010.

Library of Congress Cataloging-in-Publication Data

Fassin, Didier.
  [Raison humanitaire. English]
  Humanitarian reason : a moral history of the present / Didier Fassin ;
translated by Rachel Gomme.
    p.   cm.
  Includes bibliographical references and index.
  ISBN 978-0-520-27116-6 (cloth : alk. paper)
  ISBN 978-0-520-27117-3 (pbk. : alk. paper)
  1. Humanitarian assistance—Moral and ethical aspects.
  2. International relief—Moral and ethical aspects.   I. Title.
  HV553.F3713   2011
  174'.9361—dc22

                                                      2011011327

Manufactured in the United States of America

20 19 18 17 16 15 14 13 12 11
10 9 8 7 6 5 4 3 2 1

In keeping with a commitment to support environmentally responsible
and sustainable printing practices, UC Press has printed this book on
Rolland Enviro100, a 100% post-consumer fiber paper that is FSC
certified, deinked, processed chlorine-free, and manufactured with
renewable biogas energy. It is acid-free and EcoLogo certified.

To my parents

Contents

Preface to the English Edition

In the aftermath of the 2004 tsunami in Southeast Asia, Clifford Geertz commented with melancholy, in the *New York Review of Books* on March 24 of the following year, that "fatality on such a scale, the destruction not only of individual lives but of whole populations of them, threatens the conviction that perhaps most reconciles many of us, insofar as anything this-worldly does, to our own mortality: that, though we ourselves may perish, the community into which we were born, and the sort of lives it supports, will somehow live on." One could extend this profound insight by suggesting that the significance of such a fatality is not only about our mourning of a possibly lost world, of which all traces may even disappear; it is also about our sense of belonging to a wider moral community, whose existence is manifested through compassion toward the victims. For the attentive observer of the tsunami, the impressive magnitude of the toll, with its tens of thousands of casualties, was as meaningful as the unparalleled deployment of solidarity, with its billions of dollars of aid. We lamented their dead but celebrated our generosity. The power of this event resides in the rare combination of the tragedy of ruination and the pathos of assistance. Such disasters now form part of our experience of this-worldliness, just as do aid organizations, relief operations, and humanitarian interventions. We have become used to the global spectacle of suffering and the global display of succor. The moral landscape thus outlined can be called humanitarianism. Although it is generally taken for granted as a mere expansion of a supposed natural humaneness that would be innately associated with our being human, humanitarianism is a relatively recent invention, which raises complex ethical and political issues. This book is about this invention and its complications.

Humanitarianism has become familiar through catastrophic events, the images of which have been disseminated by the media, but it has also to do with more ordinary situations closer to us. Indeed, it is a mode of governing that concerns the victims of poverty, homelessness, unemployment, and exile, as well as of disasters, famines, epidemics, and wars—in short, every situation characterized by precariousness. It involves nongovernmental organizations, international agencies, states, and individuals. It mobilizes sympathy and technology, physicians and logisticians. Its sites of action are clinics for the poor and refugee camps, a social administration where undocumented immigrants are received and a military garrison where earthquake victims are treated. The case studies I have brought together here represent an attempt to account for this government of the precarious in its diversity during the past two decades. The first part involves policies and actors in France, the second explores scenes from South Africa, Venezuela, Palestine, and Iraq, with a transition following the transnational circulation between the Third World and Europe. This assemblage poses two questions.

First, how specific is the French case? It is true that important humanitarian organizations were founded in France, that French governments often included secretaries for humanitarian affairs, and that France played a prominent role in the promotion of humanitarian policies within international institutions, including the United Nations. It is obvious too that France has a long history of private charitable works emanating from Christian orders as well as public solidarity policies translated into social security, state medical aid, and most recently universal medical coverage, all elements that have resulted in a relatively distinct set of shared political and moral values. There is thus definitely a singularity of the French relationship with humanitarianism. However, the phenomena I describe and analyze in the case studies extend beyond the national boundaries in which they are inscribed. The tensions between compassion and repression, the problems posed by the mobilization of empathy rather than the recognition of rights, the prejudices toward the dominated and their consequences regarding the way to treat them have a high degree of generality that make them relevant in various contexts. Configurations may be different, but processes are similar.

Second, how coherent is the arrangement of such diverse geographical cases? The initial series of cases was situated in France and concerns its management of the disadvantaged, while South Africa, Venezuela, and Palestine yield three paradigmatic humanitarian scenes—that is, respectively, epidemics, disasters, and conflicts—with the final study illustrating the ambiguous links between aid workers and armed forces in military interventions such as in Iraq. The central hypothesis that holds these various worlds together is that they are inscribed in the same humanitarian governing process, whether it deals with the poor and the undocumented in the North or AIDS orphans and flood victims in the South, with comparable moral categorizations and judgments, analogous developments of moral communities and exclusions, and equivalent consequences in terms of negation of voices and histories. Examining these distant scenes through the same lens is indispensable to comprehending the larger issues at stake in our moral economies.

The argument of this book is therefore that humanitarianism has become a potent force of our world. Its dissemination is so widespread that the tears shed by the Chinese prime minister over the devastation of the province of Sichuan increased his popularity, just as the apparent indifference of the president of the United States to the tragic consequences of Hurricane Katrina demonstrated the emptiness of his campaign slogan of compassionate conservatism. Its invocation is so powerful that it can serve as grounds for military action, allegedly to protect endangered populations, sometimes foregoing alternative options as in Kosovo or forging evidence as in Kuwait, or can even be used, as in the case of Augusto Pinochet in Britain and Maurice Papon in France, to exempt individuals accused or convicted of crimes against humanity from facing justice and punishment. It is this global and yet uneven force that I attempt to analyze here.

The year 2010 began with the dreadful earthquake in Haiti, which precipitated a remarkable mobilization worldwide, particularly from France and the United States. We witnessed in fact a competition between the two countries, whose governments and populations rivaled each other in solicitude toward the victims, bounteously sending troops, physicians, goods, and money, while raising the suspicion of the pursuit of goals other than pure benevolence toward a nation that was successively oppressed by the former and exploited by the latter. This emulation was certainly triggered by goodwill, and one should not minimize the altruistic engagement and charitable efforts of individuals, organizations, churches, and even governments involved in the treatment of the injured and later in the reconstruction efforts. Yet one cannot avoid thinking how rewarding was this generosity. For a fleeting moment we had the illusion that we shared a common human condition. We could forget that only 6% of Haitian asylum seekers are granted the status of refugee in France, representing one of the lowest national rates, far behind those coming from apparently peaceful countries, or that thirty thousand Haitians were on the deportation lists of the U.S.

Immigration and Customs Enforcement Agency. The cataclysm seemed to erase the memories of the French and subsequent American exploitation of the island. Our response to it signified the promise of reparation and the hope for reconciliation.

In contemporary societies, where inequalities have reached an unprecedented level, humanitarianism elicits the fantasy of a global moral community that may still be viable and the expectation that solidarity may have redeeming powers. This secular imaginary of communion and redemption implies a sudden awareness of the fundamentally unequal human condition and an ethical necessity to not remain passive about it in the name of solidarity—however ephemeral this awareness is, and whatever limited impact this necessity has. Humanitarianism has this remarkable capacity: it fugaciously and illusorily bridges the contradictions of our world, and makes the intolerableness of its injustices somewhat bearable. Hence, its consensual force.

This morally driven, politically ambiguous, and deeply paradoxical strength of the weak I propose to call humanitarian reason.

Princeton, December 8, 2010

Acknowledgments

The studies on which the chapters of this book are based were supported by research funding from the Institut National de la Santé et de la Recherche Médicale (National Institute for Health and Medical Research, INSERM) (listening centers), the Ministère des Affaires sociales (French Ministry of Social Affairs, Research Program on Exclusion) (emergency aid for the unemployed), the Centre National de la Recherche Scientifique (National Scientific Research Center, CNRS) (legalization of undocumented immigrants), the Ministère de la Recherche (French Ministry of Research, ACI 3T) (recognition of asylum seekers), the Agence Nationale de la Recherche (National Research Agency, ANR) (immigration policy), the Agence Nationale de la Recherche sur le Sida et les Hépatites (National AIDS and Hepatitis Research Agency, ANRS) (AIDS in South Africa), Ecos-Nord (French–Latin American Scientific Cooperation Program) (disaster in Venezuela), and the Mission Recherche Expérimentation (Research Unit of the Ministry of Health, MiRe) (psychic trauma in Palestine). The research on humanitarianism was not funded by specific grants but was made possible by the organizations that opened their doors to me (particularly Médecins Sans Frontières and Médecins du Monde). The writing up was supported by a grant from the European Research Council for a project titled "Towards a Critical Moral Anthropology" and benefited, in its ultimate phase, from the serene environment of the School of Social Science at the Institute for Advanced Study in Princeton. I am grateful to these institutions for their support.

The chapters that make up this book are fully rewritten versions of previously published articles. In revising these texts, I have sought to bring a greater level of consistency to the whole, to remove a number of repetitions, to update data, and finally to correct some analyses. Several of the articles are partially altered; others are unpublished texts freely inspired by a previous article:

Chapter 1: "Souffrir par le social, gouverner par l'écoute: Une configuration sémantique de l'action publique," *Politix*, 2006, 19 (73): 137–158.

Chapter 2: "Charité bien ordonnée: Principes de justice et pratiques de jugement dans l'attribution des aides d'urgence," *Revue française de sociologie*, 2001, 42 (3): 437–475.

Chapter 3: "Quand le corps fait loi: La raison humanitaire dans les procédures de régularisation des étrangers," *Sciences sociales et santé*, 2001, 19 (4): 5–34.

Chapter 4: "The Truth from the Body: Medical Certificates as Ultimate Evidence for Asylum Seekers" (with Estelle d'Halluin), *American Anthropologist*, 2005, 107 (4): 597–608.

Chapter 5: "Compassion and Repression: The Moral Economy of Immigration Policies in France," *Cultural Anthropology*, 2005, 20 (3): 362–387.

Chapter 6: "Suffering Children, Abused Babies, and AIDS Orphans: The Moral Construction of Childhood in South Africa," in *Healing the World's Children: Interdisciplinary Perspectives on Health in the Twentieth Century*, ed. C. Comacchio, J. Golden, and G. Weisz (Montreal: McGill-Queen's University Press, 2008), 111–124.

Chapter 7: "Humanitarian Exception as the Rule: The Political Theology of the 1999 'Tragedia' in Venezuela" (with Paula Vasquez), *American Ethnologist*, 2005, 32 (3): 389–405.

Chapter 8: "The Humanitarian Politics of Testimony: Subjectification through Trauma in the Israeli-Palestinian Conflict," *Cultural Anthropology*, 2008, 23 (3): 531–558.

Chapter 9: "Humanitarianism as a Politics of Life," *Public Culture*, 2007, 19 (3): 499–520.

I am grateful to the respective publishers for their permission to reproduce these articles in this form somewhat disrespectful of the original. They have allowed me to bring coherence to pieces dispersed in different journals. The translation of the French manuscript was beautifully conducted by Rachel Gomme. The copyediting was meticulously undertaken by Linda Garat and Liz Smith. The comments by the two anonymous reviewers have been quite useful. The warm welcome of this project by

Naomi Schneider at the University of California Press demonstrated the same generosity that I received from Christophe Prochasson for the French version, which I had the privilege to publish in the series Hautes Études—Gallimard—Seuil, where Michel Foucault's lectures at the Collège de France have appeared, a company of critics of which I am happy to be part.

I would like to express my gratitude to those who, over the past ten years, have contributed to my reflection on moral economies through the exchanges we have shared: my students in seminars at the École des Hautes Études en Sciences Sociales; my doctoral students, with whom regular conversations about their work have certainly helped to build my own questioning; and my colleagues at the Institut de Recherche Interdisciplinaire sur les Enjeux Sociaux (Interdisciplinary Research Institute for Social Science, Iris), with whom I have had a continual interaction throughout the long period of writing this book. I would like to mention particularly my discussions with Alban Bensa, within the context of our workshop on the politics of ethnography; Éric Fassin, with whom I designed courses on new objects and new fields in anthropology; Richard Rechtman, who warmly encouraged me to complete this book; and Anne-Claire Defossez, for our ongoing conversation and common engagement. I am also grateful for the contributions, through meetings and discussions about some of these texts, of Athena Athanassiou, Jonathan Benthall, Michael Fischer, Thomas Lemke, Samuel Lézé, Margaret Lock, Vinh-Kim Nguyen, Mariella Pandolfi, Paul Rabinow, Peter Redfield, Nancy Scheper-Hughes, Ann Stoler, Mara Viveros, and especially Veena Das for our exchanges on the politics of suffering and João Biehl for our discussions in our course on ethnography and social theory at Princeton University. I should also mention the discussions following the presentation of some of the research brought together in this book at seminars and conferences in Paris, Toulouse, Marseilles, Athens, Montreal, New York, Princeton, Berkeley, Ann Arbor, Caracas, Buenos Aires, Johannesburg, and Hong Kong: as we all know, these often fleeting, sometimes contradictory moments of exchange can later, and often unknown to our interlocutors, prove decisive in the construction of our thinking and the formulation of our ideas.

Finally, of course, since I sought to base this anthropology of contemporary moral economies on an ethnography, none of what I have written would have been possible without the generosity of those who agreed to give me their time, supply me with documents, communicate their knowledge, and respond to the hypotheses I submitted to them. To respect the contract of anonymity and confidentiality that binds us, I have not named them where I quote from private interviews, but only when I cite extracts from their public statements or published texts. Decision makers, administrators, physicians, nurses, psychologists, social workers, members of humanitarian organizations, and also unemployed people, undocumented immigrants, asylum seekers, Venezuelan disaster victims, South African persons living with HIV/AIDS, all contributed their share to this book. They may disagree on some of my analyses, but I wish to assure them that I have endeavored to give equal value and credit to their words, even when my account is critical.

Introduction

Humanitarian Government

Everyone will readily agree that it is of the highest importance
to know whether we are not duped by morality.
EMMANUEL LEVINAS, *Totality and Infinity*

Moral sentiments have become an essential force in contemporary politics: they nourish its discourses and legitimize its practices, particularly
where these discourses and practices are focused on the disadvantaged and
the dominated, whether at home (the poor, the immigrants, the homeless)
or farther away (the victims of famine, epidemics, or war). By "moral sentiments" are meant the emotions that direct our attention to the suffering
of others and make us want to remedy them.[1] They link affects with values—
sensitivity with altruism—and some, indeed, derive the latter from the
former and morality from emotions: in this philosophical tradition, the
experience of empathy precedes the sense of good. Compassion represents
the most complete manifestation of this paradoxical combination of heart
and reason: the sympathy felt for the misfortune of one's neighbor generates the moral indignation that can prompt action to end it. Thus, encountering the man left for dead by robbers at the side of the road, the Good
Samaritan of the gospels is moved; he dresses his wounds, finds him lodging,
and pays for his care.[2] This parable inaugurates the paradigm of a politics
of compassion that feeds Western morality well beyond the domain of
Christian doctrine, which obviously has no monopoly on concern for the
misfortune of others, whether we consider the central role of compassion
in Confucianism and Buddhism or its translation as charity in Islamic and
Jewish traditions.

I will therefore use the expression "humanitarian government" to designate the deployment of moral sentiments in contemporary politics. "Government" here should be understood in a broad sense,[3] as the set of procedures established and actions conducted in order to manage, regulate, and
support the existence of human beings: government includes but exceeds
the intervention of the state, local administrations, international bodies,

and political institutions more generally. Similarly, "humanitarian" should be taken in an extended meaning,[4] as connoting both dimensions encompassed by the concept of humanity: on the one hand the generality of human beings who share a similar condition (mankind), and on the other an affective movement drawing humans toward their fellows (humaneness). The first dimension forms the basis for a demand for rights and an expectation of universality; the second creates the obligation to provide assistance and attention to others: once again we encounter the articulation between reason and emotion that defines moral sentiments. Thus the concept of humanitarian government goes beyond the usual definitions that restrict it to aid interventions in the Third World and mimetically correspond to the image presented by organizations that describe themselves as humanitarian. In fact, humanitarianism has become a language that inextricably links values and affects, and serves both to define and to justify discourses and practices of the government of human beings.

When a candidate in the French presidential election addressed "the France that suffers," he was using the same vocabulary of moral sentiments as his counterpart in the United States qualifying his own political program as "compassionate conservatism."[5] And when, under pressure from organizations providing support for undocumented immigrants, the French authorities granted residence to immigrants only on the condition that they were suffering from a serious illness that could not be treated in their home country, on the grounds of "humanitarian reason," they were using the same descriptor as the Western heads of state who called for the bombing of Kosovo as part of a military campaign they asserted was "purely humanitarian."[6] On both the national and the international levels, the vocabulary of suffering, compassion, assistance, and responsibility to protect forms part of our political life: it serves to qualify the issues involved and to reason about choices made.

It may be objected that there is often a form of cynicism at play when one deploys the language of moral sentiments at the same time as implementing policies that increase social inequality, measures that restrict the rights of immigrant populations, or military operations with essentially geostrategic goals—to take only the examples previously evoked. In this view, the language of humanitarianism would be no more than a smoke screen that plays on sentiment in order to impose the law of the market and the brutality of realpolitik. But even if this were the case, the question would remain: Why does it work so well? Thus, beyond the manifest bad faith of some and the good conscience of others—although the significance of these attitudes cannot be ignored on the level of what we might call an ethics of policy—we need to understand how this language has become established today as the most likely to generate support among listeners or readers, and to explain why people often prefer to speak about suffering and compassion than about interests or justice, legitimizing actions by declaring them to be humanitarian. In the contemporary world, the discourse of affects and values offers a high political return: this certainly needs to be analyzed.

A remarkable paradox deserves our attention here. On the one hand, moral sentiments are focused mainly on the poorest, most unfortunate, most vulnerable individuals: the politics of compassion is a politics of inequality.[7] On the other hand, the condition of possibility of moral sentiments is generally the recognition of others as fellows: the politics of compassion is a politics of solidarity.[8] This tension between inequality and solidarity, between a relation of domination and a relation of assistance, is constitutive of all humanitarian government. It explains the frequently observed ambivalence of authorities, of donors, and of agents working for the good of others, and it accounts for what has been called compassion fatigue, the wearing down of moral sentiments until they turn into indifference or even aggressiveness toward the victims of misfortune. But it also explains the shame felt by the poor, the beneficiaries of aid, all those who receive these gifts that call for no counter gift, and accounts for the resentment and even hostility sometimes expressed by the disadvantaged and the dominated toward those who think of themselves as their benefactors.[9] Many philosophers and moralists have striven to minimize this asymmetrical relationship of compassion, placing emphasis rather on the egalitarian dimension and attempting to give it the status of a founding emotion of human community: it is because we see the other as another self, they maintain, that we feel sympathy for him or her and act for his or her good.

However, the problem is not psychological or even ethical, as these writers suggest: it is strictly sociological.[10] It is not the condescension on the part of the persons giving aid or the intention of their act of assistance that are at stake, but the very conditions of the social relation between the two parties, which, whatever the goodwill of the agents, make compassion a moral sentiment with no possible reciprocity. It can of course be pointed out that the apparently disinterested gift assumes a counter gift in the form of an obligation linking the receiver to the benefactor—for example, the obligation on the receivers sometimes to tell their story, frequently to mend their ways, and always to show their gratitude. But it is clear that in these conditions the exchange remains profoundly unequal. And what is more, those at the receiving end of humanitarian attention know quite well that they are expected to show the humility of the beholden rather than express demands for rights.

Thus, if there is domination in the upsurge of compassion, it is objective before it is subjective (and it may not even become subjective). The asymmetry is political rather than psychological: a critique of compassion is necessary not because of the attitude of superiority it implies but because it always presupposes a relation of inequality. Humanitarian reason governs precarious lives:[11] the lives of the unemployed and the asylum seekers, the lives of sick immigrants and people with AIDS, the lives of disaster victims and victims of conflict—threatened and forgotten lives that humanitarian government brings into existence by protecting and revealing them. When compassion is exercised in the public space, it is therefore always directed from above to below, from the more powerful to the weaker, the more fragile, the more vulnerable—those who can generally be constituted as victims of an overwhelming fate. The concept of precarious lives therefore needs to be taken in the strongest sense of its Latin etymology:[12] lives that are not guaranteed but bestowed in answer to prayer, or in other words are defined not in the absolute of a condition, but in the relation to those who have power over them. Humanitarian government is indeed a politics of precarious lives.

This politics, which brings into play states and nongovernmental organizations, international bodies and local communities, has a history. This is not the place to retrace it, but it is worth underlining its dual temporality. The first, long-term temporality relates to the emergence of moral sentiments in philosophical reflection, and subsequently in common sense, in Western societies from the eighteenth century onward.[13] Modern identity is indissociable from the conjunction of affects and values that regulate conducts and emotions toward others and define a respect for human life and dignity.[14] The abolitionist movement, which fought slavery in Britain, France, and the United States, is often presented, in spite of its contradictions, as the epitome of this initial crystallization of moral sentiments in politics.[15] By contrast, emotional pleas and even military interventions to defend endangered populations, starting with the British, French, and Russian mobilization in favor of the Greek Revolution in the 1820s, have received little attention until recently.[16] The second, short-term temporality relates to the articulation of these moral sentiments in the public space, and even more specifically in political action, at the end of the twentieth century: while one cannot put a precise date on this phenomenon, one may note the convergence of a set of elements over the past two decades, including the creation of humanitarian organizations (which invoke a right or duty to intervene), the establishment of ministries of humanitarian assistance (in several French governments but also in other countries), and the description of conflicts as humanitarian crises (which then justifies military intervention under the same banner), to which should be added the proliferation of measures and initiatives designed to aid the poor, the unemployed, the homeless, the sick without social protection, immigrants without residence rights, and applicants for refugee status—measures and initiatives defined explicitly or implicitly as humanitarian.[17] The first temporality provides the genealogical framework for the second.

It is the latter that I am principally interested in here—the recent constitution of a humanitarian government. My aim is to offer a clear account of the reconfiguration of what can be called the politics of precarious lives over the past few decades: the studies presented here essentially relate to measures, initiatives, and forms of government (whether governmental or nongovernmental) that have been brought into operation, at the end of the twentieth and beginning of the twenty-first centuries, to manage populations and individuals faced with situations of inequality, contexts of violence, and experiences of suffering. Obviously I am not arguing that compassion is a recent invention, although it should be recognized that some historical periods, including the one under study, are more conducive to sentimentality than others. Nor do I hold that the shift that has begun is irreversible, for nothing is more unstable and revocable than the sentiment of compassion in politics, as can be viewed with the rise of the sentiment of fear related to the rhetoric of security in the first decade of the twenty-first century. Nor, finally, am I suggesting that the advent of compassion excludes other phenomena, for the social body is continually pulled by contradictory logics, particularly that of repression in the case of precarious lives. Of these multiple tensions, the case studies of this volume will provide many examples. My goal is simply to grasp the specific issues involved in the deployment of humanitarian reason in the contemporary public space and to understand how moral sentiments have recently reconfigured politics.

The social sciences themselves are not absent from the developments I am considering here. The 1990s were remarkable for the increasing importance, on both sides of the Atlantic, of what we might term a scientific literature of compassion—a body of writing relating to suffering, trauma, misfortune, poverty, and exclusion. Interestingly, two distinct intellectual geographies can be drawn. In France, the disciplines most involved are sociology and psychology. In the United States, this concern is above all the domain of literary criticism and medical anthropology.[18] Several of these publications were the result of major research programs and have been financially supported by French public and semipublic organizations and American private foundations and nonprofit institutions, respectively. In France, the grant made available by the Caisse des Dépôts et Consignations, a national savings and investment bank, for a series of studies on minor and major adversities among various social categories, from the young immigrant to the police officer, has produced the best-selling sociology book in a decade; in the United States, the Social Science Research Council has funded a series of seminars and publications on political and structural violence, from South Africa to Sri Lanka, which has had a marked influence on the scientific field in North America and beyond.[19] Thus a specular dynamic has developed whereby public bodies and private groups produce representations of the world, and the social sciences give them the authority of their theoretical reflection and the substance of their empirical research. Legitimized by politicians as well as scientists, this view is consolidated and gradually comes to be assumed as self-evident. Inequality is replaced by exclusion, domination is transformed into misfortune, injustice is articulated as suffering, violence is expressed in terms of trauma. While the old vocabulary of social critique has certainly not entirely disappeared, the new lexicon of moral sentiments tends to mask it in a process of semantic sedimentation that has perceptible effects both in public action and in individual practices, although the influence on policies and more generally on society of this scientific literature and these intellectual stances is probably greater in France than in the United States.[20] The translation of social reality into the new language of compassion is thus mirrored by a sort of epistemological, but also emotional, conversion of researchers and intellectuals to this approach to society, more sensitive to the subjectivity of agents and to the experience of pain and affliction. Studies, research programs, and scientific publications have proliferated. Within a few years, exclusion and misfortune, suffering and trauma have become commonplaces of the social sciences, lending academic credit to the new political discourse.

This novel account of the world has largely been taken for granted. Many have adopted the view that it simply reflected changes in society: people spoke more often about the excluded because there were more of them, and about suffering because its prevalence had increased; doctors and nurses, and even armies, were being dispatched to aid populations that were victims of war or disaster because our world had become more generous. Some, indeed, welcomed this development, seeing it as a sign of moral progress: in their view, public authorities and nongovernmental organizations, trade unionists and politicians, journalists and researchers were finally showing greater humanity and had more understanding of the plight of ordinary people. Others, however, derided or waxed indignant about what they interpreted as a drift toward sentimentalism, suggesting that we all now consider ourselves as victims, in a sort of frantic race to expose our misfortunes, have our pain recognized, and even claim compensation.

I take a completely different approach here, analytical rather than normative. Our way of apprehending the world results from a historical process of "problematization" through which we come to describe and interpret that world in a certain way, bringing problems into existence and giving them specific form, and by this process discarding other ways of describing and interpreting reality, of determining and constituting what exactly makes a problem.[21] Whereas volunteers eager to come to the aid of victims of conflict and oppression would previously have done so through political and sometimes military struggle, like Lord Byron in Greece, George Orwell in Spain, or Jean Genet in Palestine, today they do it via humanitarian assistance and advocacy, symbolized by Bob Geldof organizing a concert for Ethiopia, Bernard Kouchner carrying a sack of rice on the Somalian shore, or George Clooney pleading for the persecuted people of Darfur. It is not that the situation on the ground has radically changed, it is rather that violence and injustice have a different meaning for us, and more specifically, that we now justify our actions in a different way, to the extent that governments are increasingly invoking the humanitarian argument as a ground for their armed interventions. But in emphasizing this evolution in our collective understanding of the world I am not seeking to judge whether it is useful or dangerous, to determine whether we should celebrate it or be concerned about it: I am simply trying to recognize the phenomenon for what it is—and also to measure its effects, or more correctly, to interpret the issues involved with these anthropological transformations. It is for the readers, if they accept my analysis of these moral and political stakes, to draw the normative conclusions they consider to conform to their ethical and ideological view.

A new moral economy,[22] centered on humanitarian reason, therefore came into being during the last decades of the twentieth century. We continue to live within it now, in the early twenty-first century. It brings forth new kinds of responses—a humanitarian government—in which particular attention is focused on suffering and misfortune. Whether this shift stems from sincerity or cynicism on the part of the actors involved, whether it manifests a genuine empathy or manipulates compassion, is another question: the point I want to emphasize is that this way of seeing and doing has now come to appear self-evident to us.[23] However, this problematization of our societies does not go without saying. One could even state that it is in itself problematic. It requires us to examine not only the significance of the development itself but also its social and political implications, its consequences both objective and subjective. What, ultimately, is gained, and what lost, when we use the terms of suffering to speak of inequality, when we invoke trauma rather than recognizing violence, when we give residence rights to foreigners with health problems but restrict the conditions for political asylum, more generally when we mobilize compassion rather than justice? And what are the profits and losses incurred in opening listening centers to combat social exclusion, requiring the poor to recount their misfortunes, sending psychologists to war zones, representing war in the language of humanitarianism?

But how are these stakes to be understood? Social sciences and humanities have taken two main approaches in response to this question, which can be described by making a provisional distinction between humanitarian morals (the principle on which actions are based or justified) and humanitarian politics (the implementation of these actions). The first has often been limited to national territory and even to local space. The second has taken the world as its field of inquiry. The link between the two has rarely been made. This is what I intend to do here.

In the first approach—the analysis of humanitarian morals—philosophers have recently begun to examine public expressions of moral sentiments, some largely in affinity with sympathy, others on the contrary condemning its sway. The former consider suffering a lived reality that cannot be called into question (it is therefore naturalized) and frequently attempt to articulate it with a political economy (their critique thus relates to the social injustices that produce suffering). The latter see suffering as a manifestation of the modern sensibility (it is consequently culturalized), and their aim is generally to demonstrate the excesses of its public exposition (here the critique is of the sentimentality that makes a spectacle of suffering).[24] Take people who suffer seriously, say the former. Do not be fooled by the upsurge of compassion, retort the latter. Both views are seen as critique. But the realism of the first position ignores the historicity of moral sentiments and hence of the political use to which they are put, while the constructionism of the second stance ignores the subjectivation of social inequality and hence the experience that individuals have of it. The two perspectives never come together, for the first rejects the genealogy of compassion and the second turns away from the truth of suffering.

Sociology has not entirely escaped this dualism, and significantly, it was in France in the 1990s, at the point when the issue began to emerge in the public arena, that the discipline first addressed it, initially from two almost symmetrical positions. In *The Weight of the World*, Pierre Bourdieu sees suffering as the contemporary expression of "a social order which, although it has undoubtedly reduced poverty overall, has also multiplied the social spaces and set up the conditions for an unprecedented development of all kinds of ordinary suffering (*la petite misère*)."[25] The accumulation of interviews conducted by the researchers working alongside him shows that the whole of society is suffering almost indiscriminately, from the youth of the housing projects to the residents of middle-class suburbs, from immigrant workers to far-right campaigners, from police to trade unionists. The fact that suffering is also a characteristic language of the contemporary world and that compassion has become a political force escapes Bourdieu's analysis, which promotes the "intellectual love" the researcher must feel for his informants—at the risk of renouncing objectivation in his description and ultimately of reinforcing the social construction to which he unwittingly contributes. By contrast Luc Boltanski, in his *Distant Suffering*, proposes a displaced gaze, since he takes as his object the "spectator's dilemma" of those exposed to the suffering of others and caught "between the egoistic ideal of self-realization and an altruistic commitment to causes which enables one to 'realize oneself' through action," a dilemma to which the "humanitarian movement" offers a solution.[26] His inquiry thus relates to the topics of suffering and the rhetoric of pity, but in drawing on a wealth of historical cases and literary fiction it abandons almost any perspective on the contemporary world. The final section on "humanitarian action" mainly consists in a discussion of the "polemics" about the "return of moralism" to which it has given rise, and hence an analysis of strictly ideological arguments exchanged among those he ironically calls "media intellectuals." By doing so, Boltanski however risks derealizing the political stakes of this form of action and ultimately offering a mere apologia for humanitarianism.

What eludes both sociologists, in Bourdieu's case because of his denunciation of the social order and in Boltanski's because of his sociological study of denunciation, is an approach that would allow us to analyze the effects of domination expressed through suffering (which Bourdieu does) at the same time as the construction processes of which suffering is the object (which Boltanski exposes)—in other words, to consider the politics of suffering in their complexity and their ambiguity. The reason for these authors' difficulty in grasping these issues is no doubt partly methodological:

the interviews conducted by Bourdieu furnish accounts that put emotions into words without distance, while the texts analyzed by Boltanski present rhetorical figures that keep the social at a distance. In fact, whatever the richness of the exclusively discursive material collected by both sociologists, it is no substitute for the participant observation and long-term presence that make it possible to reconstruct more precisely described scenes and more broadly situated contexts, thus avoiding simplification, locating narratives and arguments within their frame of utterance, and eventually grasping the issues within which they are contained and which they contribute to constituting. Ethnography, if they had undertaken it, would certainly have made them see the world differently.

In the second approach—the analysis of humanitarian politics—international relations and political science have recently begun to scrutinize the deployment of these unfamiliar forms of intervention in zones of disaster and conflict. Political scientists and legal scholars have constructed ambitious panoramas of what they sometimes describe as the new humanitarian world order.[27] Here the scale of analysis is no longer an imaginary individual or an indeterminate collective, as in the philosophical and sociological approaches, but the world with relations of power between states, international institutions, and nongovernmental organizations—rather than a clash of civilizations. Two opposing positions emerge. Some do not question humanitarian intervention, even when it is conducted by the military in the name of protecting civilians: their analytical efforts focus on the conditions in which this action is deployed, its legality, or even its legitimacy, and sometimes include recommendations based on lessons learned from recent operations. Others make humanitarian intervention the subject of a radical critique: even while conceding that politicians may wish to defend just causes, they see the action undertaken in these conditions not only as a violation of sovereignty but also as an imposition of values and models.[28] Thus all of these studies address macropolitical configurations rather than microsocial situations: they concern international relations. The few case studies that have been conducted have until recently been carried out mainly by actors close to humanitarian organizations, who have been interested in the contradictions thrown up by interventions in which they themselves have been involved: detailed sociopolitical analyses have thus emerged from Darfur and Rwanda, for example.[29] But these are not ethnographic studies that could offer insight into the logics of actors and the justifications for their actions.

Anthropology has, in its turn, recently become interested in these far-off sites. There has been an unprecedented empirical investment against the background of a broad movement to redefine the discipline, now present at scenes of war and violence from which it had hitherto scrupulously held itself apart.[30] However, the descriptions resulting from these studies take various positions. For example, Mariella Pandolfi, who has studied the joint military-humanitarian intervention in Kosovo, presents a critical reading.[31] She decrypts the language of international organizations, particularly the notions of "complex emergency" (which amalgamates all crises, from earthquakes to war) and the "right to intervene" (used to justify operations supposedly aimed at protecting civilians, especially in extralegal situations); she puts in perspective the big hotels where the military, humanitarians, and journalists congregate and the refugee camps where these same actors invent "mobile sovereignties" as a substitute for failing state authorities. As an involved participant in the situations she observes (employed as an expert by an international organization), she delivers an implacable analysis of the humanitarian world. Conversely, Peter Redfield, who focuses on the daily life of a French nongovernmental organization in Uganda, takes a more empathetic approach.[32] Examining the humanitarian gesture closeup, he finds a convergence between the moral sentiments of the humanitarian and the anthropologist, whom he sees as "faced with the same problem," the same experience of the suffering of others and the desire to act; like the doctor or the nurse, he is concerned with the precariousness of lives, highlighted by his study of the "bracelet of life" that is distributed to babies to measure their nutritional state.

Obviously, the contexts are different. In the first case, the confusion between the military and the humanitarian reaches its climax under the lights of the media and with the background of international tensions. In the second case, the nongovernmental organization acts in a peaceful and almost forgotten region, where its members attempt to provide medical assistance. However, beyond these contrasts between the situations, the perspectives adopted by the analysts are somewhat distinct: the former gives priority to denunciation, whereas the latter remains attentive to constraints and ambiguities. The parallel between the two approaches—the critical distance of one and the empathetic engagement of the other—shows to what extent the anthropology of humanitarian government is epistemologically but also morally linked to its object, in a mirrorlike relationship that is actually difficult to avoid. Significantly, most fieldwork studies, as is the case for the two I evoked here, concentrate on the politics of distant tragedies (wars, camps) rather than the politics of nearby suffering (the poor, immigrants). Yet many elements, not least the increasing involvement of humanitarian organizations, both in distant countries and at home, and the use of the same humanitarian language in national and global politics, suggest that the two worlds need to be analyzed together and that anthropology should simultaneously address both realities.

Considering the two lines of social science and humanities research on the humanitarian question over the past twenty years, as I have summarized it far too briefly here—referring respectively to humanitarian morals and politics—my project can thus be stated simply. It is to seize morals at the point where it is articulated with politics—to comprehend the humanitarian government. This necessitates a dual focus.

First, it involves using the same theoretical approach, and the same empirical procedure, to address what is being played out in our society and in distant worlds, what is arising in both national and international arenas.[33] The moral economies in operation in a health clinic for the disadvantaged and in a refugee camp, in a listening center for the excluded in a poor neighborhood and in a trauma consultation in a war zone, in the allocation of scarce resources to the unemployed in the French welfare system or to patients in an African medical aid program have many points in common, which need to be grasped together as a whole. The case studies presented in this book therefore relate to the government of the poor, the disadvantaged, and the immigrants in France, but also of AIDS orphans in South Africa, disaster victims in Venezuela, traumatized adolescents in Palestine, and nongovernmental organizations in Iraq.[34] Each of these contexts throws light on the broader reality of the transformations being wrought through humanitarianism in the contemporary world. To grasp what is at work in this shift, one needs both to anchor empirical studies in local realities and to get a sense of the global landscape. This combination of the two scales thus avoids both monographic narrowness that delivers only circumscribed interpretations, and teleological claims that seek to identify a direction in history.

Second, I propose to base this analysis on precise inquiries rather than general propositions, to study a small number of situations that may shed some light on the question—essentially, to subject this political and moral anthropology to the test of ethnography.[35] My hypothesis is that in-depth study of specific objects, be they letters of application for financial assistance, medical certificates for the undocumented, testimonies published by humanitarian organizations, a support service in a housing project, or a military intervention after an earthquake, are more illuminating than an exhaustive analysis or a general overview in providing an intelligibility of the social world.[36] It should therefore be no surprise that we have to go by way of the casuistry of decisions on allocation of assistance to low-income individuals, the rhetoric of attestation of torture for asylum seekers, the tactics of immigrants applying for residence, in order to understand how the state politics of compassion operates in France. It is through this work at the margins that we can grasp the logics and the assumptions, the ambiguities and the contradictions, the principles of justice and the practices of judgment: the devil is in the detail. Similarly, to understand humanitarian practices in distant regions, we need to examine the images produced of children with AIDS in South Africa, the writings of psychiatrists and psychologists reporting the situation of Palestinians under the Israeli occupation, and the debates within a nongovernmental organization over whether its members should stay in Iraq under the bombs. In each case, ethnography provides insight into the convictions and doubts of the actors, their blind spots and their lucidity, their prejudices and their reflexivity: we owe our informants the respect of restoring these dialectical tensions. This has long been missing from the essays on humanitarianism and pamphlets about moralism whose monolithic theses recognized neither the complexity of the issues nor the intelligence of the actors.

The book is constructed around two series: the implementation of humanitarian reason in the politics of precarious lives in the French context, and the dissemination of humanitarian government in tragic contexts throughout the world. The nine scenes thus analyzed, covering a period spanning the mid-1990s through the middle of the first decade of this century, sketch vignettes of what we might call the humanitarian moment in contemporary history.

The first series of case studies has for background the important social, economic, demographic, and political changes that took place in France in recent decades. After what has been called in French the *Trente Glorieuses*—the thirty years of prosperity following the Second World War—the oil crisis and, more crucially, the restructuring of the economy with the industrial decline had important consequences. First, the increase in unemployment and job insecurity, concomitant with the enrichment of a minority, resulted in growing levels of poverty and inequality; as a "minimum guaranteed income" was instituted in 1988 for the disadvantaged, the language of social exclusion, with the idea that disparities were no longer vertical (up/down) but horizontal (in/out), became commonplace. Second, the immigrant workforce, which had been so decisive in the period of economic growth, became undesirable, and restrictions were brought to labor immigration, then to family reunification, eventually to any entry of foreigners from developing countries, including asylum seekers, henceforth suspected of being so-called false refugees; the rapid progression of the far-right National Front, whose candidate came second in the 2002 presidential election, was mostly based on a xenophobic discourse, which made the "immigration question" a central issue in the public debate. Third, after twenty-three years of right-wing domination—under Charles de Gaulle, Georges Pompidou, and Valéry Giscard d'Estaing—the left took power with the 1981 election of Socialist François Mitterrand, who remained president for fourteen years, the longest mandate under the Fifth Republic; however, this political change inaugurated a period of instability, with the alternation of majorities in the National Assembly, leading from 2002 to an exclusive domination of an increasingly conservative right, with Jacques Chirac and later Nicolas Sarkozy as presidents. It is in this context of profound objective change that the subjective metamorphosis I am analyzing here should be understood. The contradictions between the social, economic, and political evolution and the founding values of French democracy, the confrontation between the neoliberal policies of the governments and the moral concerns of civil society partially expressed via nongovernmental organizations, account for the emergence of compassion as an ambiguous principle underlying the politics toward the disadvantaged, not exclusive, in its actual practice, of the exercise of repression.

The second series of case studies is embedded in broader transformations on the global scene. The progressive collapse of the Communist regimes, which reached its climax with the 1989 fall of the Berlin Wall, reconfigured the international political order that had been shaped by the Cold War for several decades. These events precipitated rather than directly provoked structural changes at the level of the planet. First, the neoliberal creed appeared not only stronger than ever, but even the only viable ideology; the negotiations of the World Trade Organization established this ultimate victory, leaving open however the 2002 Doha "health exception," a compassionate measure to keep certain drugs accessible for the most severe diseases. Second, the supremacy of the Western world under the banner of the United States gave birth to a doctrine of interventionism, officially sanctioned by the adoption of the "responsibility to protect" principle at the 2005 World Summit of the United Nations; from Somalia to Bosnia to East Timor, the invocation of this moral obligation served as a justification for military interventions, with or without the legality of the Security Council vote. Third, the presence of nongovernmental actors instituted a new equilibrium of power with states and international agencies; AIDS activists such as the South African Treatment Action Campaign, charity organizations like Médecins Sans Frontières, and private foundations on the model of the Gates Foundation redrew the political map of the world. It is in this context of changing moral geography that one should apprehend the attitudes toward children in South Africa or disaster victims in Venezuela, and the stakes of humanitarian action in the Palestinian Territories or in Iraq.

In the first section of this book, I examine the policies implemented in France over the past two decades in relation to the marginal and the excluded, the unemployed and the poor, undocumented immigrants and asylum seekers through four case studies. The identification of psychic suffering resulting from social conditions led to the establishment, from 1996 onward, of so-called places of listening for marginalized teenagers and youth at risk in poor urban neighborhoods. Set up by psychiatrists and staffed by psychologists, these facilities redefined social inequality in the language of mental health; however, rather than a psychiatrization or psychologization of the social question that many prophesied, what actually occurred was the dissemination of moral sentiments in deprofessionalized spaces where presumed suffering was addressed (chapter 1). Shortly after, the abolition of emergency welfare grants for the unemployed in late 1997 sparked major protests, to which the government responded by announcing the allotment of 1 million euros on the basis of individual case assessments. Analysis of the actual procedures for distribution of this public largesse reveals the principles of justice and the practices of judgment within state services. Notably, given that applicants were required to adopt the method of petition, we can see how the exposition of their hardship results in an emotional fatigue among administrators that ultimately produces a mixture of contingency and arbitrariness in the allocation of financial aid (chapter 2). The following year, as a result of demands by charitable organizations seeking to prevent people in poor health from being deported, a criterion was introduced into the 1998 law on immigration allowing immigrants suffering from a serious illness to be granted residence. This compassionate regimen concludes a development whereby the body of the immigrant, previously valued for its labor force, is now increasingly recognized on the basis of the illness that invalidates it. A study of the practices of physicians responsible for selecting the individuals to be granted residence demonstrates the shift in legitimacy from social life to biological life (chapter 3). In parallel, the dramatic decrease in the numbers of those granted asylum, which plummeted to less than one out of five in 2000, induces a growing demand for evidence, primarily medical certificates testifying to the persecution suffered. As the condition of refugees is delegitimized, this new scenario underlines the way the applicant's word is discredited and increasingly replaced by the opinions of experts. Analysis of the attestations produced and of campaigns by support organizations shows how what appears to be a simple search for truth becomes a practice of testing veracity through the body, altering the spirit and even the letter of the 1951 Geneva Convention (chapter 4). Although oriented toward different publics, these politics of precarious life draw the moral landscape of contemporary France.

The liminality of the situation of refugees and the ambiguity of the hospitality they are provided offers a transition between the national and the international scenes (chapter 5). The controversy over the center of Sangatte between 1999 and 2001 is remarkably revealing, since it opens onto transnational issues, with the growing tension between compassion and repression in the management of immigrants and the deterrence of asylum seekers. On the border, the contradictions between the rhetoric of human rights and the practice of exception and the polarization of the world between a North to be protected and the South viewed as a threat become extreme.

In the second section of the book, I consider the implementation of humanitarian practices as a means of addressing afflictions throughout the world, again via four case studies distributed across four continents. The AIDS epidemic has affected South Africa more than any other country and since 2000 has resulted in an unprecedented political and social crisis, particularly painful in relation to children. The vulnerability of this age group is manifested through the three images, omnipresent in the public space, of the sick child, the abused infant, and the orphan. However, the empirical investigation reveals the implications of this emotional mobilization, especially the misrecognition of historical and social realities to which it contributes (chapter 6). A similar observation can be made about Venezuela, where the natural disaster of December 1999 occurred in a specific context of moral reconstruction of the nation and indeed, by a remarkable coincidence, on the very day of a referendum on the new constitution. Faced with collective misfortune, the entire society supported the declaration of a state of exception to facilitate aid to the victims. The unanimous compassion thus masked both the violence perpetrated by the police and the army, and the deep disparities in the support offered to victims (chapter 7). The same affective dimension was at stake during the Second Intifada, which erupted in September 2000, and more specifically via the emergence of a humanitarian testimony in the international public arena. On the basis of their members' experience as psychologists and psychiatrists, nongovernmental organizations exposed the wounds of the violent occupation of Palestinian territories by the Israeli army using the language of trauma.

The documents produced by Médecins Sans Frontières and Médecins du Monde illustrate the difficulties and obstacles this language presents both to articulating the historical and political context of suffering and to recognizing local forms of subjectivation of violence (chapter 8). Humanitarianism was again put to the test in April 2003 by the launch of the Iraq War, which highlighted, even more clearly than any other recent conflict, its complex relationships with the military. The heated debate in Médecins Sans Frontières about whether it should remain in Baghdad when bombing was imminent questions the meaning of such a potential sacrifice. The implications of the decision to stay demonstrate the difficulty of weighing the relative value of lives and ultimately reveal ontological inequalities rarely recognized for what they are (chapter 9). Beyond the diversity of situations and contexts, it is the logics and consequences of the deployment of humanitarian reason in these various sites that are at stake.

This book thus brings together works I have conducted over a decade. However, the project, which was outlined in my seminar on "the politics of suffering" at the École des Hautes Études en Sciences Sociales in the early 2000s, has progressively shifted and been refined over time. My initial intuitions have been confirmed for some and corrected for others. This is why I decided to publish the texts, many of which were not easily accessible, that marked this journey, but to rewrite them completely to give my argument the coherence that is now apparent to me. It is usual when collecting papers for a volume to leave them in their original form, partly through a concern for authenticity, partly because of the difficulty and length of any revision that transcends the purely cosmetic. I go against this custom here in order to make sense of a project that only became completely intelligible to me when I reached the end of it—an end that is of course in itself provisional. Via a series of studies on apparently disparate subjects and geographically diverse locations, it is an endeavor to grasp humanitarian government in the diversity of its expressions, to explore the complexity of contemporary moral economies, and therefore to contribute as an anthropologist to the moral history of the present.

PART I

Politics

1. Suffering Unveiled

Listening to the Excluded and the Marginalized

> Efforts to reduce suffering have habitually focused on control and repair of individual bodies. The social origins of suffering and distress, including poverty and discrimination, even if fleetingly recognized, are set aside.
>
> MARGARET LOCK, *Displacing Suffering*

The 1995 presidential election campaign in France was dominated by the theme of "social fracture." In a context where unemployment had finally come to be recognized as a structural fact of French society rather than a temporary result of a particular set of economic conditions, as it had long been held to be, a gnawing anxiety had developed around what was termed, during the 1980s, "new poverty," and from 1990 onward, "social exclusion." During this period when sociologists asserted that society was no longer organized as a vertical hierarchy but rather divided with an inside and an outside, the idea that the old inequalities between classes had been replaced by a new and radical social line between included and excluded appeared attractive to many politicians, researchers, intellectuals, and journalists.[1] Jacques Chirac made it the leitmotif of his campaign for the presidency, declaring, in a foundational speech on February 17, 1995: "Economic certainty and a secure tomorrow are now privileges. The young people of France are expressing their helplessness. There is a deepening social fracture, the burden of which is being borne by the nation as a whole." Many commentators saw this strategic choice as key to Chirac's victory, which was, it has to be said, unexpected, since he appeared to be trapped between two other candidates, one Conservative and one Socialist, who left him little ideological space: his success was therefore interpreted as the result of a skillful right-wing candidate campaigning on what was generally seen as a left-wing issue.[2] Following his election, the new president kept his promises, at least nominally: the government formed by his prime minister Alain Juppé included, in addition to the traditional Ministry of Labor and Social Affairs and the by now customary Department for Emergency Humanitarian Action, a Ministry for Social Integration and against Exclusion, and a Department for Housing Projects, renamed "neighborhoods in difficulty." The most innovative measure, introduced after a cabinet reshuffle, was the establishment of support centers, which received the remarkable label *lieux d'écoute* (literally: places for listening).[3] A number of reports had highlighted the new phenomenon of "psychic suffering," particularly among teenagers and young adults, whom these facilities, offering welcome and a listening ear, were intended to serve. A preliminary circular appeared on June 14, 1996:. it instituted "reception centers for youth aged between 10 and 25" and aimed to "respond to teenagers' distress." It is worth noting that it was signed by both the minister for labor and social affairs, Jacques Barrot, and the secretary for emergency humanitarian action, Xavier Emmanuelli; the involvement of the latter was thus set within the context of an at least partial reorientation of the missions of the major humanitarian organizations from international causes toward the disadvantaged within French society.[4] A second circular was published on April 10, 1997: this one related more explicitly to "listening facilities for young people and/or their parents" and sought to meet "their need to express their problems"; it was signed by the minister for urban planning and social integration, Jean-Claude Gaudin, and the secretary for urban integration, Eric Raoult; it was something of a surprise to see the latter's name at the bottom of this document as he was better known for his harsh discourses on public order issues. Thus the new support centers were the result of an unprecedented coupling of humanitarian and security concerns.

In the months that followed, these facilities proliferated throughout France.[5] One of them, in a town of Seine-Saint-Denis—a *département* (that is, administrative territory) known to be especially hard hit by economic difficulties, but with a high level of social and political engagement—was led by a psychiatrist with a team of psychologists. The municipal administration had wanted the team to be based in a *cité* (housing project), but the mental health professionals, fearful at the prospect of spending their working days among a population with which they were not familiar, had argued for what they euphemistically called a "neutral setting." They had therefore taken possession of an elegant building in one of the town's old neighborhoods. They gained in peace of mind, but certainly lost some of their most disadvantaged clientele.[6] Yet the activity report they submitted to their board of management suggested that the situation was worrying:

> Faced with the climate of insecurity and anxiety generated by the lack of stability in work, training and family, young people with no reference points form a vulnerable group. The explosion of violence and crime among youth, and the increasingly young age of those

involved, result in teenagers becoming stigmatized and provoke mistrust and even fear. How do we establish a link with these young people who, even when they are experiencing psychic suffering, cannot formulate a plea for help? [7]

This alarming observation thus confirmed the politicians' analysis: the combination of instability and insecurity generated both the suffering that translated into violence among young people and the mistrust that developed into fear among adults, a vicious circle for which the listening center was the solution.

The picture presented in the facility itself was very different. Teenagers sped there enthusiastically after school for a snack before settling in small groups to play Monopoly or hang out in the IT room. There were certainly arguments and sometimes fights, but little more than one would expect on a school playground. Looking at these adolescents, it was difficult to recognize suffering, even disguised as violence. But as we have seen in the excerpt, the psychologists had a ready answer to this objection: the suffering was usually invisible to the inexperienced eye of nonspecialists; teenagers' failure to express it simply became a confirmation of its existence. Yet the statistics of the center indicated that only 6% of the youths had been referred by psychiatric services, 6% by child protection services, and 5% by education services, while at least 80% came of their own volition and often with pleasure. This did not prevent the psyche experts from imagining that they had "major problems," thus revealing much more of their ignorance of this environment, socially so distant from their own, than the after all fairly ordinary reality of the schoolchildren: "When you arrive here, it feels like another planet," admitted one of the support workers, unfamiliar with the verbal and corporeal expressions of these teenagers. But over and above this gap between psychologists belonging to the Parisian upper middle classes and the adolescents of immigrant descent from the disadvantaged neighborhoods of Seine-Saint-Denis, what interests me here is the form of government that translates social inequalities in terms of psychic suffering and proposes listening to the distress of working-class people as a response to their social difficulties.

Toward the end of the twentieth century a new language emerged in France to describe social problems, their effects on individuals, and the possible solutions for them. The problems were related to exclusion, the effects were interpreted in terms of suffering, and the solutions put forward revolved around the activity of listening. We could describe a set of notions that are constructed together and complement one another in order to account for a social reality, as a semantic configuration. "Exclusion," "suffering," and "listening" constitute just such a semantic configuration for the 1990s, one which we might qualify as compassion based. These notions make it possible to articulate what sociologists have called a "new social question"[8]—that is, both what causes "the social" to exist as a problem, between economics and politics, and how it is constituted as an "issue" through a problematization that is specific to a moment in history. Every historical period can be characterized by the semantic configuration that best expresses the way the social question is understood at that moment: in the 1970s, for example, the problem, its consequence, and its solution were articulated respectively in terms of "maladjustment," "poverty," and "integration," in a context where the great political themes that are familiar to us today, such as unemployment, immigration, and insecurity, were yet to be fully formulated.[9] But in any given period, a number of semantic configurations may develop in parallel, finding resources in different spaces and sometimes even competing to become established as the legitimate definition of the social question. Thus in the 1990s a set of ideas constituted around "housing projects," "urban insecurity," and "zero tolerance" gradually emerged until at the beginning of the following decade this new semantic configuration, which can be described as security focused, became overwhelming during the subsequent decade.[10] It is therefore essential to consider these commonplaces that characterize a period as fluid and dynamic networks.

But a semantic configuration does not appear out of nowhere. It originates in a specific social world—professional, institutional, cultural—which at a given moment becomes to some extent recognized as an authorized describer of social facts and a competent provider of social responses. In France during the 1990s, the field of mental health played this role. It found the words to articulate social disarray. Society, or at least major elements within it that were involved in addressing the new economic realities, from government officials to social workers in poor neighborhoods, adopted the vocabulary of mental health to implement policies around inequality and deviance, poverty and crime—issues that were now seen more in terms of exclusion and suffering that called for assistance and listening. In emphasizing this development, I am not suggesting that the traditional tools of the state were dismissed: welfare services were maintained and sometimes expanded, technologies of repression were used and even refined, but other responses also appeared, responses to which psychiatrists and psychologists contributed their theoretical and practical tools, which proved all the more efficacious because the ground had been prepared for them by the social sciences, various politicians, and the media. What I am attempting to grasp here is the social innovation introduced in and by the world of mental health, understood both as a body of professionals and as a body of knowledge. The analyses frequently advanced that see this phenomenon in terms of psychologization, or even psychiatrization, of the social give only a very partial account of it. Once we go beyond official statements to examine discourses and practices as implemented in national and local policies, particularly the policy promoting these listening centers, we find that rather than a unilateral determination of direction and emphasis, what we are witnessing is a crystallization of representations and ideas around a series of words and notions.

THE EMBODIMENT OF THE SOCIAL

On October 15, 1999, in a fringe meeting at the Sixth Bayeux International Festival of War Correspondents and Photographers, a French journalist, commenting on changes in the market for reports and images that relate and illustrate the world's events, observed: "I think we have gone beyond the stage where it had to be bodies and blood. What is required today is suffering—particularly the suffering of women and children, because it moves and mobilizes people more easily." The host of the radio program *Pot-au-feu*, interviewing this journalist for the France Culture channel, commented soberly: "The Pietà rather than the Crucifixion, then." A striking formulation indeed. This shift was starkly illustrated by the controversy around the tragic photograph of the desperate Algerian mother who, on the morning of September 23, 1997, learned that her eight children had been massacred the day before in Benthala, along with four hundred other people.[11] What the global press published on their front pages about the slaughter was not the image of the lifeless or mutilated bodies of the victims, but the representation of this woman's pain. Thus the reader became a spectator of suffering rather than of violence, and the emotion to be felt was compassion rather than terror.

But suffering was not only portrayed in pictures, it was also put into words. By the end of the 1990s it had become ubiquitous in the world of work. A magazine, reporting on the proliferation of protest movements, ran the headline: "Suffering Comes Out onto the Streets." A sociologist, Danièle Linhart, explained: "Social workers and occupational physicians stress how badly people who work are doing in many sectors. Before, colleagues used to pass on union cards; now they exchange antidepressants." She went on to deplore this development: "There is more talk about suffering, but it is still often expressed in individual terms. . . . Listening to one another, sympathizing with one another's troubles, identifying with their suffering is one thing. The issue is in coming back to a collective focus." Social relations in industry and changes in the organization of production were increasingly described in the vocabulary of psychopathology. ".Changes in Working Conditions Generate New Kinds of Suffering" ran the headline in one national daily newspaper, above a long article commemorating the centenary of the law on accidents at work that quoted a number of psychoanalysts and psychologists at length. Their account was unequivocal, summed up by Damien Cru, a specialist in occupational psychopathology: "Previously, suffering was confined to the workers, and they kept quiet about it. Now these phenomena affect all professional categories, including managers and researchers."[12] In other words, whereas previously the worker was championed, now everyone in the world of work, even the most privileged, was pitied. Above all, what was previously stated in terms of economic exploitation was now expressed in the vocabulary of mental health. Where before trade unionists condemned the conditions in which professional activity was exercised, now the occupational physician cared for psychic distress. Of course, this development should not be overstated, as the earlier language was not entirely replaced by the newer, but almost more significantly and somewhat ironically, the discourse of protest began to find its most effective resources in the lexicon of suffering.

Moreover, suffering was starting to become contagious. In other words, people were affected not only through their own situation but also because they were faced with the condition of others. Empathy itself was becoming pathogenic. This contagion could be direct, in face-to-face encounters with the person suffering, or indirect, via the mediation of images or words that expressed suffering. In the first case, health care and social welfare professionals were obviously the most at risk. The Society for Therapeutic Training of General Practitioners, for example, introduced a program for doctors on "the limits of care or compassion." The organizers asked "why the suffering of health professionals is so disregarded," and invited public authorities to "instigate assessments for stress, not just skills." To help participants recognize "the doctor's suffering" they distributed a self-assessment questionnaire among the group, the "Malasch burn-out inventory," helping them to establish whether they were indeed affected by "professional exhaustion" or even "depersonalization."[13] Indirect contagion seemed particularly to put television viewers to the test. A study by the Public Debate Observatory on the reception of news as distilled on television each evening and watched by an average of twenty-three million individuals revealed that "French people experience their television news as suffering." According to the director of this marketing research organization, "Watching a television news broadcast is a psychological and physical ordeal that produces a sort of vertigo, deriving from both quantity and diversity, which becomes a source of anxiety." The editorial work of the presenters is then to act as "psychological counterweight," helping to "attenuate the disaster"; through their commentary, which "reassures even as the images raise anxiety," they "make it possible for the viewer to stay present with all this horror."[14] Instead of Hannah Arendt's opposition between compassion with those close to one and pity felt at a distance,[15] here we have a form of generalized closeness to suffering that allows empathy to be expressed almost identically whether one is face to face with the person or thousands of miles away.

The inflation of suffering can be approached in various ways, which have taken mainly two forms in the French context. First, this discourse can be considered a description of reality, accepting both that there is more suffering than before and that people are more exposed to the suffering of others. We might call this first approach naturalist. Thus, commenting on a book on "social suffering," Jackie Assayag writes: "We are living in an age haunted by suffering. Not the suffering to which religion and literature accustomed us. No past tradition has prepared us for this spectacle of atrocity and terror. Although it is unequally shared but widely distributed, 'social suffering' has ultimately colonized our future with its nightmares. The political sociodicies of disaster have now taken over from the old theodicies."[16] This is what philosophers, anthropologists, and journalists express more globally, in their writing on the violence and injustice of the twentieth century. It is also affirmed, on the scale of everyday experience, by sociologists, psychologists, and physicians who report their observations on psychic distress caused by new forms of organization of work.[17] The second approach, conversely, rejects the discourse on suffering as a sort of artifact that merely reveals the current tendency for complaint to become routine. We might call this the ironic approach. In his study of depression, Alain Ehrenberg argues that our era offers "an excellent opportunity to suffer," and speaks of "the fashion for suffering." Quoting an official report stating that psychic suffering has become the most prominent symptom of precarious lives, he notes that "this focus on suffering, and also on the cognitive use of it to understand and define social problems, is quite recent."[18] This is, in a slightly different form, the line taken by a series of philosophical reflections and literary essays that often condemn and sometimes deride the contemporary tendency to produce victims and victim discourses, to feed on compassion and extol compassionate attitudes.[19] If we take the first position, a question still remains: insofar as it is difficult to imagine that earlier generations did not experience psychic suffering as a result of their living or working conditions, why are the social sciences, and more broadly society, prepared today to investigate realities that they would have dismissed before? If we take the second position, a different question arises: if psychic suffering is merely a vague signifier of the confusions of our time in a booming market in compassion, why does it express them so well, and above all so consensually? I therefore believe a third approach is needed. I qualify it as critical. It consists in taking psychic suffering seriously as both a lived reality and a public discourse, considering the combined presence of the two as a social fact characteristic of the moral economy of contemporary societies.

How is this approach to be described? I would say that it emerges from an astonishment: How has suffering become so firmly, yet so easily, established in our semantic world? But it also stems from a shift: Should we not see what seems taken for granted—the fact that people suffer from their misfortunes—as the product also of a cultural operation bringing into existence precisely that which could not hitherto be formulated in the public sphere? It is not a question of contesting the reality of suffering (although we can have a sense of how hard it is to compare the genocides of the present era with the exterminations of past centuries, the psychic distress of contemporary workers with the painful experiences of nineteenth-century proletariat). Nor is it a matter of underestimating the temporal variations of discourse on suffering (though we cannot limit ourselves to this assessment if we ignore the social and political effects it produces in the management of international conflicts and the government of dominated populations). We need to consider suffering as a language of the present and to explore the meanings and implications of this—admittedly partial—reconfiguration of our vision of the world. It is this exercise of surprise and displacement that Ian Hacking engages in relation to memory:[20]

> My curiosity is piqued exactly when something seems inevitable.
> Why are such diverse interests grouped under *memory*? One senior
> American philosopher, Nelson Goodman, as committed to the arts as
> to the sciences, has called himself skeptical, analytical, and construc-
> tionalist. I have those tendencies too. I wonder skeptically: why has it
> been essential to organize so many of our present projects in terms of
> memory? I wonder analytically: what are the dominating principles

that lock us into memory as an approach to so many of the problems of life, from child rearing to patriotism, from aging to anxiety? And I wonder, what constructions underlie these principles? I am not looking for the trite wisdom that there are different kinds of memory. I wonder why there is one creature, "memory," of which there are so many different kinds.

Something that seems to go without saying—who would imagine denying the reality of suffering or the existence of memory?—cannot be considered as such by the historian who, like the anthropologist who knows that things are not the same everywhere, is well aware that it was not ever thus. For both historian and anthropologist, the investigation begins with a question: Why is it like this here and now?

Returning to suffering, the question becomes: Why do we believe today that the "social" makes people "suffer" when we were unaware of it before? To put it another way: How has this come to seem self-evident to us? And finally: What are the consequences of this representation of the world through pain?

THE BIRTH OF A QUESTION

For a "transient mental illness" to exist in a particular society at a given moment in time, Ian Hacking argues, it must find what he calls, using a biological metaphor, its "ecological niche," the point where the combination of circumstances through which a new kind of pathology can emerge is brought together. This is how he accounts for the emergence and decline of hysteria, mad travelers' syndrome, and more recently, multiple personality disorders.[21] According to the Canadian philosopher, there are four elements to this niche: a medical classification that provides a diagnostic framework; a normative polarity that makes it possible to distinguish positive from negative; the possibility of observing the phenomenon, making it visible and measurable; finally, the opportunity to resolve a social problem that finds no other solution. Thus transient mental illness can exist so long as it fulfills these four conditions. Of course, in the case I am considering, suffering is not exactly a mental illness, it is rather a psychic symptom; moreover, we can hardly claim that it is transient, since this would presuppose that once having emerged, it would soon disappear, a potential evolution we ignore of course. If we are willing nevertheless to approach suffering from the point of view of phenomenology or hermeneutics but simply from that of political sociology, or even moral anthropology, the question is how—that is, in what specific historical conditions—it became social.

In France, the 1980s were marked by the development of the "new poverty" and the explosion of "urban violence."[22] The concentration of these phenomena within specific areas (the *banlieues,* or poor neighborhoods, and their *cités,* or housing projects) and in specific categories (the working class, especially of immigrant origin, which was especially affected by the changes in the job market) resulted in terms of affirmative action rather than universal approach, reparative rather than distributive justice: policies of economic integration for the unemployed (*politiques d'insertion*) on the one hand and policies in favor of housing projects (*politiques de la ville*) on the other. Above all, the linking of the two realities in the public space perpetuated the association between poverty and crime, between the disadvantaged and the dangerous classes, that has characterized attitudes toward the social question since it first arose in the nineteenth century, and hence also the remedy for it, oscillating between compassion and repression. But this moral polarization is unstable. From the late 1980s, the compassionate register began to take over from the repressive. The development of policies of damage reduction for drug users, which focused almost exclusively on the poor neighborhoods, offers a significant indication of this process. Whereas up to that point action had been based almost entirely on public order, centering around the police and justice (with a few specialized psychiatric departments involved in drug withdrawal), the new approach highlighted the two issues of endangering one's own life (with the risk of AIDS and hepatitis) and psychic pain (of which drug use was seen as both consequence and aggravating factor).[23] This reversal of the representation of drug users, from feared and ostracized criminals to threatened and suffering beings, formed the prelude to a radical restructuring of public action in which what was now conceived as "care," in terms of reducing risk and promoting treatment, became a central axis of local government policies in the poor neighborhood.

More broadly, the attitude to the social question became more closely aligned with those considered as victims. As the number and above all the visibility (particularly in the media) of the unemployed rose, a shared feeling of empathy and a moral imperative for solidarity seem to have taken over from the previous tendency to stigmatize behaviors.[24] The "economic crisis" came to be seen as the source of all these problems; the unemployed, the poor, and the youth of the projects were its victims. Moreover, the introduction of the *Revenu minimum d'insertion* (minimum guaranteed income, RMI) in 1988 instituted new contractual obligations between the recipients of this benefit and the support institutions: in exchange for the guaranteed income they were granted, the recipients had to do everything they could to find a job, and the institutions were to do all they could to help them in this process. This contract implied exposure of the self through personal narratives and good intentions.[25] Not only did those receiving the benefit have to present themselves at job centers, give an account of and justify themselves, they also had to devise a plan for recovering their place in the social world on the basis of this account: in other words, they were required to link their past and their future around an uncertain present.

In the early 1990s two new terms emerged that anchored public action solidly in the compassionate register: "exclusion" and, above all, "suffering." In both cases the state administration and the social sciences played a pivotal role and came together in legitimizing these new categories politically and intellectually. "Exclusion" appeared first in texts produced by the Commissariat Général du Plan (General Planning Commission), notably in two reports produced under the direction of Philippe Nasse in 1991 and Bertrand Fragonard in 1993, which developed the concept and normalized its use in political circles. At the same time, it was theorized by sociologists of the self-named "second left" (non-Marxist, close to the Commissariat), such as Jacques Donzelot and Alain Touraine, who asserted the existence of a new form of social differentiation, radically different from the inequalities of the preceding period of industrialization.[26] Though interpretation varied somewhat from one report or one author to another, there was a broad consensus in ascribing exclusion to a new social order that was no longer "vertical" but "horizontal," with an "inside" and an "outside," and with a growing proportion of the French population lacking *lien social* (social links)—an expression that soon became a cliché. Although the analyses that gave rise to this new description were based on few empirical studies and thus offered no picture of what the experience of the so-called excluded might be, the terminology of exclusion evoked more concrete realities than did the language of inequalities. The media adopted the term widely, using personal stories and images to show that the problem was no longer restricted to the margins of society but affected the whole: no one was safe any more, everyone was at risk of falling into the "other side." Opinion polls confirmed that a large proportion of French society felt in danger of exclusion. Very few commented on the fact that the risk of unemployment or short-term employment was closely linked to social category[27] and was, for example, six times higher among unskilled workers than among professionals.

The convergent views of experts, media, and public opinion were confirmed by the investigations (here based on empirical research) conducted by teams working with Pierre Bourdieu, within the framework of collective research supported by the Caisse des Dépôts et Consignations, a public savings bank involved in social development programs. While the notion of suffering was not really conceptualized in the collective volume published in 1993, it was situated at the core of the theoretical project and above all was demonstrated through each reported interview and each situation described.[28] The intention had been made clear by Bourdieu two years earlier: "Concerned to identify and understand the true bases of social suffering that is expressed only through opaque and obscure signs and symptoms, we chose to interview people who are 'not well in themselves,' as the common phrase goes, because they are not well in their social position." To make sense of this suffering, researchers had to work through a "form of active and equipped listening that requires an apparently contradictory stance: on the one hand, complete openness to the persons interviewed, total submission to the singularity of their individual case, which may lead one, through a sort of more or less controlled mimesis, to adopt their language and enter into their perspective, feelings and thoughts; on the other, a methodical questioning backed up by knowledge of the objective conditions common to a whole category and attentive to the effects of the survey relationship."[29] This research therefore established a relationship between social condition and personal experience (people are "not well in themselves" because they are "not well in their social position") and defined the place of the sociologist quite clearly (as the only analyst capable of a form of "listening" that is sensitive to both the subjectivation and the objectification of misfortune). Therefore, on the basis of the sociologist's authority, social suffering acquired official status and empathetic listening became a legitimate tool, with the social sciences acting as a model for social work—and all the more because the book's success was partly due to the fact that unlike previous studies of exclusion, it showed that everyone was or could potentially be affected by suffering. Rather than perpetuating the idea of a social world divided between excluded and included, as the sociologists of the second left asserted, Pierre Bourdieu, who can be seen as representative of the "first left" (neo-Marxist), revealed that everyone suffers, presenting a mirror in which all could recognize themselves.

Thus, when Jean-Marie Delarue, the interministerial commissioner for urban affairs, appointed Antoine Lazarus, a professor of public health, to head a working group on "city, mental health, precariousness, and exclusion," everything had been set in place for the analyses and proposals that resulted, two years later, in the publication of the most influential report on the topic.[30] The "ecological niche" of social suffering had been established—

or at least three of its conditions of possibility had conjoined. First, by offering both an interpretation and a response, social suffering suggested a political resolution in a socioeconomic situation that the government admitted it had not got a purchase on. Second, in being validated by official bodies and attested by the social sciences, it became observable and even quantifiable. Third, by privileging compassion over repression in the management of the social question, it provided a positive moral axis. All that remains therefore is to examine the fourth dimension—how psychiatric taxonomy gave it recognition.

THE CLINIC OF EXCLUSION

As has been recognized since Austin's lectures, utterances may be "constative" or "performative"—that is, they may say something about the way things are or produce things by saying them. However, words uttered in the public arena may be both constative and performative at the same time, being presented as a pure observation of facts while contributing to bringing these facts into existence: to speak of insecurity as a mere description of reality is to participate in bringing the feeling of insecurity into being. But for the discourse to function socially—in other words, for it to be recognized as true—it must obey certain rules that can be determined from opposite cases, starting with the "doctrine of infelicity conditions," when one or more of these conditions are absent.[31] Thus uttering a constative or performative phrase is not enough for it to have effect. There must be a procedure recognized by convention and brought into operation by the appropriate people and in the appropriate circumstances. Suffering only became an efficacious notion in the definition of public policy at the point when it was addressed by psychiatrists and set in a legitimate institutional framework.

In his introductory remarks at the 1997 conference organized by the Observatoire Régional sur la Souffrance Psychique en Rapport avec l'Exclusion (Regional Observatory on Psychic Suffering Related to Exclusion, ORSPERE), its director, Jean Furtos, a psychiatrist at a public asylum in Lyons, recognized what he and the entire "social body" owed to the report, asserting that it "was fundamental" because it "forced us to understand and act" by revealing a suffering that until then had been allowed "to fall into the abyss of denial, indifference or contempt." Three years earlier, at another conference that marked the beginning of a major mobilization of psychiatry, he had even drawn on a personal memory that suggested how long it had taken

his own discipline to identify the problem: "In the early 1980s a few of us, from very different regions and with very different theoretical backgrounds, were invited to reflect on the theme of psychiatry in the year 2000. In my perhaps unreliable memory, there was no one who thought it likely that psychic suffering related to poverty, precariousness and exclusion would become one of the challenges of the third millennium. Yet social distress was evident. It had not yet been exposed as it is now: the Lazarus report was yet to lift the veil on it."[32] In other words, 1995 represents a watershed in the emergence of the notion of socially determined suffering. More precisely, this discovery that it is possible to suffer from social conditions derived not from a deep internal shift in psychiatry, which then seized hold of the problem and brought it into the public sphere, but from the meeting of one of its marginal currents (that of social awareness and activist practice) with a set of actors involved in urban policy and working within a context where sociology was a core influence.[33] Thus in the early 1990s there was close, although not always direct, interaction between the social sciences, government expert advice, and mental health. In this context, in order to explain the success of the report on social suffering, two as yet underappreciated directive interpretations need to be taken into consideration.

First, the Lazarus report shifts the traditional object of psychiatry, asserting that the psychic disorders observed in the poor neighborhoods are not a matter of mental pathology: "If it is not sickness, it is suffering," the report maintains. This is a logic that Robert Castel had described earlier as "promoting the psychological for its own sake," that is, "beyond psychiatry."[34] Effectively, the report expresses the abandonment of the split between the normal and the pathological that psychiatry introduced into the realm of medicine in the nineteenth century. With suffering, the normal is brought into the field of mental health: individuals living in precarious situations are not sick; the psychic distress they experience represents the appropriate response to their socioeconomic situation. Their suffering is in no way pathological: on the contrary, it demonstrates that they are functioning well psychically. The new horizon of public action in this domain is therefore not psychiatry, in the sense of treating mental pathologies listed in a traditional nosography consisting of depressions, neuroses, and psychoses, but literally mental health in the sense of taking care of those wounded by the ordeals of life.[35] However, the authors of the report did not immediately hit on the term "suffering," which has since become the sole legitimate designation. Among the professional networks working on these issues, which formed the backbone of the working group, experts would rather speak of "ill-being" (alternately *mal-être* and *malaise*—terms found throughout this document).[36] But the word "suffering" probably better describes an experience that anyone might share, which explains why it was brought to the fore in the report's title, not without literary aspirations. It therefore became the accepted term in public policy, social work, and mental health.

Second, the Lazarus report reverses the approach to the psychic problems encountered in the poor neighborhoods by focusing on the actors assigned to care for disadvantaged groups before even addressing these groups themselves: "The distress of those who intervene to assist these populations forms the point of departure for our reflection," states the report in the introduction. General practitioners, social workers, teachers: all of these professionals are emitting a "call of distress" that needs to be heard without delay, we are told, for there is "an objective urgent need to address their problems." They feel resourceless and impotent in the face of the situations they are encountering, resulting in all the phenomena of exhaustion that are observed among them. This analysis draws on a central element of the psychodynamics of work, which played a pioneering role in revealing suffering and was becoming increasingly popular at that time. The 1998 publication of *Souffrance en France* (Suffering in France) by Christophe Dejours, the instigator of this school of psychoanalysis, triggered a plethora of reports in the press and special issues of journals. In his book, Dejours showed that "the irreducible gap between the prescribed organization of work and the actual organization of work," between ascribed objectives and real outcomes, was the major source of suffering for salaried workers, from the lowest-ranking employee to senior managers.[37] This was precisely what all those studying the professions involved in social care had been observing—the gap between collective expectations of social workers in particular and professionals dealing with disadvantaged groups in general, and their capacity to find solutions for the populations they were supposed to help, whether in the form of financial assistance, housing, employment, or education.[38] But over and above this issue of the painful experience of powerlessness, what was identified in the suffering of professionals was the logic of compassion contagion: they suffered in their contact with those who were suffering, simply through the force of empathy.

Thus it was established, first, that the social could make people suffer without it becoming a pathology, and second, that this suffering affected both users and providers of services. It followed that in the wake of this report, on the premises of its analysis and on the basis of its proposals, what the psychiatric team in Lyons called a "clinic of the psychosocial" became established. This was of course not the only place where a mental health practice developed around exclusion.[39] Nevertheless, it merits particular attention in view of the public visibility it brought to psychic suffering.

The two new avenues opened up by the 1995 Lazarus report's innovations reappeared in this psychosocial practice. On the one hand, a new reality was being addressed: "This suffering, which is by definition psychic because it is experienced in the singularity of the individual, is not of the 'object' of psychiatry," wrote Jean Furtos. "Rather than speaking of etiology, a concept more appropriate to causalist medical thinking, I would say that we are witnessing an existential pain with a social topography: one can 'have pain to one's social link' just as one can have myocardial pain." The medical metaphor virtually paraphrases Pierre Bourdieu's formula ("not well in themselves"/"not well in their social position"). More precisely, according to the director of ORSPERE, "the field of psychosocial practice emerges in the two zones of objective loss of social objects"—that is, aid (which manifests a form of dependency on social action) and exclusion (which manifests a breakdown of all social links). Both situations are matters of "mental health" as opposed to pathology. On the other hand, the suffering of service providers themselves, faced in their practice with the suffering of users, must be taken into account: "The excessive sense of urgency returns them to a feeling of distress and powerlessness," Furtos asserts. "It is important to recognize this feeling of urgency, to honor it as such without trying to respond with omnipotence or haste; otherwise what results is bitterness and disappointment, we will call it failure and will become exhausted."[40] Significantly, moreover, ORSPERE's activity focused mainly on service providers, notably in the form of "working groups made up of social workers" employed in the fields of social assistance, job-seeking support, and housing, in order to analyze the "problems encountered" in collaboration with them. Psychosocial practice, thus defined and deployed, was admittedly not recognized by all mental health specialists—and many of the professionals I encountered in the course of my research in the Paris region did not make reference to it, or even dismissed it as irrelevant—but it did define a frame of reference that is all the more difficult to ignore given the high level of legitimacy it enjoyed among public authorities and the organizational skills it demonstrated in the burgeoning field.[41] With its observatory and its network, its journal and its conferences, the clinic of exclusion was extending its institutional influence.

Within the course of several years suffering had become a routine object of public policy. Emerging from academic circles, recognized by a few clinicians on the fringes of psychiatry, benefiting from a context where the exposure of intimacy and recognition of subjectivity gave it a sort of shared self-evidence, it was only constituted politically at the point when actors authorized to speak of mental health gave it not only the sanction of their authority but also the resources of their profession. The addition of the adjective "psychic," which appeared only in the mid-1990s, represented the symbolic gesture that authenticated this new notion and permitted the provision of care for these new patients. The psychiatric description of a "psychic suffering" caused by a social situation or position therefore functioned as a performative utterance that justified the entry of the concept into the domain of public action. Admittedly, the actors involved were not the most established within the mental health system, since they included neither professors nor scientists, but the success of their enterprise was guaranteed by the convergence of their logics with a political world that had become aware, through expert reports to senior levels of government but also via the daily coverage of the media, that exclusion and its consequences were not only social but also political issues. The creation of listening centers was one of the consequences. It marked the official entry of social suffering into the lexicon of public action.

BEYOND WORDS

Language is what enables us to have access to the world and communicate the meaning of what we apprehend, but Wittgenstein's analyses remind us not to take the word for the thing, and the proposition for the reality it only claims to name.[42] The "critique of language" that he asserts as the root of all philosophy has two implications for the social sciences. On the one hand, we must ask to what extent the words used contribute to forming (and transforming or even deforming) the objects that constitute the world, and on the other, we must examine the way actors take hold of words to manipulate them (make them their own, misappropriate or contest them) in their everyday activity. In other words, we need to grasp the movement whereby language imposes a reality and at the same time the real resists language. This means that it is essential to study the concrete introduction of the vocabulary of suffering and listening into French public policy during the 1990s. We need to take seriously the effect that words have in the representation of the social world (speaking of exclusion rather than inequality or poverty, of suffering rather than injustice or violence, of listening rather than equity or sanction), and equally what actors do with it (when they speak or act).

The two ministerial circulars of June 14, 1996, and April 10, 1997, that instituted listening facilities are interesting from this point of view, because what they state differs from the reality to which they refer. The first circular opened with the problem—the subject of intense media focus at the time—of "marginalized youth taking up begging." The second highlighted "the use of toxic substances, entry into crime, the gang phenomenon." In both cases, problems of public order were the apparent justification for the initiative. But the solution remarkably consisted in listening to "the distress" (according to the first circular) or "the needs felt" (in the words of the second). This approach to marginal youth and drug abuse represents a remarkable translation of a social reality into a public problem and public policy: deviance was recognized as suffering, and the response prioritized listening over repression. At least this was the political account. Institutional practices and social usage would take a few liberties. The unspecific nature of the circulars; the necessity to facilitate rapid application of the measures, which favored structures already in place that had been conceived with distinct logics; the diversity of professions represented in the facilities, albeit with psychologists being in the majority; and the heterogeneity of the target populations, who ranged from well-integrated high school students and runaway teenagers to the long-term unemployed and illegal migrants: all these elements contributed to making the operation of the listening centers far removed from what the ministers who signed the circulars, but also the promoters of the project, imagined.[43] There is nothing particularly remarkable in this, one might think, for the reality of public policy never marries its stated intentions. But in the case of these centers, the ambiguities and lack of definition were constitutive of the very project that conceived them.

Suffering itself, which the facilities were supposed to address, remained problematic. In practice the actors involved in listening centers constructed it practically in terms of a range of logics, depending on the psychoanalytic and sometimes the political tradition to which they adhered, but also on the aims and the users of the center where they worked. Some highlighted it and portrayed it in excess: any unexpected manifestation, any untoward element of language or behavior, a complaint but equally a silence, could testify to a suffering that the individuals deemed to be affected need not necessarily have recognized or validated, precisely because those who suffered often failed to acknowledge their suffering for what it was. Others criticized the notion and rejected the political instrumentalization of their discipline: in their view, social difficulties did not always generate suffering, and conversely, suffering had sources other than social ones; above all, they objected that psychologists and psychiatrists were not there to act as a sort of mental police by treating the psyches of individuals whose problems were social. Many, however, considered suffering a self-evident fact that did not need to be questioned: they used the term as if it went without saying, and some even refined the meaning of it by introducing a distinction between psychic suffering and social suffering.

Moreover, there was not simply the question of what suffering is, but also of who suffers. A psychological support unit had been set up in Paris to provide assistance to recipients of the minimum guaranteed income when the "referring" social workers considered they presented psychic disturbances that hindered their search for work.[44] Thus a consultation with a psychologist became part of recipients' "job-seeking project," and refusal to attend could theoretically result in their monthly income being reduced or withdrawn. At his first meeting, one benefit recipient could not hide his surprise at finding more social workers than disadvantaged people at the listening center: the former had come to participate in one of the working groups set up around the theme "suffering of professionals and burnout in relation to aid," which apparently generated more interest than the sessions for the latter. "It's a bit strange for an organization like this," he commented. This anecdote points to a general fact that, as we have seen, originated in the premises of the 1995 report: the social workers faced with the suffering of others, sensing their powerlessness to remedy it, experience vicarious suffering.

In these conditions, it is easy to understand why the argument that "the social" (as it was frequently referred to in a reified way) was being "psychiatrized" or even "psychologized" was so often used, especially among actors working in listening centers or in mental health more broadly, to condemn, if not the reality, at least the risk of developments in psychiatry and psychology focused on managing the poor. While not contesting this potentiality, we need to take the true measure of it in light of the inverse processes, much less frequently raised, of under-psychiatrization and de-psychologization, if I may use such unrefined formulations. These processes emerged in two very distinct ways. Under-psychiatrization, on the one hand, was the result of disaffection on the part of psychiatrists—already few in number, particularly in the most disadvantaged areas—for working in the public sector and the standard-fee private sector: they were choosing instead the free private sector or charging top-up fees, effectively putting their services out of reach of patients with low incomes. For example, psychologists in Paris treating unemployed patients approached fifty psychiatrists in the city to ask if they could refer the most difficult cases to them;

they were refused by all but one. The reason given each time was that their profession was not social work, and some more honestly admitted their concern that the presence of such patients in their waiting rooms would make their usual clientele uncomfortable. The putative danger of psychiatrization of the poor, except in the restricted context of the institutionalization of some pathologies, was therefore unlikely: it served principally to justify the failure of the majority of psychiatrists to engage in areas they knew little about and considered unrewarding. De-psychologization, on the other hand, derived from an almost opposite demographic reality. The surplus of psychologists on the job market led to increasing numbers of them working in a range of spheres—particularly that of social assistance, where they competed with social workers for the less specialized posts, including in the listening centers. However, rather than exporting their practice, as they would have liked to do, they found themselves forced to engage in activities often far removed from their training and habitus. In one of the centers under study, a psychologist who was effectively working with youth complained that she had been employed for anything but what corresponded to her skills. Yet this should hardly be a surprise: the ministerial circulars were clear about the need to "demedicalize and deprofessionalize" the new facilities. The poor were not mad, and suffering was not a pathology; hence care should "reforge the link," it was suggested, rather than "treat patients" who were actually not sick.

It was thus psychiatrists on the margins of their profession who gave psychic suffering its official status, while psychologists seeking work were recruited to listen to the weight of the world, but noticeably the majority of the former took good care not to venture into this new terrain, while the latter were usually called on not to do the work for which they were trained. In short, suffering was too broad a signifier to be entirely appropriated by mental health specialists, and listening a practice too ill defined to establish a real professional practice. But this suited public policy makers all the more since, in their view, the point was to address a social issue and therefore, despite appearances to the contrary, to manage neglected regions and marginalized groups rather than hearing the complaints of the excluded, to pacify rather than to treat. Social suffering is not just a psychological category: it is also a political construction.

Suffering is a recent invention. It is not, obviously, that people have not always suffered, nor even that anyone could say they were less aware of it before: it is just that suffering remained an essentially private matter, or else something set within the framework of religious experience and the redemptive suffering of Christianity. Suffering is therefore a recent invention to the extent that it has entered the public sphere and become a political issue. Considering the French case, twenty-five years ago the worker subjected to intense pressures on a production line, the unemployed man unable to find a job, the immigrant victim of racial discrimination, the teenager failing at school, and even the social worker faced with professional contradictions probably suffered. But we did not know about it and they did not say so. There was no legitimate place to express it: suffering did not exist socially. Today we recognize it. The idea that social conditions such as poverty, exclusion, marginalization, and even social position, in the sense of the gap between expectations and reality, tensions between goals and limitations, should be sources of frustration, humiliation, distress, or torment has become familiar—in short, natural—to us. It is now a commonplace of political and trade union discourse, of commentaries on high schools and housing projects, of analyses of the economic crisis and the state of the world. The "social"—a vague essentialization of inequality, violence, and deviance—makes people suffer, and that suffering must be heard. It should even be listened to, and this was the aim of the policies introduced in the late 1990s.

A history of suffering should probably begin from Charles Taylor's observation in his genealogy of the modern moral identity.[45] Our conception of human respect is based on avoiding suffering, he underlines, pointing to the public punishments imposed on criminals in the past, and the scenes of popular excitement they aroused, as something that has become foreign to our sense of humanity.[46] He concludes: "We are much more sensitive to suffering, which we may of course just translate into not wanting to hear about it rather than into any concrete remedial action. But the notion that we ought to reduce it to a minimum is an integral part of what respect means to us today."[47] In the *longue durée*, his analysis is correct. But looking specifically at the contemporary period I am analyzing here, two significant inflections need to be added: one relates to the definition of suffering, and the other raises a paradox about the exposition of it. First, suffering is not just a physiological or psychological fact; it is also a social construction. When Taylor thinks of suffering he probably has in mind bodily pain, but suffering has recently been redefined and considerably broadened to include a whole range of affects assumed to be present in individuals facing difficult social situations, and hence imputed to an immaterial agency. We are witnessing an extension of the domain of suffering. Second, suffering is no longer something that should be hidden from others or concealed from oneself: it is something that can legitimately be described in others and revealed in oneself. Where Taylor saw a refusal to hear about suffering, we must now emphasize the collective concern to expose it; not only is suffering displayed in images, stated in discourse, and recounted in interviews, but listening to it now forms part of public policy, and more particularly of the social aspect of policy, on the same basis as medical care for sick people in precarious situations and financial assistance for those facing economic hardship. The question, parallel to that posed by Michel Foucault about sexuality,[48] thus becomes: Why today are we so attached to both showing and talking about suffering?

This verbal and visual display of our compassion has been the object of a range of contradictory appreciations. Some condemn the mawkishness of our sentiments and the complacency of our listening: we are in an era of victims where everyone pities themselves and others. Others, on the contrary, applaud the attention finally being given to what hitherto went unrecognized and remained a hidden, illegitimate, unheard pain. Finally, many are content to take it for granted that we are suffering more and that this is why we talk more about it; this position originates sometimes in naivety or, conversely, in instrumentalization, but usually derives from a moral conviction that social links have broken down. Rather than adopting one or other of these positions, I have tried here to answer not the philosophical question of *why*, but rather the sociological issue of *how*. What happened over the past few decades that led us to recognize social subjectivity? And what is happening now that institutions have been set up to respond to this suffering? Nikolas Rose was certainly one of the first to grasp this question:[49] "The self is a vital element in the networks of power that traverse modern societies," he writes. "The regulatory apparatus of the modern state is not something imposed from outside upon individuals who have remained essentially untouched by it. Incorporating, shaping, channeling, and enhancing subjectivity have been intrinsic to the operations of government." It is this practice of government that interests me, as it is embedded not only in discourses and regulations but also in structures and actions. In France, one of the least egalitarian countries in the West in terms of income, taxation, education, or health, and in an era in which social inequalities have continued to deepen, the normalization of social suffering in the public arena and the institution of a national policy of listening do not derive only from new forms of subjectivation resulting in the manifestation of a concern for the misfortune of others; they are also modes of government that strive to make precarious lives livable and elude the social causes of their condition.

Let us return to the premises of this policy. In his manifesto for the presidential election campaign, published on January 10, 1995, Jacques Chirac anticipated the risks of "social fracture" and the resulting "disarray," predicting, like a prophet of social suffering and its damaging consequences: "A soft terror holds sway in the disinherited neighborhoods. When too many young people see on the horizon only unemployment, or pointless training courses following ill-defined studies, they end up rebelling." Ten years later—following a period during which inequalities had continued to deepen—France's "disinherited neighborhoods" erupted in the most violent riots of the past three decades. The talk then was no longer of social suffering: rather, a state of emergency was declared. It was the end of an era. Security had taken over from humanitarianism.

2.   Pathetic Choice

Exposing the Misery of the Poor

> We cannot know why the world suffers. But we can know how the
> world decides that some suffering shall come to some persons and
> not to others.
>
> GUIDO CALABRESI AND PHILIP BOBBITT, *Tragic Choices*

How was "1 billion francs" to be distributed efficiently and fairly to the
poor? This was the question faced by the French state following Prime
Minister Lionel Jospin's announcement, in January 1998, that he was to set
up a *Fonds d'urgence sociale* (Social Emergency Fund, Fus) as a political response to "the movement of the unemployed and the precarious" (to use
the phrase that quickly became accepted). Over the preceding weeks, this
social conflict had emerged not only as the most pressing issue the new
Socialist government had confronted since it came to power, but also as the
problem of greatest concern in the view of public opinion, which had been
sensitized by the media's focus on the theme of poverty as Christmas holiday season was approaching.[1] The protest had started after the announcement of the suppression of social funds from the UNEDIC (the unemployment
insurance system), which provided support for those of the unemployed who
were in the greatest difficulty and which in December tended to be seen as
an automatically allocated Christmas bonus.

To compensate for the loss and above all to stop the social mobilization,
the prime minister and Martine Aubry, minister for employment and
solidarity, decided to release a sum that, although slightly lower than the
usual total of those funds, had a symbolic value—a "round" billion francs,
or 150 million euros[2]—and commissioned local authorities to distribute it,
in place of the local offices of the ASSEDIC (the unemployment insurance
local agencies), which had fulfilled this task for the old social funds. At the
time, there were officially 3,114,000 people seeking work in France, representing 11.8% of the population of working age, one of the highest rates in
recent years and, moreover, considerably above the European average.[3] The
ministerial circular addressed to prefects (the representatives of the state

in the local administration of the *département*) on January 12 stated that the government's initiative was intended to benefit "people and families in severe distress who, even with the existing provision, are at serious risk of being unable to support themselves." Armed with this instruction, which left a great deal to their interpretation, and faced the day after the televised announcement of the establishment of the fund with a flood of applicants, the officials responsible for implementing the measure were forced to improvise responses, imagine procedures, and invent principles in order to ensure equitable distribution of the state's largesse. This was a delicate exercise of meting out local justice for which they were unprepared, and they were to discover the extent to which their decision could dramatically influence the situation of the people concerned.

The allocation of a scarce resource poses a now classic problem that sociologists describe as a "tragic choice."[4] Much has been written about this issue, mostly in relation to its medical implications, and particularly concerning organ transplants, which present a paradigmatic situation since the supply of organs is much lower than the demand from suitable candidates and criteria therefore have to be established so that this scarce resource can be distributed fairly. The decision is clearly tragic because it concerns commodities whose effect is to prolong life or improve its quality.[5] Emergency financial aid is of course a very different situation. Its distribution may appear to raise much less troubling questions because it is assumed not to affect the physical existence of potential beneficiaries of this aid, and to be a matter of the more prosaic everyday provision of social support.[6] But reading the applications submitted by those requesting aid, with the details of their income, duly attested by written documents, and the letters listing the reasons for their needs, suggests that one would be justified in taking the opposite view and considering that poverty also puts individual survival at stake, albeit in a different way. The following passage, written by a thirty-five-year-old French man who had been unemployed for a year, was divorced with five children, and had a monthly income of 325 euros with fixed monthly expenditure of 357 euros for his rent and the alimony he paid to his ex-wife, gives an idea of the content of the appeals submitted to regional government offices in the hope of obtaining the emergency aid:

> I just can't cope anymore, I worked in Italy as a molder and stratifier for eight years because my ex-wife lived there, there was no relationship problem between us, I had to come back to live with my parents in R. it's not working out there either because I've been trying to get

away from my stepmother since I was a kid all I've got to live on is the RMI [*Revenu minimum d'insertion* (minimum guaranteed income)] and I send 150 euros to my children, I've never asked for help but now I'm not ashamed to any more because I don't know what to do, believe me it's really hard. The social worker in R. helped me get a room at the Sonacotra [social housing for immigrants] hostel in V. because I was supposed to have a job there but it didn't work out, what's more I haven't paid the hostel deposit which is 400 euros and I'm worried I'm going to end up on the street because I can't go back to my parents now I'm living from day to day I've got no one I can count on except your help, I've got nothing to eat, I've sold the few clothes I had at the flea market to get something to eat I don't know what more I can say I'm counting on your help Thank you

It might be thought that this situation (with its unavoidable expenses exceeding available income) is exceptional. It is not. The statistical analysis I carried out with the services of the Direction Départementale des Affaires Sanitaires et Sociales (Directorate of Health and Social Welfare, DDASS) in Seine-Saint-Denis (the *département* where I conducted this research) shows that, of the twenty thousand individuals who submitted an application to the Social Emergency Fund, one-third of the unemployed receiving the corresponding benefit, one-fifth of those on minimum guaranteed income, and one-tenth of salaried workers had fixed costs greater than their regular income: in other words, to use the quite surprising but particularly expressive terminology of social action, they had negative "rest for living."[7] Thus whether they were unemployed or in low-paid work, receiving unemployment benefit or social security, people were at risk—to varying degrees, but always substantially—of having unavoidable expenses higher than their regular income and of being able to survive only by going into debt. The problem of the tragic choice was therefore effectively posed, because there was a limited quantity of a disposable good to be allocated to those whose material—and even biological—conditions of existence were at stake.

The politicians' rhetoric of "vital needs" that had to be met located the issue of this government-instituted financial assistance clearly in the register of "survival," a language that the applicants used in their letters. As the plea quoted here and many others testify, there was an issue of damage not only to people's dignity but also to their bodily integrity. By stating the aim of this emergency fund as being to address "the most difficult situations" that could not be resolved through "social security," the government was clearly indicating that its intervention was somehow below the level of social justice, in the simple arena of "maintaining the conditions of existence."[8] The members of the committee for allocation of the fund said that they had "discovered" that they were dealing with "food poverty," and stated that they thought the aid they granted would allow recipients to "get their head temporarily above water." In their view, the decision whether to grant aid and what amount did indeed represent a tragic choice, in the sense that it had a decisive impact on the conditions of existence of those seeking financial support. This choice was nevertheless unusual because people were asked to justify their application in a short text explaining the reasons for their request. They were invited to recount their misfortunes and their poverty, looking for words that might move and win over their readers. More than tragic, the choice was pathetic, in the sense that applicants attempted to provoke emotions. Harking back to the traditional form of a petition addressed to the sovereign,[9] institutions were calling for an exposition of the applicants' suffering and needs.

To understand the responses to these petitions, my research was conducted through a series of interviews and the analysis of a sample of applications.[10] If it is true, as Harold Garfinkel argues,[11] that "the person defines retrospectively the decisions that have been made," which suggests paradoxically that "the result precedes the decision," then it can be understood that this method allows for the rules stated at the outset to be compared to the subsequent decision outcomes. I therefore focus first on analyzing the principles of justice brought into play, as justified by the members of the committee in the interviews I had with them, in order then to test these principles against the practices of judgment as evidenced by examination of the case files. Through this confrontation, I endeavor to understand what moral evaluation actors were making when they decided to grant aid to some rather than others, thereby alleviating the suffering of some people and not others; but I also seek to analyze, in counterpoint, the efficacy of the applicants' arguments and the rhetorical choices they made in their attempt to move the officials. To do this, I must proceed via a precise analysis of the state's reasoning that lay behind the individual decisions. It is only by examining the detail of the calculations made or corrected, focusing on the crossings-out and underlining, that we can understand what is at stake in their choices. I hope readers will forgive the sometimes wearisome nature of this investigation: it is the price for making the practice of public charity intelligible.

THE REST FOR LIVING

There is an important difference between the distribution of financial aid and the classic cases that the concept of the tragic choice has been applied to in the field of medicine. In the case of financial aid, the resources available can in theory be divided as desired, which is clearly not the case with organs for transplant or even drugs to be administered. We could imagine the extreme case of a formally egalitarian system of allocation where the same sum would be granted to all applicants, following the model of the distribution of "Christmas bonuses" to the unemployed, thus eliminating any possibility of choice: this is in fact how the aid was allocated in Marseilles. However, applying this principle runs contrary to the spirit of the measure as clearly stated in the ministerial circular and fully internalized by the members of the committees: the point was not to supplement income in order to remedy the shortfall of social protection, which would have meant appearing to cede to the demands of the unemployed workers' organizations, but to ensure that "aid is at a level high enough to provide assistance appropriate to the situation of each individual, and adjusted to the cases of distress identified." "Appropriate" and "adjusted": this is clearly a scarce resource that not all can benefit from, but it is unusual in that the amount allocated can be set on the basis of criteria left up to the devolved services of the national state—in other words, the local Directorates of Health and Social Welfare. The procedure of judgment brought into play relates both to eligibility (who should receive aid?) and to the amount (how much should be given?). Thus the decision has two aspects, like that which juries in France are called on to make in determining the guilt of the accused and the penalty to be inflicted; this leads to a retribution that is easily modulated.

Moreover, as we have seen, the persons allocating the aid were not simply informed of the applicants' objective situation, as in the case of decisions on organ transplants or the allocation of drugs, but were solicited by the subjective account of each applicant's request. This statement was an essential element of the application file, and the "description of financial difficulties and reasons for the request," as it was labeled, was even designed as a way of circumventing the usual assessment by social services, for reasons both practical (saving time) and ideological (to avoid what was seen as the normative view of social workers). The fundamental principle of the new procedure, according to a senior manager of the local administration, was "not to base the allocation on social assessment but to recognize individuals' autonomy and their ability to express their needs clearly."

This option put applicants in the position of having to justify their request in a text, with the conviction that the final decision would depend on this justification. Hence the energy that applicants invested in laying out their story and their suffering, which led one director of health and social welfare to comment coldly that her officers were "crying along with the disadvantaged." Compassion could therefore be an important element in the procedure.

Before embarking on an analysis of the decisions, we need to get a sense of the sums involved. The initial amount of 150 million euros was fixed by the government on the basis of the downward adjusted total of the social funds distributed by ASSEDIC, which had averaged 213 million euros over the preceding three years. This figure exuded a powerful symbolism (the "billion francs" for the unemployed and the poor), serving to demonstrate the goodwill of the government and contain the anger of those out of work, even though it was modest in comparison with the 300 billion euros (a sum two thousand times greater) devoted annually to the "nation's social program." The Ministry for Employment and Solidarity then distributed this sum to the ninety-five local administrations on a pro rata basis in relation to the number of registered unemployed and of persons on minimum guaranteed income, two figures considered valid indicators of poverty. Thus the Seine-Saint-Denis *département* was to receive 4.5 million euros for distribution; comparing this sum to the 1 billion euros distributed in child allowances and other social benefits by the Office for Family Allocations in the same year gives an idea of its relative significance. The amounts in question were indeed fairly modest.

In practical terms, distribution of the sums was the task of the "allocations committee" set up by the Social Emergency Commission, under the authority of the Préfet. The committee, chaired by a senior officer of the Directorate of Health and Social Welfare, also included representatives of the elected local assembly (Conseil Général), of the Office for Family Allocations, and of the Unemployment Insurance Agencies. It had sole power of decision regarding the twenty thousand applications submitted over a period of just under six months. It met four or five times per week, often for half a day, and usually involved senior officers of these bodies. The committee met a total of 115 times, and in some of the sessions in March and April assessed more than four hundred applications. This was a remarkable process, in which the everyday management of one-off assistance was entrusted to an assembly of directors of regional institutions carrying out a task normally devolved to social workers or administrative officers. It was nevertheless a process that was ill-suited to the idea of individual assessment of cases, because even at such a fast pace the average time devoted to each application was around one minute—and still less when the workload was the heaviest. By the end of the process, grants had been allocated to 72% of applicants, significantly below the national average of 80%, a discrepancy all the more noteworthy considering the fact that Seine-Saint-Denis is one of the most disadvantaged *départements* of the country and had to deal with a considerable number of applications: as we will see, this was the consequence of the disqualification of part of the immigrants and of the development of a form of compassion fatigue. What interests me is the process of decision and, even more specifically, this virtual encounter between the members of the allocations committee and the physically absent applicants, when emotion and reason concur to the decision.

The Ministry of Employment and Solidarity's guidelines for establishing criteria for this decision are at once politically precise and technically vague. They effectively formulate two political requirements. First, the response to each application should be personalized, in line with the individualized approach to the social that had become the new government doctrine.[12] Second, it must address emergency rather than simply supplementing insufficient resources, in the manner of the traditional logic of aid.[13] These two criteria emphasize the fact that the assistance must never be presented as a "due," a principle that one of the chairs of the allocations committee made baldly clear, asserting that the "logic of the aid" was to "get away from the 450 euros demanded by the unemployed" in their calls for a minimum benefit. In offering personalized emergency assistance under these conditions, national solidarity was to be distinguished from the demands of the unions and workers' organizations: neither automatically granted "Christmas bonus" nor improvement in the overall level of "social benefits," the Social Emergency Fund was to give to each poor individual according to his or her situation and his or her needs.[14] Charity is not without hidden political agendas.

As in most *départements*, the Seine-Saint-Denis allocations committee did not adopt preestablished rules, but gradually built up a "doctrine," as the senior administrative officers termed it. The overall principles of the procedure were formulated during the initial meetings: decision on the basis of the information presented by the applicant, and thus without assessment by social workers; individualized approach integrating objective and subjective account of difficulties; response essentially corresponding to financial emergency; advice as to other resources available if appropriate. However, no principle for defining eligibility was established. According to one of the committee chairs: "The criteria were never completely defined, and never set out clearly. But we realized empirically that we were calculating a residual income on the basis of income minus fixed costs, which we divided by the number of individuals in the household in order to determine the per capita rest for living. When this was below 150 euros, we gave a grant." Nevertheless, this method is perhaps less the fruit of chance than this might suggest. The calculation of family income based on the same principle was already being used by the children's welfare service in the allocation of temporary benefits for families in difficulty. In effect, the "rest for living" was no doubt more noteworthy as a linguistic invention than as a technical innovation: it expresses perfectly the minimalism to which administrative language was reduced in the operation of aid programs for groups whose living situations were illuminated by the crude light of statistics, showing that almost one in four individuals had negative residual income—they had literally nothing to live on and therefore could not avoid falling into debt.

While the procedure for calculating the monthly sum available per person resulted from a simple adaptation of existing tools, the way the maximum income level for eligibility—150 euros for a single person, for instance—was determined calls for explanation. Two reasons were generally put forward for this choice. The first relates to custom, as this amount was already in use in "social assessments" without ever having really been formalized. The second reason emphasizes the magnetic effect of the "round sum of a thousand francs." However, one of the committee chairs, casting back to their initial working sessions, offers a third, unexpected but striking, interpretation:

> There were a lot of applications from immigrant workers living in hostels. To start with we were turning them down. Most of them were receiving minimum income, and with what they were paying in rent they had a residual income of about 150 euros. So we thought: they've got a roof over their heads, they can afford to eat, they don't fall within the strict framework of the circular, because its aim is not to combat poverty but to respond to situations of distress. And they were often asking for aid for their families, who'd stayed behind in their country, but the fund wasn't set up for that. So since we wanted to treat everyone in the same way, the 150 euros came from that. Yes, that's where we got that figure from.

While it is impossible to discern which of these three explanations is the correct one, it is nevertheless worth noting that the first two relate to a relatively anodyne generality that allows for a rationalization both effective and plausible, while the third on the contrary expresses a form of invisible discrimination at the heart of the state administration: on the one hand, it gives exceptional status to migrants living alone in hostels, because their situation appears never to be classified with the common lot of serious distress; on the other, it maintains the appearance of equality, masking this exclusion by establishing a discriminatory rule in the name of an apparently universal principle. Of course, this exceptional status can only be combined with the principle of equality on condition that the fact that immigrants living in such hostels regularly send money back to their families, thus usually reducing their actual income below the established threshold, is not taken into consideration. This can be seen from the account of one Malian applicant, father of six children who he does not say are not living with him, though the committee assumed it, given his hostel address: "I only get the minimum income and I have a family to look after. I haven't had any work since '95 because of my age. I'm 57. And yet I've worked in France for 33 years. That's why I'm asking for exceptional financial assistance to get my financial situation into balance." However, this automatic rejection applied only to migrants living alone in hostels, and many immigrant families did receive assistance, sometimes substantial.

Whatever the reasoning behind them, the choice of criterion and the threshold established seem to move away from the ministerial guidelines. First, they replace the charitable reasoning recommended in the circular with a reference to a basic arithmetic standard. Second, they divert the aim of relieving emergency situations by operating simply as a palliative for insufficient income. There are two points to be made about this difference in relation to official policy. On the one hand, the principle of examining each case individually was systematically maintained, despite the institution of the standard income threshold. The committee scrutinized every case and read all the applicants' letters. Based on assessment of each situation, the individualized approach allowed for the possibility of reversing the automatic decision to grant or refuse aid that would have been triggered by income above or below the fixed threshold. Thus one of the committee chairs was justified in asserting that "applications were examined very individually," even if the indicator chosen played a greater role in decisions than had initially been envisaged. But on the other hand, making the decision on the basis of an everyday budget evaluated simply by subtracting costs from income rendered the notion of social emergency meaningless. The calculation revealed a trivial but obvious point, that the few dozen euros left over once the rent, water, electricity, and telephone bills were paid could not be enough to provide for the subsistence of the households in question, which included four out of five of those granted unemployment

TABLE 1. Social distribution of the "rest for living" per person

Residual income (euros)	Unemployed*	Minimum income*	Poor workers*	Applications granted**
Less than 0	34 (30)	21 (19)	10 (7)	86%
0 to 75	26 (23)	26 (24)	14 (10)	86%
76–150	22 (20)	28 (25)	37 (36)	93%
151–300	16 (5)	21 (11)	27 (11)	42%
More than 300	2 (0)	4 (0)	12 (1)	6%
Total (proportion of grants)	100 (78%)	100 (79%)	100 (65%)	74%

* The first figure indicates the total number of applications, the figure in parentheses shows the number of applications granted (expressed as a percentage in the last line): for example, 34 registered unemployed people had a negative residual income per person, and of these, 30 received assistance; 79% of those on minimum income received assistance.

** The proportion of applications granted measures the efficacy of the "rest for living" criterion in distinguishing between applications and thus guiding the decision: for example, when residual income was negative, assistance was granted in 86% of cases.

insurance, three out of four of those receiving minimum salary, and almost two-thirds of workers who had "rest for living" below the threshold (table 1). The civil servants' discovery of this "chronic poverty" refuted assumptions about temporary financial difficulties that would justify exceptional aid. This was pointed out by a high-ranked administrator, who said that "there's no real social emergency, except in the case of people who haven't got any housing or anything to eat"—a fairly rare situation. As some commentators did not fail to observe, the emergency the fund was really addressing was political rather than social.

The calculation of the "rest for living," and its use as a criterion for determining the committee's response, can ultimately be considered as a way of constructing an objective marker for the institution of local justice. This tool constituted a practical means of effecting the initial selection on an empirical basis that had been validated in other sites of distribution of public money. The selection proved globally effective: eight out of nine applicants living below the threshold received assistance, whereas two out of three living above the threshold were denied—this difference indicating that decisions were more often adjusted toward generosity.

A reading of the applications similarly shows that although it was initially taken merely as an indicator, the fixed threshold quickly became a psychological boundary. Several of the applications in which the disposable sum per person is a few euros above the crucial level show the trace of a rectification, with initial agreement being replaced by an ultimate refusal, indicated to the applicant through the formula: "Your situation does not meet the conditions set down by the circular issued by the Ministry of Employment and Solidarity on 12 January 1998, i.e. 'persons or families in situations of serious distress at serious risk of being unable to maintain subsistence.'" However, this formal justification often contradicted the applicants' letters. For example, such a negative response was provided to a man living with the minimum income whose application nevertheless indicated that he did fall within the framework of the circular:

> I've been renting since January 1996 and I've always prioritized paying my rent, just that I can't manage to pay all my expenses for December 1997. I've never asked for help before in spite of the difficulty I have at the end of each month. I put a lot of effort into finding a job and that costs me a lot of money and now I'm forced to go into debt for the first time and it's making me really anxious. I made a payment arrangement of 30 euros per month with the Seine-Saint-Denis Finance Department. Under the terms of my job-seeking contract, I have to do a training course that I'm really interested in, and I don't want my financial difficulties to get in the way of my plans for finding work.

The exceptional circumstances described in this text, and the applicant's demonstration of his good intentions, were only transitorily sufficient to overcome the mathematical effect of the threshold. The sum of 450 euros initially granted was then crossed out because his income was over the limit: his "rest for living" had been recalculated to 170 euros, putting him just over the threshold. Here reference to the norm operated as a decisive factor. But it was subject to almost ridiculous checks. In this case, for example, the applicant's income was 322 euros per month and his fixed costs were 265 euros, giving him a disposable sum of 57 euros, which should have meant his application lay below the threshold. He was rejected however because the committee adjusted his calculation to exclude the transport costs and debt repayments described in his statement, thus rounding the sum subtracted from his income down to 150 euros and causing him to lose the advantage of financial assistance. This observation illustrates the care taken in evaluating the "rest for living," as well as the absurd result to which it could lead. Not only were supporting documents required, but figures and calculations were checked, in some cases to determine the monthly figure for a cost covering several months or the whole year, in others to subtract a sum not deemed to qualify as part of fixed costs, and in still others to exclude a person considered not to belong to the household and therefore not to be taken into account in the calculation. There were nevertheless limits to the minute detail of this accounting, attested by the handwritten figures the officers added to the applicants' sums.

In effect, the applicants' own accounts of their situations contained aporia that made it virtually impossible to maintain complete consistency in deciding between them. For example, a thirty-year-old French man on minimum income declared that his only cost was the 120 euros he paid each month to his mother, with whom he lived. He had no other expenses, but noted 1,200 euros of debt resulting from fines for traveling without a ticket. This was why, he explained, "I would like to be able to travel by public transport with a valid fare to look for work." Obviously, the monthly train pass he was unable to pay for did not figure in the account of his fixed costs. However, it was the lack of it that had caused his debt, and which, now that he feared being caught again, contributed to his difficulties in finding a job. If, rather than expressing his wish to buy a ticket, he had been able to actually do so, the calculation of his residual income would have gone in his favor, because it would have been below the threshold; but he had not and was denied aid. Similar situations arose in the case of homeless people who could not afford to rent a room or stay in a cheap hotel and hence, lacking regular costs and sometimes living in the streets or squatting in empty apartments, paradoxically ended up above the threshold. This was the irony of aid: assessment of the person's economic circumstances did not include expenses that could not be incurred because of poverty, yet which would have made it possible to acquire goods or services indispensable in the search for a job.

The institution of an arithmetical criterion of eligibility derived from a concern for ease of decision as much as for equity in the distribution of aid. While retaining the possibility of generating a different decision in light of individual circumstances, especially in relation to the applicant's written statement, the committee members adopted a decision-making tool that was at least outwardly simple and reliable. Hence the success of this criterion, attested by both the concern for systematic checking of the calculation and its rapidly generalized use at the committee's sessions. Nevertheless, in use it proved more complex and less robust than had been imagined. Because economic assessments of households were always delicate and the instrument was applied hurriedly, without precise adjustment, but also because situations of poverty were particularly difficult to assess and minute variations in interpretation had irrevocable consequences for decisions, the use of the "rest for living" figure revealed its limits—limits of which the actors involved were not fully aware when a few euros above or below the threshold guided them toward rejection or acceptance.

SHARING OUT POVERTY

But the committee members did not only have to decide who was to receive assistance. They also had to determine the sum to be granted in such a way as to offer "an appropriate, proportionate response." In this respect, the total amount of the fund made a degree of generosity possible (an average of 321 euros for each of the 14,298 applications granted), at least compared to what the social services typically distributed in terms of aid. The sums in fact remained relatively modest, both in comparison with the levels of debt acknowledged (38% of applicants had debts above 1,500 euros) and in relation to the levels of need expressed (22% of applicants had fixed costs higher than their income). The head of the social services thus reported happily: "For the first time we had serious funds to respond to the need of people in difficulty for additional resources: instead of giving them a few measly euros to tide them over, we had substantial amounts that made it possible to give real assistance." She concluded with a tautology that nevertheless says a lot about the way aid works on the everyday level: "If we have very little money there's no point. What makes an assistance fund effective is if there is money." This relative financial affluence, compared to the aid normally distributed, was a source of satisfaction for all members of the committee, even though some added that their greatest pleasure was being able to restore a right to an applicant who until then had none, by pointing them toward the appropriate service. In this context, aid granted was never less than 150 euros. The average in the sample considered here was 335 euros; the highest amount granted was 840 euros. This shows that substantial adjustment was possible.

Two principles came into competition in the allocation of aid: the fixing of sums in relation to the roughly assessed composition of the family, and the case-by-case ruling based on specific criteria for each individual. The first established an economic scale that set "single people" against "families." The second sought to send a "signal" to applicants, by a sort of social semaphore. According to one of the committee chairs, the latter prevailed: "The sum granted aimed to cover part of the debt contracted or the fixed costs. We could either grant an amount that would provide general aid or an amount that had some meaning for the person to pay off a particular debt, for example to the electricity company, or to meet an unforeseen cost like a broken-down boiler, or to finance a one-off project like sending a child on holiday. As much as possible, we tried to grant assistance that people could identify. We avoided at all costs to just supplement their income." In the version provided by another committee chair, the order of priorities was inverted: "There weren't really tariffs as such, but more like norms. In principle we gave 150 or 200 euros for single people, 450 or 500 euros for couples or those with children. Unless there was something in the application that justified a specific amount: a debt, some life event, a specific project. In that case, we chose the sum to send a message to the applicant. But in the vast majority of cases it was impossible to identify a specific sum." This contradiction between the two versions—specific signal versus determined sum—reveals not so much a divergence in analysis as a real difference in the two committees' practices. Their respective chairs set their personal mark on the decision, one seeking to personalize aid to communicate different "meanings" to each applicant, the other trying to proceed through "norms" that were identical for all.

However, these declared preferences were not necessarily manifested in the decisions, as the following two examples illustrate. The first involves a French woman, mother of a young boy, unemployed, and living on a "rest for living" per person of 85 euros. Her account states: "Partner left leaving me with debts for unpaid rent and his car bills. A 3-year-old child who's often ill. Difficulty looking after myself and buying clothes for my son." The committee chair, who had asserted that he preferred to allocate an amount that the recipient could identify, nevertheless granted 450 euros in this case, a sum that simply corresponded to what he normally granted families with children. But in order to make his intention clear he wrote in the margin, "insurance, hospital + water"—a note about which the recipient would obviously never be aware because she would receive a standard letter with no indication of what the sum was supposed to represent; moreover, it was all the less "readable," in fact, because it was rounded up. The second case concerns the application of an Algerian man, married with five children, living on minimum income and family allowances, with a "rest for living" per person estimated at 100 euros. His letter explained: "I can't manage anymore. The children are leaving school and there's no work and that means they're staying at home so as not to be homeless and I also have to feed them and buy them clothes." The committee chair who said when interviewed that he operated a scale of grants did not apply it in this case, but instead allocated a sum of 403 euros that corresponded to "one month's costs," according to the handwritten annotation. However, he clearly changed his mind, crossed out this conspicuously exact sum, and eventually granted 400 euros.

In both these cases, as in many others, the notes in the margin, the additional calculations and deletions reveal the careful attention paid to setting the amount of aid. But while the "message" was directed toward the applicant, the precise sum allocated has a meaning mostly for the person making the decision. Paradoxically, the applicants would know nothing about the "signal" addressed to them, except perhaps in the 4% of cases where a singularly precise grant might give them an inkling: receiving a sum of 163 or 574 euros might suggest that the figure corresponded to a specific reality that they might still have to detect behind the calculation that had resulted in it. But in more than two-thirds of the decisions where a note indicates that the committee sought to enable the applicant to repay a debt, overcome a difficulty, or realize a project, the rounded-up sum rendered the subtle choice imperceptible: thus in the two examples just given, the intention, which was explicit in the notes in the margin, was invisible to the recipient. Contrarily to what they imagined, the administrators were in fact talking to themselves.

Setting an amount that could be identified by applicants was not in any case opposed to the idea of a scale: the two situations described, which are fairly similar in socioeconomic terms, resulted in similar sums being granted, whatever the reasoning behind the calculation. In many cases, it appears that the final sum was fixed in relation to the signal the committee sought to communicate, but around a value corresponding to an established norm. A Moroccan woman who was earning the minimum wage for a part-time job, who was mother of a young child, and whose income after fixed costs amounted to 75 euros per person, was first granted 450 euros, in line with the scale; this was then adjusted to 425 euros to make it "readable," with the note "rent" indicated in two places on the file. In that case, she lost only 25 euros in this process of recalculation. But sometimes there was a wide gap between the two principles, as in the example of a Senegalese couple whose expenses were above their income: their supporting statement noted that their financial situation had resulted in a two-month delay in payment of wages, amounting to 700 euros. Rather than allocating the standard rate for this situation, the committee granted them the very exact sum of 204 euros for "3 months' residual rent," calculating the amount not in relation to the sum owed, but on the basis of the difference between the amount paid and the housing allowance they were receiving. For this couple, the loss resulting from the committee's application of the principle of legibility compared to the use of the scale was nearly 500 euros. Sending a "message" to applicants could therefore result in penalizing them. Instead of being pedagogic it was merely punitive.

In general, the tension between the two principles (scale and signal, norm and meaning) was resolved in accordance with a logic that prioritized "meaning," but on condition that the "norm" was not exceeded. The "message" sent should not cost too much, either in financial terms or from the point of view of the moral of the signal. Ideally, the two principles converged. Such was the case of a young Moroccan woman living with her two children and their father, on 126 euros per person, who received 433 euros, a sum corresponding exactly to her stated debt. When the sum deemed identifiable was below the scale rate, the lower amount was always granted. A French couple with a young child, living on 143 euros per person after costs had been deducted from a single wage, was granted 164 euros, a sum corresponding to their debt. A Tunisian single mother of one, earning a half-time minimum wage with a residual income of 91 euros per person, was awarded one month's rent, or 182 euros. In both circumstances the sum was well below what they might have received if the scale had been used.

When the sum the committee wished to set in order to make its response meaningful was too far above the scale, however, it was the scale rate that was applied, but in this case the contradiction was resolved either by abandoning the idea of sending a message or by adapting it. The first option (abandoning the message) is illustrated by the example of a Peruvian couple with one child, whose resources amounted to 107 euros per person after deduction of costs: the committee initially decided to grant them the equivalent of "half the rent arrears," or 730 euros, and then revised its decision in the light of the large amount, eventually authorizing the 450 euros that corresponded to the scale. The second option (adapting the message) corresponds to the situation of a French single mother with one child, whose costs exceeded her income and whose accumulated debts from her previous accommodation the committee wished to clear; since the sum was too high, she was awarded 600 euros, with a note at the bottom of the page: "arrears from Nantes, excluding housing tax (electricity, telephone, hospital, rent)." Through such complex adaptations, the committee members maintained what appeared to them as coherence in the principles of justice, combining universal rules with subtle reasoning.

These principles were, on the one hand, a principle of equality, setting an identical sum in relation to objective, albeit crude, criterion (number of people in household, with only two options—single person or more than one), and on the other, a principle of equity, giving to applicants according to their needs (effectively responding to one of three grounds: debt, unforeseen

---

General measure: the scale

Fixing of a "standard rate":
150–200 euros for a single adult, 450–500 euros for a family

Individualized measure: the signal

Identification of a "specific message" to send:
repayment of debt, resolution of a difficulty, realization of a plan

Final decision:

Signal resulting in cost above the scale value: "standard rate" is selected (*equality*)

Signal resulting in cost below the scale value: "specific message" is selected (*equity*)

Figure 1.   Reasoning behind the amount of grant awarded

circumstances, and one-off projects). In the general logic just described, equity prevailed, provided that it did not pose a threat to the principle of equality by suggesting too high a sum (figure 1). Reviewing the figures, it would appear that the scale was more widely applied than the signal: 58% of grants amounted to fixed sums; we have seen, though, that the reality of intentions is more complex, since an amount corresponding to a scale rate could be awarded with a particular intention. Sometimes the sums fell outside of this logic: only 150 euros was awarded in 11% of cases, particularly for single persons living with their parents; but generously 600 euros was granted in 4% of cases, often to large families.

It is nevertheless surprising that, given the care taken in calculating the "rest for living" for the purposes of determining eligibility, this calculation was never used in setting the amount of grants. The monthly residual sum available per person had no influence in the distribution of resources. Committee members never mentioned referring to this criterion. Moreover, analysis of the application files does not indicate that it played any part in the decision-making process. The committees did not give more to those who had less. Once applicants fell below the 150 euro threshold that made it highly likely they would receive assistance, they entered a different evaluation system. The level of per capita disposable income did not predict the grant received any more than it did eligibility, as I have noted. Just as a household with negative "rest for living" had no greater chance statistically of receiving aid than a household with between 100 and 150 euros per person, similarly the first household could not expect to receive more. In short, the Christian parable of the eleventh-hour laborers was being applied in the domain of aid. Once they entered the moral space of aid, individuals were no longer judged on the basis of their level of poverty when it came to determining the remedy for their problem. They were to be assessed only in relation to a basic scale and a semantic procedure whereby the authorities demonstrated their command of the rules of the game.

However, local justice cannot be described solely in terms of the rules by which those involved accounted for their decisions. Beyond the principles of justice underlying the distribution of aid—principles that were not formulated in advance to form a basis for decision making, but rather articulated by the actors after the fact to justify their reasoning—it was everyday reasoning, affective reactions, and moral positions that determined the acts of judgment.

COMPASSION FATIGUE

If the decision had rested exclusively on the calculation of an indicator and the establishment of a threshold (for the purposes of eligibility), and on the dual principle of keeping to a scale and sending a message (for the purposes of setting the amount of grants), the "description of difficulties and reasons for applying" submitted by applicants would have been of no more use than the "sums requested"—the sole value of which, as we have seen, was to demonstrate to the officers the reasonableness of poor individuals' expectations of public support. If this were the case, the individualized treatment of situations advocated by the government and claimed by the committee would have meant nothing. But this is not the case. A number of indices combine to demonstrate that committee members did not limit themselves simply to applying more or less explicit rules. Before examining these indices, it is nevertheless important to describe in detail the procedure for allocating resources. Being aware of the dual constraint of individualization of approach (with each case being presented separately) and limited time (an average of one minute per application), we can take the measure both of the significance of the rules and of the level of freedom committee members took on within these rules. Three elements testify to this maneuvering space the committees allowed themselves.

First, committee members' insistent highlighting of individual stories, which they combine with appreciations and sentiments about both the situations described and the decisions taken, shows the subjective importance of the administrative casuistry: "We were happiest when people living on social welfare had received a real blow and we were able to help them, for example when their washing machine had broken down." In another case: "There was this student exchange trip to Spain for the daughter of a Malian man who was bringing her up on his own and bleeding himself dry for her." The high-ranked administrators' interest in the accounts written by applicants was not only functional, using them to determine the petitioner's eligibility and the amount to be awarded. For some it also had an ideological aspect, testifying to the pointlessness of standard social assessments but not without a paternalistic tinge. "People are perfectly capable of formulating their request themselves. What struck me was the quality of expression and even the sensitivity of their letters. It was always very clear. That confirmed our initial analysis that people are autonomous," one regional officer in charge of social services remarked, in pleasant surprise: she did not know that "her poor" were gifted with such remarkable social competences.

Second, statistical analysis of the sample clearly indicates the maneuvering space the committee allowed itself in formulating decisions. In the assessment of eligibility, 53 decisions went against the preset threshold: 24 were harsher than the norm and refused aid to people whose residual income was below the 150 euro rate, while 29 were more generous and granted aid to households whose residual income was above the fixed limit. It is more difficult to quantify the reasoning for the decisions on the amount to be granted, as the justification is not always indicated: however, only 96 of the 224 favorable decisions were based exclusively on the scale; in the other 128 cases, personal data influenced the decision, with clearing debts noted in 31 cases. In general, the degree of freedom the committee allowed itself with regard to a universal norm such as a threshold or scale was greater when determining the amount than when assessing eligibility, if only because the stated principles explicitly included taking into account a criterion of "meaning" that covered multiple possibilities for choice.

Finally, qualitative analysis of the application files reveals a wide variation in decisions, particularly in the setting of the sum to be granted. The applicants' statements are often the decisive factor in these variations in judgment. A single man earning 1,070 euros per month and with fixed costs of 690 euros, whose income was thus 150% over the threshold, received 225 euros, with the note "in view of the debts and the context" written on his file. His "debts" actually amounted to 6,350 euros, the equivalent of one and a half years of his residual income, and his letter, which was no doubt what moved the committee, described the "context" as follows: "I live alone in a 2-bedroom apartment, until last month I was getting housing assistance benefits. I haven't got enough to live on properly, too many debts to repay. I can't get any money out of the unemployment insurance and my contract ends on 09/17/98. After that nothing. I want to start again, free of debt, without owing anything. I'm paying for mistakes when I was younger, now I'm 27 and I've got no future. No one wants to or can help me, maybe you can do something for me."

In retrospect, we can conclude that applicants were wise to take particular care in formulating their statement. In this justification exercise, their skills in arguing their case allowed them to pass a test. In the absence of true social assessment, the written account was deemed to recount an authentic story. The committee members' positive appreciation of the quality of these texts related less to their literary value or grammatical accuracy than to clarity of exposition and truthfulness of testimony. It was not enough for the account to move the reader, it was supposed to do so accurately, in a context where suspicion could result in an application being denied. However, when the committee's notes expressed doubt, this nearly always related to missing documents, whereas the statements were viewed as tangible proof of truthfulness. Two outcomes were possible.

In some cases the narrative convinced the committee, even if objectively the application was not very credible. In this circumstance reservations tended to be expressed through the amount granted, which would be below the level envisaged in the scale. A young French woman with two children stated that her income was 330 euros and gave a few more or less precise figures for her fixed costs, without providing any supporting documents. It was therefore impossible for the committee not only to verify her expenses but also to calculate the sum available per person. Nevertheless, her account convinced the committee because she was granted aid: "I've been on a training course from 2.27.98 to 5.28.98 = RMI = 330 euros with no wages: 0000F. Cost of transport meals clothes = 200 euros/month. I have expenses for clothes for the children canteen child-care fees and all the rest of the costs and as soon as I've finished my training I'm going to be working thank you for your understanding."

However, in many cases the statement was not sufficient to reverse a poor impression made by an application. The suspicion that arose when a disturbing detail was discovered could thus negate all the applicant's demonstrations of good faith. A young Peruvian single mother of two children, with a one-year residence permit, declared a wage corresponding to a part-time job paid at minimum wage, with costs exceeding her income. The bills she attached to her application, though, were in another name, as the examining officer of the application noted in two places: next to the statement of debt was written, "No! not in name of applicant"; then next to the final decision was noted, "electricity, telephone, rent bills in name of Mr. N. (same address) Mr. N. not included in the list of members of household!" Yet, closer reading of the application might have lifted the doubt, or at least identified that this discrepancy attested to its truthfulness: as is customary in Latin America, the children went by the family name of both parents, so that "Mr. N." could be identified as their father; the bills under the name of "Mr. N." indicated that the young woman had not changed the account name after he left, probably because of the precariousness of her residence status. The lack of supporting documentation with regard to these elements paradoxically argued in favor of her honesty—she restricted herself to simply outlining her needs, without imagining that suspicion of the documents submitted would lead to her being refused assistance: "At the moment I can't pay my electricity or phone bills and I can't feed my children properly and my wages aren't enough. I'm also in debt to my friends and my financial situation is difficult because I'm not getting child welfare or housing assistance benefits."

In contentious situations like these there was one element that was always decisive: if a social worker had been involved, by supporting the application with a comment, signature, or stamp, and sometimes by also helping to complete the form. The value attributed to this external sanction, especially when it demonstrated a clear opinion, obviously reveals the acknowledgement of skills ascribed to professionals, but also indicates that social assessment, despite being disparaged by some committee members, retained real legitimacy. Often a comment judiciously adapted to the logic of aid supported the request—for instance, for a French family with two children obtaining a sum of 600 euros, well above the scale: "The parents want to repay their debts. Don't dare tell us the amount." Sometimes a more directive statement was provided, as in the case of a Malian family with nine children who received the sum requested, beyond the standard rate: "The father received two huge bills in December: a reminder for one year's water costs, and rent for 1997. Can he be allocated financial assistance of 750 euros to help him pay these two bills?" Rarely, the intervention became more insistent, especially where there was an appeal against a prior decision. When a twenty-five-year-old French woman receiving the minimum income was twice refused aid by the committee because of insufficient "elements (grounds for application and supporting documents) to allow even a basic assessment of your situation," the social worker at the Roma Support Unit took on the application herself. Her vehement protest overcame the reservations of the committee, which was probably tired of resisting and awarded her 300 euros:

> You sent Miss F. a letter regarding your refusal to grant the financial assistance she had requested through me. The reasons for this refusal were the lack of documents supporting Miss F.'s account of her situation which could thus justify allocation of aid. I have put the application together myself in order to support her request and her personal and family situation have been clearly explained. Miss F. is registered disabled with an incapacity level of 80%, but she is waiting for her disability benefit to be renewed and in the meantime RMI is not always enough to cover her needs. She lives alone and is isolated following the accidental death of her mother in October 97; her father receives minimum state pension and lives alone; her brothers are on minimum income and live together but move around the whole of the Paris region. She still has to pay off some of her mother's funeral expenses, a sum of 900 euros, and she doesn't know what to do. Therefore given Miss F.'s very precarious personal and family situation, I am asking once again on her behalf for a grant of 900 euros from your organization.

Society has always had certain expectations of the poor—what they are and what they should be, how they behave and should behave. This is indeed a sociological fact that extends to anyone:[15] the representation we have of others tends to become a yardstick against which we judge their discourses and their actions. However, a particularly strong moral dimension is evident in relation to the poor, much more than to other social categories; this derives from the meaning that each society ascribes to poverty in the establishment of a just order. The detractors of social assessment on the committees took up the criticism often addressed to social workers: that of acting as agents of this normalizing ideology. "We wanted to get away from moralizing," said one of them emphatically. Their success remains to be established.

In fact, when writing their statement, applicants to the Social Emergency Fund tried to persuade their readers. Their primary means to this end, and to eliminating the physical and social distance between themselves and the decision makers, was to move them—in other words, to establish, through the statement, a relationship of proximity that could allow them to share a common humanity. In this attempt to create a link of sympathy that would make them virtually and transiently present in the space where decisions were made, they were obviously unaware of the principles and criteria applied by the committee (with reason, it might be added, because the committee itself only discovered these as it progressed through assessment of applications). Nevertheless, they had some idea of the way they would be

TABLE 2. Effects of rhetorical figures on committee decisions

	Tropes			
	Need	Justice	Merit	Compassion
Style	Factual (52%) 67%	Vindictive (4%) 83%	Dignified (20%) 89%	Imploring (24%) 77%
Register	Accountancy (32%) 65%	Protestation (9%) 83%	Virtue (20%) 83%	Sympathy (39%) 76%
Argument	Poverty (61%) 71%	Iniquity (10%) 75%	Integration (14%) 77%	Misfortune (15%) 87%

Note: The percentage shown in parentheses refers to the frequency the rhetorical figure occurs in the body of texts. The percentage shown in italics refers to the committee's rate of award of grants. Thus the factual style, observed in 52% of statements, resulted in aid being granted in 67% of cases. The parenthetical figures total 100% on the line (not the column). The figures in italics do not add, since the complement to 100% represents the denials (33% of applicants using a factual style were refused aid). For a detailed commentary on the meaning of each rhetorical figure and the methodology used in categorizing them, see Fassin (2000). Discussion within this chapter provides illustrations.

judged (even if only because of the multiple contacts most of them had previously had with welfare services).

Their rhetoric was grounded in four tropes of justification: need, justice, merit, and compassion, each of which was expressed via style (expressive tone), register (type of evidence submitted), and arguments put forward (nature of the facts referred to). There are two methods we can use to evaluate the influence of these texts on the committee's decisions. The first is statistical, calculating the rate of favorable response in relation to each rhetorical figure identified (table 2). This approach produces an exhaustive reading of applications and subsequent decisions generated but is limited in that the effects of each element of the account cannot be considered "all other things being equal." The second method is a case-by-case analysis of individual decisions, which is useful because for any given application it makes it possible to take into account, within the logic of the procedure adopted by the allocations committee, all the elements involved in the application, and even sometimes to make comparisons between similar situations. The limitation of this exercise is the individuality of each case and each decision. Both methods were used here. Before outlining the results, I describe the four tropes.

Need is expressed in a factual style, in the register of financial accounting, with the texts mainly reiterating data on income, costs, and debts, resulting in a double statement of insufficient resources and failure to meet needs: it thus appears largely redundant in relation to the administrative documentation, offering only a few elements of explanation or justification here and there, and has little effect on decisions. For example, a thirty-two-year-old married French woman with a residual income of 50 euros expressed her request in a sober tone:

> I'm asking you give serious consideration to my insecure situation.
> Been unemployed for more than 3 years, my husband's social security
> benefit has ended without renewal since February 97, he's not getting
> any income any more even though he's sick, he had his third operation
> recently, he doesn't get disability benefit and he can't work. We've been
> living on 430 euros that I get from unemployment insurance for a year
> and a half, with a rent of 300 euros per month plus our expenses. I'm
> sure you can imagine what it's like living in this situation. I hope you
> can help.

The theme of need is both the most frequent configuration and the only one that results in a lower-than-average rate of award. When a distinction is made, among the arguments put forward, between those that describe insufficient resources or financial difficulty and those that evoke the risk that their essential needs such as food, housing, or protection against the cold will no longer be met, the former received aid in only 67% of cases, while the latter were awarded grants in 80% of cases. The argument of need thus appears less effective, except when it presents a tragic statement of a threat to survival.

The theme of justice employs the style of vindication and the register of protest, either collective on behalf of the poor as a whole, or individual in reference to a personal wrong suffered at the hands of an employer or a government institution. A forty-six-year-old Algerian woman, bringing up four children on her own with a monthly residual income of 82 euros per person, says: "My current situation is as follows: I have 4 children to look after and my only income is 550 euros per month, I owe the state 9,600 euros, and I don't know how to clear it. I can't make it no more, I've got too many debts and I'm really disappointed that the government won't increase social security because that would really help poor families."

Justice represents a minor theme in the applications, noted in only one in ten of them: in effect applicants fall in with the role they imagine they are required to play within the structure of an application to the authorities, and only rarely express themselves in terms of demand; this argument therefore had little influence on the committee's decisions. Although we should be cautious in making this evaluation, given the low number of cases, it is notable that accounts highlighting social inequality in general or the unfairness of a particular situation were effective in 83% of cases: the only negative element was if the tone was threatening or, surprisingly, when suicide was evoked, since it was viewed as blackmail. Therefore, contrary to what applicants believed, the committee found their condemnations of social injustice legitimate.

Merit, which is manifested through a dignified style and in the register of virtue, seems to have been particularly persuasive for the committee. While not often employed, it was usually decisive. The virtuous poor have long been perceived as the deserving poor. In the form that applicants ascribe it to themselves, merit relates as much to the economic order (involving efforts to find a job) as to the social order (rejecting deviant practices) and to the moral order (putting forward family responsibilities). In the statements it is generally expressed with reference to these three orders. First, the desire to reintegrate into society through work is a recurrent motif that has been firmly internalized by applicants. One single man receiving unemployment benefits was awarded 225 euros, representing almost double what he requested:

> This is my social position I was doing health care training at L. hospital then I had to look for a job again I was getting unemployment benefit in the meantime I did a training course to get the certificate of professional capacity which I got no problem so I'm trained to drive coaches. So in that job I got work no problem in a halfway house. But now I have to buy a uniform and safety shoes that I have to have. That's why I'm asking you again if possible to give me a grant from 120 to 150 euros.

The promise to manage one's meager resources well also acts as an important pledge of goodwill, given that the administrative officers see debt as virtually a deviant practice. A jobless single man recounts: "The money problem and it's hard to live, especially to buy food. Because I've got a lot of expenses to pay as well as child support for my two children. I'm still living on the street. So I'm asking if you can help me pay off my debts and to get food." Justifying the decision to grant him 150 euros even though his net income was 175 euros, the committee chair noted: "Makes real efforts to balance budget."

Finally, concern for children or for aging parents, could stimulate the committee to look favorably on an application. A divorced father of two children who did not live with him, whose residual income was assessed at 200 euros, indicates: "I've got my children every other weekend, and half of the school holidays. I have to feed them, and myself. My motivation is to get back to better health, and get a job in my profession. I'm currently doing a training course in L. to get myself back on track. When I've got a bit more money I'll be able to provide better for my children's education and for them to visit more often, for them to be more comfortable." Combining plans for professional development and family care, his argument was heard: he received 225 euros.

But judgment as to merit can also be deduced by default, either in refusals, though this is rarely expressed as such, or in subtle deductions made in calculating the grant. One instance of a rejection on moral grounds is the case of a young French man receiving the minimum income who applied to help support his family, comprising his widowed mother and his two brothers, one of whom was working and the other in high school. His application contained all the evidence needed to calculate his residual income, which was 112 euros, in principle giving him the right to support. However, the committee was reluctant: the sum of 150 euros, which was initially allocated, was subsequently deleted. The problem was the man's declared debt—not the amount of it, but the specifics: "three-piece leather living-room suite," from a cheap store. The committee considered this an unacceptable reason. The attempt to reject the application hinged on three types of argument, although normally only one reason would have been sufficient: first, the committee reevaluated the expenses, but this did not raise the applicant's income above the eligibility level; then his income was questioned, through reference to "lack of detail about the applicant's situation," despite the fact that his situation was clearly described and supported with evidence; finally, the committee fell back on an alternative, suggesting the applicant be "directed to the Office for Family Allocations," which clearly was not appropriate for this case. In the end, the young man received nothing.

One example of moral deduction is the case of a Malian mother whose residual income per person was estimated at 56 euros and who described her situation in this way: "We are asking for financial support to pay a fine and an electricity bill. We are bringing up and educating three children in my school and my sister, whose guardians we are. We have to pay all our household expenses out of just minimum income and family allowances." The sum applied for was 309 euros. The amount granted was 240 euros, with the annotation "electricity/gas bill." Despite the modesty of the request, which was well below the standard rate, the fine of 70 euros was deducted from the amount awarded: in the eyes of the administration, this represented an unworthy debt.

Compassion, the remaining of the four rhetorical figures adopted in applicants' personal statements, employs an imploring style and is cast in the register of sympathy, often describing a misfortune or an accumulation of difficulties in precise detail. It forms part of the traditionally instituted relationship of the poor within social work and aid institutions. Because this emotion is produced in the interaction between the suffering of one and the gaze of the other, a common humanity can emerge despite the gap that separates the long-term unemployed individual and the officer charged with assessing his or her situation. Emotion is a powerful driver in the exercise of charity, particularly because it plays on two levels: empathy with the unfortunate individual, and the satisfaction of helping him or her. For both the civil servants and the social workers involved in completing the applications, as well as the committee members who made decisions about the aid to be granted, this dual dimension cemented a collective experience, which everyone talked about at length in the interviews. Hearing them describe their feelings about the misfortunes of the poor and the symbolic benefit of delivering even partial relief to them, it might be assumed that compassion would overwhelm the moral space of judgment. But this was not the case, and neither the imploring style that reiterated expressions of desperate supplication nor the register of sympathy that attempted to establish a relationship of proximity through concrete and painful detail had any effect on the rates of award of grants, which at 77% and 76%, respectively, were around the average. It seems that only the description of poignant ordeals (the onset of an illness or an accident, death of a partner or parent, or a divorce—but not loss of work, which was too common in this context) was likely to increase the proportion of positive responses from the committee.

There is a simple reason for this insensitivity, which might initially appear unexpected in a process that, through the applicants' own account of their situation, prompts an empathetic search for suffering. It is the recurrence in these statements of the same themes of misfortune, unemployment, illness, frustration, failure, and discouragement. Sympathy for the unfortunate thus became a sort of routinized affect that permeated decision making but operated on it rather indiscriminately. The committee's increasing strictness over the course of the months testifies to this phenomenon. The evolution is evident in both the proportion of applications granted and the sums allocated, despite the fact that the available sociodemographic data do not indicate any change in the profile of the applicants and no specific financial constraints intervened to make the decision makers less forthcoming. Out of the 19,726 applications submitted, the rate of favorable response fell from 75.1% in January–February to 70.5% in March–April and 62.5% in May–June. Similarly, out of this total of applications, the average amount granted to each successful applicant decreased from 406 euros in the first two weeks of the committee's activity to 286 euros in the last two weeks it convened. Over time, compassion became dulled through constant contact with the hardship of the applicants. Contrary to what might have been imagined and to what applicants themselves must have assumed, the description of suffering had only a small impact regarding the decision. A woman who, with her husband and two children, had a "rest for living" of 50 euros per person, writes: "My husband's been out of work with no benefit since September 96. We get a bit of minimum income and my maternity benefit + family allowance. There's never a month when we can make it even. Every month is really really difficult for us once we've paid the expenses and debts we haven't got anything left. Our children didn't have a Christmas like all the other children because we didn't have the money." This moving account had no effect. Aid was granted, but only on the grounds of the residual income threshold, and just 375 euros, corresponding to the lower level of the standard rate for a family. The committee was not swayed by supplication.

However, this iron law was not immutable. A single man with a "rest for living" calculated at 63 euros described his situation in the following way: "Having been seriously ill and in hospital in November 1995 for 3 months and seeking work since 2/2/96 and separated from my wife since 11/29/96 I'm only getting minimum income and despite all my efforts and going without as I do I can't make ends meet in the hope of finding a job to get back on track I'd like to be able to pay off as much of my debt as possible to have a payment holiday and prove my intention to pay off my debts." The committee, chaired by the same director of welfare service, awarded him 375 euros, double what the scale prescribed for a single person. The accumulation of misfortune (sickness, unemployment, separation) offers a reasonable explanation for this generosity, given that there is also demonstration of merit (seeking work, repayment of debts, showing goodwill). But a reading of the full set of applications suggests a different, circumstantial interpretation, which is confirmed by the interview the director gave me: in contrast with most high-ranked administrators who privileged families, this male official recognized that he was more sensitive to the condition of single men.

These differential effects in the mobilization of compassion, of which there are numerous examples, emphasize the shifting nature of the criteria for judgment, both between different committees and within a given committee, as in the example cited here. It is therefore important to examine the limits of this exercise of local justice as regards both the norms it declared explicitly and the values to which it implicitly refers.

THE ARBITRARY AND THE CONTINGENT

However much actors responsible for allocating scarce resources aspire to fairness, and however precise the criteria they adopt to standardize their choices, their decisions cannot entirely be brought down to objective rationalizations (conforming to norms—in this case the eligibility threshold and principles of distribution) or even subjective interpretations (adhering to values, such as merit, or moved by emotions, such as compassion). Many of the decisions taken appear to escape the rule both of reason and of sentiment. They simply relate to the exercise of power. No justification seems able to account for them. They do not even claim to be fair.

These apparently incomprehensible decisions are in fact of two different types, which I propose to qualify as arbitrary and contingent.[16] The arbitrary describes a decision in which the power of the decision maker is revealed above and beyond the rule, in an almost gratuitous form. The contingent refers to the idea of particular circumstances that play a determining role in relation to the rule. Thus overall, for the decisions where application of an explicit rule or reference to a powerful reason cannot be detected, we can speak of the exercise of authority without reference to the principles or values of justice. I will call these decisions arbitrary when they relate simply to the will of the decision maker. I will term contingent those where a form of chance prevailed over intention. The former represent an excess of power. The latter reveal a default of power. In both situations, authority is exercised unjustly.

One particular form of unjust decision relates to a lack of expertise in the committee. Ignorance of social policies and administrative rules could lead the committee to apply the opposite response to that which would have been made had they been fully informed. A married Serb man with two children and a negative "rest for living" was suspected of cheating, with the chair indignantly noting on his application: "Resources missing: minimum income at 265 euros!" He was not granted any aid because he was considered as not having declared the totality of his resources. The committee failed to take into account the fact that, because he was receiving other benefits, his minimum income had been diminished. Had the committee better understood the functioning of welfare, it could have avoided suspecting the applicant of duplicity and, given his negative "rest for living," would certainly have granted him aid. The unfair decision in this case resulted from incorrect application of the rule. Rather than whim, it was simply a question of incompetence. Although specific, this example derives from general conditions: ignorance only resulted in injustice because public generosity toward the poor is always dispensed against a background of suspicion as to the reality of their situation and the truth of their declarations. Those unfair decisions, in the sense that they did not derive logically from universal principles (even questionable) or specific rules (at least regularly applied) occurred mainly on three levels.

First, they relate to the calculation of the "rest for living," which as we have seen was the determining factor in obtaining aid. Variations in the rigor of this exercise are observed in three different elements: the inclusion of some costs (notably transport, debt repayments, local taxes, and amounts paid to parents), the account taken of the family situation (an adult son is sometimes considered external to the household; conversely, an absent father may raise doubts), and finally the amount of attention devoted to checking the applications (lack of documentary evidence might or might not disqualify an application, figures might or might not be reworked). Thus differences in modes of calculation prompted contradictory decisions, even for two consecutive applications within the same session.

We have seen how excluding travel costs and debt repayments from the evaluation of costs led to the residual income of one man on minimum income moving above the decisive threshold, depriving him of the assistance that his statement convincingly justified. Shortly afterward, the same committee examined the case of a young French woman also receiving minimum income. Her declared costs included 150 euros for room and board paid to her parents, for which she produced no evidence, and a monthly train ticket. In this situation these two amounts were subtracted from her income. Although her resources were identical to those of the man in the previous case, and her declared budget was virtually the same, the subtraction kept her below the threshold. The committee granted her 300 euros. Such microdecisions to include or exclude a sum in the amount to be divided—or a person in the number among whom it was to be shared—may seem trivial. But they have serious consequences if we consider that in this case, the amount granted to one and refused to the other constituted almost a month's income for each.

Second, injustice affected the assessment of applicants' eligibility. It was of course manifested in the exceptions to the 150 euro income rule—exceptions that ran counter to the principles regularly applied. In the case of the homeless, whose net income was paradoxically often above the threshold since they had no or very low regular expenses, some received assistance but for others the threshold effect was strictly applied. Applications from young adults living with their parents were generally turned down, as they were not considered a full household, although they were sometimes granted assistance for reasons that were not indicated and could not be interpreted from the file. A high level of debt sometimes caused rejection of the application, which would then be referred to the Overindebtedness Committee, but in other cases it simply acted as a contributing circumstance in obtaining aid.

The two following examples are illuminating. A couple with two children, the husband a technical adviser in the construction industry and the wife unemployed, had a residual income per person of 58 euros. Their 9,860 euro debt covered three months' medical expenses. Their statement explained the efforts they had made to "reduce our costs, pay our debts and meet our most basic everyday needs"; there was even mention of a "promise of part-time job." The application was rejected, although the "rest for living" was below the threshold; it was merely referred to the Overindebtedness Committee. The letter of rejection sent to the applicants contained the standard wording informing them that their situation did not correspond to that of "persons or families at serious risk of being unable to support themselves"—one wonders how such a denial would have been received by a family of four overwhelmed by debt and living on 230 euros a month. For another couple, also with two children and one employed adult (in this instance the wife), their income had been below their expenses since the husband had lost his job. There was a major debt with a repayment plan, a copy of which was supplied. Acting as a pledge of the couple's serious intentions, this document resulted in them receiving 450 euros in aid. In this case, debt was not an obstacle. In general, the granting of aid to a person who was above the threshold, or conversely the rejection of an application where income fell below the threshold, related to choices hard to systematize.

Third, unfairness arose particularly in the determination of the sum to be granted. The variations might be quantitatively wide but at the same time based on the most subtle of reasons, either because the decision makers sought to send a message to some but not others, or because they were influenced by one or more details included in the applicant's statement— elements that varied depending on the composition of the committee and the mood of the moment, and resulted in some cases in incomprehensible strictness and in others in unexpected generosity. Unfair decisions could work in applicants' favor or to their disadvantage. A single woman with two children, who had a residual income of 143 euros per person, explained her situation as follows:

> Living in a two-bedroom apartment and having to buy furniture for my children because my 3-and-a-half-year-old daughter is still sleeping in a crib and my son on a mattress I got into debt through borrowing from a close friend. The problem is I can't pay her back, What's more I've had to give my bedroom to my daughter because she's 5 years younger than her brother. So I've had to buy a fold-out bed and I'm sleeping in the dining room in a bed I still haven't paid for. You can understand that with 628 euros a month I can't manage: repaying the loan from my friend + 225 euros groceries a month and that's without the rent that's always different but it can be as much as 137 euros with the electricity. I haven't even got enough to buy decent clothes for my children or myself, just now I'm looking for a job. I've no money to buy a monthly ticket so I keep paying for more expensive daily tickets. And then there's the state of my son's room that needs redecorating. And then I haven't even got the money to pay for them to go to the recreation center.

She asked for 750 euros. The committee, which initially allotted 375 euros, amended this sum and eventually granted her 822 euros for her "furniture debts." This was the highest amount awarded among the three hundred applications under study. A few weeks later the committee, chaired by a different administrator, assessed an application from a woman similarly receiving the minimum income and also bringing up two children on her own, with a residual income per person of 91 euros. Her debts were comparable to those of the woman in the case just mentioned. She wrote modestly: "On my own with two children to look after, it's difficult for me to meet my needs. I've got ten months of rent arrears. Therefore even the most minimal assistance would be welcome." The aid she received was certainly minimal, since the committee only awarded her 225 euros—about half what the standard rate would suggest and only just over a quarter of the grant given in the previous case. Charity is always discretionary.

Under these circumstances, there is something disturbing in the fact that applicants were asked to fill in a box indicating the "amount of aid requested," which 226 of the 300 in the study did. In not one single case, however, was this suggested figure followed up by the committee, even though one official of the social services commented with satisfaction on the "modesty of the sums requested": in fact, the median demand was 690 euros; one-third of applicants suggested only 450 euros or less and only 14% asked for more than 1,500 euros, generally to meet major debts. When a couple with a precarious work contract and a residual income of 12 euros per person solicited 300 euros, because of a recent debt for electricity and gas rounded up by 10 euros, they were awarded only 290 euros, supposedly to send them a clear signal of the intention to limit aid to that sum. For another couple with two children, who calculated a residual income of 136 euros per person and asked for 450 euros, a sum corresponding exactly to the amount of their debts, they received only 150 euros, even less than the 182 euros that their letter indicated as an essential expense for eyeglasses for the wife, who had already lost sight in one eye; no explanation was given for this decision.

Through these systematic refusals to accede to requests that the forms yet specifically invited, the committee seemed to want to remind applicants that the decision was entirely its prerogative. In the first of the two cases cited here, the principle of sending a "message" to the applicants (clearing the debt) was applied, probably without their realizing, since in the month that elapsed between submitting the application and receiving the check, the couple's debt had almost doubled (we know this because, no doubt impatient at not having received anything, they submitted a second application four weeks later). In the second, still more telling, case, where the sum granted could have been matched to the dual logic of the scale and signal (since the amount of the debt was precisely the level prescribed in the scale), the committee officers chose not to take this route. There could be no better indication that only the committee knew what was good for the poor and that it intended to make that clear to them.

However, the arbitrary and the contingent, as they are expressed in decisions here considered unfair, should not be seen as the manifestation of an anomic justice (figure 2). Rather than an absence of norms, what is exemplified here is the multiplicity of norms from which the committee can choose, with no systematic preference given to one or another. The fact that when setting the amount they may give priority to the general scale in one case and to a specific need in another, that in the latter case the signal they choose to send the recipient may relate to a debt in one case and to a project in another, and that some are more generous toward the disadvantaged families while others favor homeless men, is sufficient indication that the arbitrary and the contingent result from an excess, rather than a lack, of norms. It is therefore not surprising that this analysis of the unfair decisions reveals all the ingredients of principles and values that were previously described. The arbitrary does not run counter to the norm, and nor does the contingent contradict moral principles: unfair decisions result from the unpredictable and sometimes unjustifiable application of one or the other. What the arbitrary and the contingent have in common is that

	The arbitrary	The contingent
Definition	Injustice in the application of the measure—i.e., inconsistent application of more or less explicit rules	
	Intentional	Unintentional
Mechanism	Goodwill or unwillingness	Good luck or bad luck
Consequence	Penalization or satisfaction (refusal or award of aid, amount reduced or increased)	
Structural conditions	Regime of obligation: a. Aid is not a social right of those receiving it. b. A grant of aid implies a social duty on the part of those giving it. Individualized treatment: a. The applicant has to use skills to justify the application. b. The person distributing the aid has to apply values to make a decision.	
Reinforcing factors	Multiplicity of principles (fluctuating hierarchy) Vagueness of criteria (empirical construction) Shifting guidelines (oral transmission)	
	Justice based on moral principles with concern for meaning	Variable membership of committee
Attenuating factors	Establishment of an eligibility threshold (with exceptions) Institution of a scale of allocation (concurrent with messages) Internalization of an ideal of the just decision (nevertheless ambiguous) Possibility of appeal indicated in writing (rarely used)	

Figure 2. The arbitrary and the contingent: Common features and differences

they both derive from inconsistent application of more or less explicit rules. What distinguishes them is that the former is intentional and the latter fortuitous.

This boundary is more difficult to trace than it might appear, though: when we find that in the cases of two men receiving minimum income, with negative "rest for living," the committee awarded one, who had not written a supporting statement, 380 euros, and the other, who had presented his justification in the dignified style, 150 euros a few days later, we may reasonably assume that this results simply from the fluctuations of everyday bureaucracy, but it is impossible to eliminate completely a conscious determination to assert a difference. Except when it is explicitly indicated through reference to a moral or didactic value, or when it contrasts strongly with the expected decision or the average sum granted, it is often difficult to determine whether the satisfaction of requests and the penalization that results from unfair decisions are due to goodwill or ill will on the part of the committee, or to the fortunate or unfortunate consequences of members' fatigue or mood of the moment.

The common root of these two figures of injustice is composed of two main elements. First, aid relates to a regime of obligation. Public generosity does not institute citizens reclaiming what is due to them from national solidarity, but poor people beseeching the state's benevolence. This has two consequences. On the one hand, the "obliged" cannot assert a social right or demand precise rules: they submit to the modalities imposed on them, of which they know nothing. On the other, the "obligers" feel they have a duty toward the society whose resources they are spending and the state whose charitable mission they are executing: the involvement of senior public officials throughout the operation clearly indicates how seriously the matter was taken. Second, the decision derives from the individualized approach. In seeking to take into account individual features, the empirical reasoning generated tends to shift from common and transparent principles of justice. Here too there are two consequences. On the one hand, the "obliged" must draw on social and rhetorical skills to justify their request, and this generates unequal treatment in comparable situations. On the other, the "obligers" use moral norms to form a basis for their decisions, demonstrating the added value ascribed to merit and misfortune, or rather to their verbalization in applications.

These two structural forms of injustice are augmented by elements specific to the modalities applied in the working of the committee, the effects of which reinforce the overall logics of unfairness: the rules are multiple and concurrent, with no clearly defined hierarchy; the criteria are imprecise, giving rise to variations in the calculation of budgets or the application of a scale; because the guidelines do not exist in written form, there is no listing of principles that could be transmitted from one meeting to another. One factor contributing to arbitrariness in the establishment of norms is the desire to signify, to send a "message" to the recipient of aid, often implying an evaluation of the person's merit or the legitimacy of their debt. We have seen how the "meaning" intended, which is in fact rarely interpretable to the recipients, usually leads to a reduction of the sum that simple application of the neutral but approximate principle of household resources or composition would have determined. Conversely, the variation in committee membership can be seen as a factor contributing to contingency. The chances of escaping the effect of the eligibility threshold or receiving a higher sum varied, depending on which committee assessed an application and on the criteria or values applied by its chair. One chair might be sensitive to the distress of single mothers, another to single men. One might give priority to the scale of standard rates, seeing it as more in line with equality; another might emphasize message, for the sake of its didactic value.

But symmetrically, the arbitrary and the contingent are limited by a set of elements that attenuate their effects: first and foremost existing rules, such as the eligibility threshold and the scale of grants, which even if they are not strictly adhered to, are applied; but also self-constraints, such as the internalization of an ideal of the just decision by the officers dispensing resources, and social controls, such as the institution of a procedure of appeal for rejected applications. Thus the decisions taken reflect not an absence of justice, but a multitude of variations on the theme of what appears as a specific regime of justice for the poor.

The publication of Frances Fox Piven and Richard Cloward's book *Regulating the Poor*, in 1971, sparked intense debate among English-speaking social historians.[17] The authors showed how improvements in public assistance to the poor served to control social unrest during periods of economic difficulty and how, conversely, periods of stability in the production of wealth made it possible for greater pressure to be exerted on the workforce, thereby enabling a reduction in social protection provisions. Historians of welfare criticized this Marxist reading of the "history from below," arguing that social progress was essentially the result of progressivism on the part of government or business elites, motivated not by the fear of popular unrest but by increased awareness of the degraded living conditions of the poor. In the continuation of this debate, the institution of the Social Emergency Fund in France, although a minor development in the history of aid, certainly provides ammunition for historians of conflict rather than the historians of consensus. The primary aim of the fund was not to relieve the hardship of the poor but rather to forestall a protest movement that was beginning to spill out beyond the "movement of the unemployed and the precarious." Notwithstanding the government's declarations justifying the measure on the ground that it wished to "provide more substantial assistance in the most difficult situations," as the prime minister put it, the decision to distribute "one billion" is an exemplary illustration of public charity's perennial function of social regulation.

Those who applied for financial aid from the state clearly understood this. The analysis of the applications reveals the rarity of statements making demands, in contrast to the frequency of accounts that portray hardship and aim to arouse pity—a fact that is all the more noteworthy because the provision of emergency aid was the response to a social mobilization. In the street, the poor asserted their rights to justice. On the forms applying for aid, they appealed to the obligation for assistance. In so doing they gave credence to the local representatives of the state who told me they wanted to "clamp down on militancy by trying not to grant the sum demanded by the unemployed workers' movement," and who expressed satisfaction that through their involvement in the implementation of the Social Emergency Fund, "the voluntary organizations took off their campaigning hat and put on their social workers' hat." For them, as for the nineteenth-century social economists, the distinction between the right of the aided and the obligation of assistance lay at the heart of public charity: in no case should the obliged assert a right; the issue was social control of the working class.

Thus, echoing the usual processes of objectification of poverty, of which the social assessment study undertaken by social workers provides the model, the deployment of a mechanism for exposing suffering can be interpreted as an imposed exercise of subjectivation of the poor—that is, of the construction of the self as a subject of aid. However, the apparent success of the exercise (since in their supporting statements, the applicants are much less likely to demand justice than to present themselves as deserving or appeal for compassion) does not tell us anything about the subjectivity of the applicants. Were they really submitting to the injunctions of the state services, or were they simply demonstrating a skill acquired via years of contact with the bureaucracy of assistance? Obviously, we cannot know—insofar as this distinction itself has any meaning, considering the ambivalence on both sides of the aid line.

What then was the impact of the state's gesture? What was the significance of its agents' strenuous efforts to distribute, in accordance with more or less elaborated principles of justice, sums that were relatively modest in relation to the social action and family policy budgets? For the financial support offered by the Social Emergency Fund, and the structure for allocating it, could well be deemed of little import. Granting two or three hundred euros more to this or that individual was a drop in the ocean given the difficult and sometimes extreme social situations that applicants for the public largesse faced daily. In these conditions, the committee's decisions can seem rather anodyne, and the microsociology I propose here might appear excessively detailed in comparison with decisions that have limited consequence and short temporality. However, while this one-off assistance was indeed simply an episode in the long history of charity, it nevertheless reveals more general phenomena and wider transformations in the treatment of the poor—and even perhaps of the dominated in a broader sense.

Whether they are asylum seekers or foreigners seeking residence, poor people visiting clinics in disadvantaged neighborhoods or attending local job-seekers' centers, applicants for assistance from regional bodies or from humanitarian organizations, individuals applying to overindebtedness committees or rent arrears support committees—in other words, anyone for whom recognition of a right is never separated from a reminder of the debt to society they are thus contracting—they are expected to produce the same narrative tropes and forms of argument to justify their request, and the same procedures of evaluation and judgment are used to decide if they can legitimately be granted the precious commodities of residence permits, medical or social services, financial assistance, and debt rescheduling. In return for the gift of fragments of their life, they receive the counter gift of a means of survival. This is the structure of the exchange organized by the management of the poor. In this transaction of symbolic and material goods, the mediators are the administrative officers, social workers, health professionals, and staff of charitable organizations. They have more or less potential to modulate the resources at their disposal. The choices they make are more or less poignant, but they are based on principles of justice and bring into play practices of judgment that express both the ethos of public action and its arbitrariness. There is therefore reason to consider that the lessons learned from studying the distribution of the Social Emergency Fund have a greater relevance than its transitory existence might suggest.

Historical parallels might be helpful to apprehend this signification. The small Austrian town of Marienthal experienced remarkable economic expansion during the second half of the nineteenth century, thanks to the establishment of a prosperous cotton manufacture. As a result of mechanization of the factory, followed by economic crisis, the manufacture closed in the late 1920s and most of the town's inhabitants became unemployed. As mentioned earlier, in 1931 the sociologist Paul Lazarsfeld and two assistants carried out a study focusing on the aid distributed by the municipal authorities at the end of the year. They noted: "Thanks to all these additions, life is a little easier at Christmas. But the only truly effective aid would of course be work." Sixty-six years later, when the Social Emergency Fund was launched, almost the same could have been said—with two significant modifications, however. First, today even those who work are not necessarily safe from poverty, and in the cases I studied one in six of those applying for emergency aid had work. Second, and perhaps more important, in the past, aid was given unconditionally, whereas now applicants are required to expose their suffering. The accounts of everyday hardship that their petitions offer us thus speak both of their precarious living conditions, described in these narratives, and of our moral economies, as revealed by the administration's decisions.

3. Compassion Protocol
Legalizing Diseased Undocumented Immigrants

> Is not medical language expressing, in its own way, the general situation of immigrants? If it is so determined, it may be no more than a variant on the commonplace discourse on immigrants and the immigrant condition. The immigrant is no more than his body.
>
> ABDELMALEK SAYAD, *The Suffering of the Immigrant*

One of the first initiatives of the new left-wing government resulting from the French parliamentary elections in 1997 was the publication, on June 24, of a circular from the minister of the interior, Jean-Pierre Chevènement, reconsidering the situation of various categories of illegal immigrants. Though at the time it went almost unnoticed, except by immigrant support organizations, the most remarkable aspect of this document was the automatic granting of residence rights to "any foreigner habitually resident in France and suffering from a serious condition requiring medical treatment, and for whom deportation would result in exceptionally serious consequences, provided that he or she would be unable to receive appropriate treatment in the country to which he or she is returned." According to this paragraph of the circular, which was confirmed as Article 12b11 of the law of May 11, 1998, one of the many rewritings of the ordinance of November 2, 1945, relating to "the entry and residence of foreigners and the right to asylum," the ill individual would receive a residence permit together with a work permit.[1] The recognition of this ground for legalization, which resulted from persistent campaigning by immigrant support organizations, marked the culmination of a development in state local administrations through the 1990s, whereby a place was increasingly made for what the authorities at that time called "humanitarian reason." In a period when restrictions on residence rights continued to be extended and the number of undocumented immigrants increased in line with the hardening of legal conditions for the entry and residence of foreigners, illness—provided it was sufficiently serious and treatment deemed inaccessible—opened new avenues and, ambiguously, new hopes.

It is in light of this evolution that the following appeal, excessively deferent and grammatically awkward, submitted by a Senegalese man in the late 1990s, should be read:

> To the Préfet. By the powers granted to you under Article X of the decree of 1945, and humbly beseeching your goodwill, I am reiterating my application following the unexpected rejection that was no doubt due to misunderstanding during my interviews with the DDASS [Direction Départementale des Affaires Sanitaires et Sociales (Directorate of Health and Social Welfare)] medical officer. Contrary to what I expected, she asked me no questions, but chose among the few negative results that bore no relation to what I am suffering from. Admittedly I did not come to this country for medical reasons. However, after six years of irregular treatment for the same illness, and now with the granting of my sickness-benefit which will finally allow me to undergo regular care, I would have liked and wished to be admitted under this provision. In fact at the time, as I was a member of a group on the students' committee in Dakar, threatened and sought by the police among others, I was afraid that I would end up like many others, forgotten in the prisons. Hence my unplanned arrival in France. Since my father was wounded in the war serving with the Senegalese Tirailleurs [infantrymen incorporated into the French colonial army who fought alongside the regular military during the Second World War], and also having been the only source of income for my family apart from his military pension which is paid very late and is not sufficient, for all these reasons, it is clear that return in these conditions is impossible for me. However, exceptionally, I ask you, sir, to grant me authorization to stay simply to allow me to receive treatment. I look forward to a favorable response and I hope you will believe in my sincerity.

Having exhausted all administrative avenues for legalization, as well as all possible justifying arguments, this individual invokes the need to seek treatment as a last resort in his appeal to the prefect, who represents the state in the *département*. Although he mentions the risks he runs in his home country because of his political activities (which might have warranted examination of his application on grounds of asylum), points out the date of his arrival to demonstrate that he is settled in France (the circular allows for the possibility of legalization after seven years living in the country), and finally, makes reference to his father's military service with the French army (which would have given his father residence rights and might have influenced his own situation), these elements are used more to give a globally favorable impression, and as far as possible enhance the credibility of his request, than to claim a right: that he has not asked for refugee status, probably would not be able to claim residence based on length of stay, and refers indirectly to his father's meager war pension suggests that he has little faith in these three supporting elements. Illness has, one might say, become his last hope. His body is finally the only social resource capable of arousing a compassion that has been translated into law and would perhaps allow him to be granted permission to remain. Conversely, were he feeling well he would no longer have any hope of obtaining residence rights. Exposing his suffering, he thinks he might still have a chance.

In this chapter I focus on this development of the law and the concrete ways in which it was applied.[2] What is the nature of this remarkable humanitarian procedure that the French state invented during the 1990s? How was it put in place, and how was it implemented? What is this new moral order that makes the sick body a superior criterion for evaluation of the grounds for a request for legalization? I first analyze the historical transformations that affect the body of the immigrant and their translation into a rapidly evolving legislation. I then look at the activity of the public medical officers scrutinizing requests, which can be interpreted as a moral work of identifying legitimate foreigners. And I finally present some of the tactics deployed by immigrants to defend their rights and sometimes manipulate the law. I thereby hope to unveil the contradictions of this last resort, which I propose to qualify, in reference to medical language,[3] a compassion protocol.

THE BODY OF THE IMMIGRANT

In 1980 the Franco-Algerian sociologist Abdelmalek Sayad, in a lecture that has been republished several times since, attempted to define "the illness of immigration" as follows:[4] "Because the immigrant has no meaning, in either his own eyes or those of others, and because, ultimately, he has no existence except through his work, illness, perhaps even more so than the idleness it brings, is inevitably experienced as the negation of the immigrant." He went on: "The importance of what is called the 'language of the body,' or, to put it a different way, the organic importance of the body, is, basically, nothing more than the importance of the body as organ, or in other words, first as labor power, and only then as a form of self-presentation." In those times, one would be tempted to say, since the era in which demand for foreign labor made immigration a social necessity seems now so remote, the immigrant's body was entirely legitimized through its function as an instrument of production, the performance of which was interrupted by illness or accident. The "closure of borders" announced in 1974 had admittedly sounded the death knell of what was termed "labor immigration," but the popular representation was still one of the "immigrant worker" whose usefulness was confirmed by the factories and whose precariousness was underlined by the hostels: coming from southern Europe or Africa, the immigrant helped create national wealth but endured an indefinitely renewed provisional legal status. The body of the immigrant at that time was a productive body, assumed to be in good health. Any physical impairment would constitute a breach of the relationship contracted with the "host" society. Inability to work because of illness or an accident was a source of suspicion on the part of the social welfare bodies, which presumed simulation, and of the medical world, where the term "sinistrosis" circumspectly articulated doubt as to the organic reality of the suffering.[5] The impaired body, the body unable to produce, was socially illegitimate, then.

Times have changed. We deal today with a different configuration of the social space—a configuration in which the rise in unemployment and the restructuring of industry since the 1970s have made the immigration of unskilled labor undesirable, despite the fact that some sectors of the French economy continue to rely on it, either through temporary contracts (in agriculture and wine making) or in the form of illegal employment (in construction and the garment industry). A configuration in which the category of immigrant has gradually been replaced in the public arena by that of foreigner, marking the shift from a logic of supply, in which production capacity regulated the need for immigrant labor, to a logic of demand, in which the disappearance of that need has paved the way for a regime of solicitation on the part of foreigners. A configuration, finally, in which the immigrant, who is three times more likely to be out of work than the average in France, appears as the archetypal form of "the useless in the world" that Bronislaw Geremek describes, while the foreigner emerges on the social stage as the "undocumented," the figure of radical exclusion.[6] In this new state of the social world, the body of the immigrant has become illegitimate as labor force, since it is always suspected of deleteriously affecting the job market, but the body of the foreigner has found a new source of legitimacy through illness, which, under certain conditions of seriousness and impossibility of receiving treatment in the country of origin, makes it possible to obtain a residence permit on "humanitarian grounds." Through a complete reversal in outlook, pathology, which previously aroused suspicion, has therefore become a source of social recognition.

Provisional authorization to remain for medical treatment, a practice that was initially very loosely institutionalized and left to the discretion of each prefect, then inscribed in a ministerial circular on the legalization of un-documented immigrants, and finally translated into the law on entry and residence of foreigners, is of course only one of many regulatory provisions covering the granting of permits. But it nevertheless tells much about the changes that have taken place, both because it has been so successful (it was under this provision that the number of residence permits rose most rapidly during the 1990s, at a time when successive legislations were restricting virtually all the other avenues for obtaining permission to stay) and in terms of its significance (it instituted a new form of relationship, which may be qualified as compassionate, creating some categories of foreigners who are only legitimately present on French soil because their physical or sometimes psychic integrity is at risk). "The immigrant is no more than his body," Sayad wrote. Sometimes the foreigner, too, is no more than his body, but this body is no longer the same: useless to the political economy, it now finds its place in a new moral economy that values suffering over labor and compassion more than rights.

THE LAWS OF HUMANITARIANISM

"Unless his presence constitutes a threat to public order, any foreigner habitually resident in France whose health is such that he requires medical treatment the lack of which could lead to exceptionally serious consequences, and provided that he is effectively unable to receive appropriate treatment in his country of origin, will be granted a temporary residence permit validated 'for private and family life' ": so runs the ordinance of November 2, 1945, stipulating the conditions under which foreigners may enter and stay in France, as modified by the law of May 11, 1998 (known as the Chevènement Act, which repeated the terms of the 1997 circular virtually word for word.[7] For the legislator, the aim was to bring regulations into line with Article 8 of the European Convention on Human Rights, following several rulings against the French state both in French courts and in the European Court of Human Rights, but also to do away with the category of foreigners "who can be neither deported nor legalized" that had been created by the law of April 24, 1997 (known as the Debré Act, named after a right-wing former minister of the interior). The latter had introduced protection against deportation for "foreigners suffering from a serious health condition" without giving them the right to a residence permit, creating a legal and political imbroglio. Thus, as the logic that combined the introduction of increasingly restrictive immigration laws with the strict application of repressive measures led to a growing number of undocumented individuals being deported, including some suffering from serious conditions (primarily AIDS), a humanitarian exception was enshrined into law.

The concern for the plight of ill undocumented immigrants began to emerge in the late 1980s. Campaigns for immigrant's rights by nongovernmental organizations, the establishment of private and public free treatment centers where the undocumented formed the majority of clients, and eventually the protest by official bodies in charge of public health issues progressively made the government aware of the problem.[8] During the early 1990s a number of prefects took the initiative to grant three-month residence permits on a case-by-case basis. In the absence of any legal framework, these were granted by the discretionary power of the local government on the basis of a report from the medical officer at the local DDASS—an arrangement that subsequently became generalized throughout France. If the prefect's office refused to issue the residence permit, an appeal could be made to the national Directorate of Population and Migration, or even to the Ministry of the Interior. Issued by dispensation, these permits almost systematically prohibited the recipient from engaging in paid work, and gave no right to any social welfare benefits. In Seine-Saint-Denis, the *département* that, along with Paris, dealt with the largest number of applications for legalization, an average of approximately two hundred temporary residence permits for the purposes of medical treatment were granted each year.

The incorporation of health status in the provisions of the law, initially as a block to deportation, and subsequently as grounds for granting residence, marked a watershed. The first mention of illness in French legislation appeared as the result of an amendment adopted by the Assemblée Nationale (the French Parliament) on February 27, 1997, during the parliamentary debates on the Debré Act. However, this amendment merely stipulated that foreigners "suffering from serious illness" were not to be deported, and did not introduce provision for granting residence. In other words, the dominant logic remained one of repression, with provision for discretionary exemption. It was in fact the circular of June 24, 1997, signed by the Socialist government, that made illness a criterion for legalization in its own right. This circular reiterated the terms of the law on protection against deportation, making reference to the serious medical condition in question and the impossibility of receiving appropriate treatment in the country to which the individual would be returned. This time there was a new element: the permit was associated with a right to work if the patient and the doctor so requested. This new logic was affirmed in the Chevènement Act. Legal recognition of the suffering body had been established. Available statistics—which are few and difficult to obtain—testify to this change.[9] The application of this criterion was particularly striking at *département* level. In Seine-Saint-Denis, the number of applications for temporary residence on health grounds was 737 in 1997, 757 in 1998, and more than 1,000 in 1999, representing a fivefold increase over previous figures corresponding to the period when there was no state regulation on this issue. At the national level, the figures for residence permits not merely requested but actually issued for the purposes of treatment show a similar trend. The data are available only since 1998, when the law came into effect, but in that year the total was 1,045, rapidly increasing to 3,605 in 1999 and 4,795 in 2000.

Three different time frames can consequently be distinguished in the application of humanitarian reason in the management of immigration (table 3). Before 1990, serious illness was an exceptional circumstance for the purposes of granting permission to remain, with no specific reference in legislation, and left purely to the discretion of the prefect's office. Between 1990 and 1996, it gradually became more and more routinely used in administrative practice and was consolidated in regulations through the provision for appeal, but it remained within a regime of dispensation in which the prohibition on employment reminded foreigners that the state's relationship to them was one of obligation. From 1997 onward, serious illness was established in law: it opened the prospect of obtaining a residence permit as of right, was accompanied by permission to work that was in principle automatically granted, and created a legal status and even a social condition of the sick foreigner.[10] Thus, from being suspect, the suffering individual was first temporarily tolerated, and subsequently acquired full legitimacy.

What is remarkable is that outside of the deep ideological divides around the theme of immigration that were expressed throughout this period (as revealed by the parliamentary debates on the various legislative acts), the recognition of the sick body generated very few of the partisan splits that habitually mark policy about these controversial issues. It was a Conservative majority that voted in the prohibition on deporting foreigners suffering from serious illness, while at the same time ratifying a text that in all other respects was stricter than previous legislation. And it was the Socialist government that issued the circular and introduced the law granting sick immigrants temporary residence permits. The two measures are of course not equivalent (the introduction of the notion of the right to residence and the authorization to work representing a major advance in

TABLE 3. The three periods of humanitarianism in the management of immigration

Era	Regime	Period	Regulation	Rights	Numbers
Suspicion	Exception	Before 1990	No reference to illness in law	No specific rights	Very few
Toleration	Dispensation	From 1990 to 1996	Protection against deportation and no right to work	Temporary residence for the purposes of treatment	150–250 per year
Legitimation	As of right	From 1997	Right to remain with authorization to work	Residence permit valid for "private and family life"	700–1,000 per year

Note: These figures are for the Seine-Saint-Denis *département* only.

recognition of the status of sick immigrant), nor were the positions of the two sides the same (the transcripts of the sessions of the parliamentary Commission on Clandestine Immigration and Illegal Residence of Foreigners of 1996 reveal that a few right-wing representatives contested medical assistance to illegal immigrants and even called on social workers and health care professionals to inform on them when they sought medical care), but in neither case was there any real challenge to the specific benefits awarded to seriously ill aliens. Humanitarian reason became generally accepted as a just cause, or at least as a cause that could not be challenged publicly. Yet at the same time, conditions for family regrouping or for political asylum, to cite only the two categories for which the international norms are most firmly established, were bitterly contested, giving rise to virulent attacks that sought to question the application and even the grounds of these principles.

By analogy with the therapeutic measures applied at the end of life for patients suffering from illness deemed incurable, we can describe the measures and the procedures devised to allow foreign patients without residence rights to stay in France, receive treatment, and have their living costs paid, as a compassion protocol. The measures were inscribed in the texts of legislation, ministerial circulars, and decrees relating to application of the provision. The procedures comprised the medical examination and expert opinion, the administrative decision, and the channels for appeal. My analogy with the medical compassion protocol is based on two factors. First, the law reserves this sad privilege for extreme circumstances, since it specifies that the measure should only be used in the case of a health condition in which the lack of treatment would result in "exceptionally serious consequences": it could not be made clearer that this is a logic of extremity. Second, the justification for the legislation is couched in an emotional register that places the member of parliament voting for it, or the official in the prefect's office applying it, in a relationship of empathy with the suffering being, a relationship that transcends the rational arguments and ideological prejudices that could be raised against it: appeal is made to the sentiment of humaneness. The compassion protocol is thus a procedure of the last resort that derives from a form of sympathy evoked in the face of suffering. It demands the right to keep alive individuals who have nothing except their mere existence.

This is, at least, the way things were presented in the world of principles and ideas, where the law is debated and stipulated. However, as mentioned earlier, there can be no measure without corresponding procedures: the protocol presupposes both texts to serve as a frame of reference and concrete situations in which they are applied. It is into the gap between these two, where actors are embodied and decisions become effective, that the inquiry on the field delves.

THE JUSTICE OF THE EXPERT

"Should we accept 'getting our hands dirty' by agreeing to work with the immigrants' service of the prefect's office on the difficult issue of deportations?" asked Charles Candillier, a medical officer in the Seine-Saint-Denis Directorate of Health and Social Welfare, in an internal memo.[11] His answer is crystal clear: "Although we recognize the ethical ambiguities of the situation, we did agree, on the grounds that our intervention could only be beneficial in helping to prevent arbitrary expulsions." He adds: "Moreover, our experience has shown that this intervention was effective. The actual technical problems are much smaller than this report suggests. There should be no discussion in most cases. Where there is uncertainty, the person at risk of being expelled should always be given the benefit of the doubt. These expert opinions give us more credibility on the issue of deportations, enabling us to intervene more fully through contacts with the prefect's office and support organizations." However, this analysis, based on the experience of a public health professional called on to rule in several hundred cases each year, was by no means unanimously shared, as the wide variation in the opinions of medical officers shows. According to a survey conducted throughout the Île-de-France region, medical officers reported that between 5% and 50% of the opinions they issued were unfavorable.[12] This is confirmed by the study of three thousand applications drawn from three of the seven *départements* in question. It establishes that in 1997 and 1998 the proportion of applications proposed for legalization by the health department was 42.7% in Hauts-de-Seine, 74.5% in Seine-Saint-Denis, and 96.7% in Val-de-Marne. Before examining the significance of these variations in medical expert opinion in greater detail, I describe the evaluation process.

The concrete procedures for granting temporary permission to remain on health grounds were for a long time left to the discretion of each prefecture, as we have seen: this stemmed in part from different statistical realities, since the least active among them had to deal with only a few applications each year, while others received several hundred. Gradually, a system became established whereby a state medical officer was responsible for assessing requests, but before the publication of the circular on June 24, 1997, many prefects continued to use the services of approved doctors who were paid by the state on a case-by-case basis. This circular made the medical officers the cornerstone of the process, with their opinion communicated to the prefecture's immigration service, and followed if it was favorable, except in specific circumstances wherein the law indicated a danger to the public order. There were substantial variations between *départements*, however, in terms of requests for an independent opinion that might help clarify the decision (some sought to make these compulsory, while others were satisfied with the evidence submitted by the patient), the scrutiny of individual situations (some merely assessed written applications, whereas others required each applicant to be interviewed), and the way the final decision was taken (some were adjudicated by an individual, and others by committee). These procedural differences clearly influenced the ultimate decision, although the effects cannot be mechanically deduced: for example, a letter from a doctor treating the patient might supply evidence that objectified the seriousness of the condition, or conversely might relativize the pathology; when the adjudicators met the applicants their presence engendered a proximity that encouraged benevolence, but sometimes aroused suspicion or caution. A decree and a circular specifying the procedures were therefore issued in an attempt to standardize practice.

Yet the variation in medical opinions observed was due less to the form of the procedure than to the use the medical officer made of it. These physicians, who are employed by the state, have various trajectories, some having worked in Africa with the Ministry of Cooperation, others having exerted their activity in hospitals in France without getting a post, and still others being disappointed by private practice. To obtain the official title of médecin inspecteur de santé publique (public health physician inspector), they undergo two years of training at the National School of Public Health in Rennes. Subsequently, they can be appointed to any state position, either in the ministry or in a directorate. In the *département*, they are under the authority of the prefect and have various missions, including working as medical experts for the immigration service. There are four factors—professional, political, deontological, and ethical— underlying this practice, deriving both from the distinctive features of the profession and from the specific problems posed by the opinion to be given: the latter two elements distinguished the administration of this local justice from other medical practice.

Professionally, the medical officers were subject to specific rules, since their role was not to concern themselves with individual cases but to manage public health. Some agreed to play the game of the new regulation and strove to identify those applicants who met the legal criteria; others considered that examining patients or assessing their applications was not part of their job and often tended to give almost systematically favorable opinions. Politically, the medical officers belonged to the civil service, presupposing a neutrality and an independence that they defended all the more vigorously given that questions were sometimes raised about the amount of pressure they were thought to be put under by prefectures. Nevertheless, they could not entirely escape the ideological issues around immigration in French society: this led to varying assessments of the legitimacy of granting documents to sick foreigners when they were evaluating not cases of pathologies that were life threatening in the short term, but the much more numerous cases where there might be debate as to the seriousness of the condition. Deontologically, the medical officers were caught between the duties mandated to them by the public institution that employed them and those their profession required them to respect, even though, surprisingly, they were not required to register with the Ordre des Médecins, their professional organization. While the conflict between these two principles never escalated to the turning point reached by some civil servants, who abandoned professional secrecy to denounce the criminal activity they observed in the exercise of their duties, there was still a tension between the imperative of the state, which reserved the residence permit for exceptionally serious cases, and the obligations of medicine, which maintains a principle of precaution. Ethically, medical officers applied a conscience clause that cannot be reduced simply to the physical or even the medical dimension: their deliberations often took into account the psychic or social repercussions of their decision, as well as biographical information. Although these elements had no direct link to the clinical condition, they could support the legitimacy of the request—as, for instance, when rejection risked destabilizing a psychic condition or isolating the individual socially.

These four dimensions combined in various ways to result in the three ideal-typical positions for medical officers, as illustrated in the three *départements* of Hauts-de-Seine, Seine-Saint-Denis, and Val-de-Marne (table 4). Strict legalism, which consists in rigidly adhering to the prescribed regulation and hence limiting the number of favorable opinions, corresponds to a strong internalization of the mission of representing the state: medical officers see themselves primarily as civil servants entrusted with rigorous application of the law. Unconditional liberality, which results in approving almost all applications, makes reference to the autonomy of the profession in relation to both clinical practice, since the issue is about managing populations rather than ruling on individuals, and the state, the aim being to

TABLE 4. Three models of local justice in the granting of temporary residence permits to sick foreigners by medical officers of the prefectures

Ideal type	*Dominant frame of reference*	*Status valued in priority*	*General principle applied*	*Rate of favorable opinions*
Strict legalism	Authority of the law	Civil servant	Reason of state	Low
Unconditional liberality	Autonomy of the profession	Officer	Public health	High
Tempered generosity	Professional ethics	Clinician	Intimate conviction	Moderate

distinguish the medical officers' role from the threatening function of health police: the role of public health officer is prioritized. Finally, tempered generosity, which involves an individualized and in-depth approach to each case, appeals to a sort of professional ethics that leads the clinicians to deliberate carefully on each case on the basis of their intimate medical conviction: here invocation of medical humanism is the dominant factor.

Of course, like any typology, this one provides only a schema for interpretation that cannot definitively enclose actual practices in a formalized framework. However, examination of the figures for the three prefectures shows that it is effectively manifested in the practices of the various medical officers. The chances of sick foreigners being granted residence permits certainly varied depending on where they lived—or where they chose to submit their application, since they sometimes employed tactics seeking to increase the likelihood of legalization by using a different address. Because the allocation of a scarce commodity was locally managed, there were wide disparities in the treatment of applications and hence inequalities of access to a right from place to place.

Moreover, medical officers were not the only physicians to operate a variable local justice. Their colleagues working in private practice or in hospitals, who were often asked to submit a report on the pathology suffered by the immigrant patient, were also subject to contradictory pressures. From the prudent withdrawal of some from a task they did not view as their job ("It's not up to us to decide about residence permits") to the political instrumentalization of the measure by others, who saw it as an opportunity to perform a just act ("If we can help people in difficulty this way, we should do it"), all positions were possible. The following cases, taken from my field notes in the early years of the first decade of the 2000s, illustrate these two extremes:

> A young Algerian man illegally resident in France for nine years sought hospital treatment for the long-term consequences of polio, manifesting in deformation of the lower limbs, a limp, and pain. In a letter addressed to the man's doctor, the orthopedic surgeon recommended a series of operations to correct the deformation, accompanied by a prolonged period of rehabilitation, after which satisfactory functional recovery might be achieved. In order to complete this course of treatment, the patient obviously needed to have entitlement to public insurance benefits; authorization to remain on health grounds would guarantee him this. The orthopedic surgeon was therefore asked for a report in support of the young man's application to the prefecture. At this point, however, he refused, asserting that the surgery was not recommended and that he could not draw up a certificate, as requested: "treatment will be limited to the prescription of orthopedic footwear," his letter pusillanimously concludes.

The surgeon's medical evaluation thus altered when he was required to commit to stating it to the authorities: there was no longer a question of remedying the disability, but only of recommending minimal equipment that did not suggest authorization to remain was justified, to the utmost despair of the patient, who could not understand why his doctor had changed his mind. Other physicians sometimes took a very different position:

> A 45-year-old woman from Benin sought permission to remain for treatment. She had come to France ten years earlier with her young son, who had been diagnosed with a rare muscle tumor and required a long anticancer treatment. Following his recovery the son returned to Benin, but his mother stayed in France to work in order to support her children. With no residence permit, she survived in extreme precariousness and supported her family on the income from undeclared cleaning and child-care jobs. Her main concern was to continue to be able to bring her son over to France once a year for a medical check-up. When she was seen in hospital, her only health problem was moderate arterial hypertension, which was kept well under control by simple treatment. Yet the general practitioner, sensitive to her story, drew up a certificate for the prefecture that referred to a "serious illness that might be life threatening if she returned to her country."

The physician's assessment amounted to asking for documents on medical grounds by proxy: obtaining them for the mother, who was affected by a routine and controlled condition, made it possible to treat the son, who was suffering from a serious disease.

These represent two contrasting approaches to the doctor's civic responsibility. However contradictory, the differing positions nevertheless reveal, each in its own way, how these professionals situated their medical expert opinion in a political space where the deontological points of reference had become blurred. Thus the issuing of a diagnosis and a prognosis—an everyday act for the clinician, in principle involving no difficulties other than technical ones—became a problem of conscience that seemed to involve ideological or ethical issues, both for the doctor who refused (when it would have been enough to produce a descriptive medical report that drew purely on his medical competence), and for the one who overstated the seriousness of the condition (when he was only required to state a clinical condition). Between these two extreme positions—the refusal to state an opinion, and the excess of justification—the first of which appears to be more frequent than the second, all variations are possible, not only from one expert to another but also from one moment to another for the same practitioner. The administration of local justice derived equally from the application of clearly stated principles and from an interplay between the arbitrary and the contingent, as we saw in the case of emergency financial aid. The arbitrary manifested the whim of the expert (strictness or generosity dispensed at his discretion), while contingency pointed to the effects of chance (variations in judgment depending on mood or the time). But the reason that these variations on the theme of local justice are possible is because, contrary to what the regulation suggests, the very object of the deliberation—in particular, the seriousness of condition and the accessibility of treatment—remained open to interpretation.

THE FRAMES OF JUDGMENT

The law, later detailed in a circular to prefects, cites three conditions that must be present when humanitarian rationale is invoked. One relates to residence, and the other two to the medical situation itself. However precise they may appear—each word of the text having been carefully weighed, as the minute variations in wording from one version to another indicate, and the struggles of nongovernmental organizations to have this or that term modified confirm—the three conditions produced varying interpretations, and hence civil servants were faced with the need to generate rulings on the basis of moral values rather than merely technical criteria. This is true of all official medical expert opinions, but particularly so in situations that involve not only a threat to life (for the patients, for whom deportation may be a death warrant) but also political issues (for society, which has a highly sensitive relationship with immigration). Truth ordeals arise between the clinical expert and the immigrant patient—ordeals in which what is deemed the just decision is formed, and sometimes negotiated, word against word.

The first criterion is that the beneficiary must be an "alien habitually resident in France," which the circular following the May 11, 1998, law suggested should be "assessed flexibly," though it added that "only in exceptional cases should length of residence be less than one year." Clearly, this criterion aimed to prevent people who came to France solely for the purposes of getting treatment for their illness from also acquiring a temporary residence permit and free health care under the medical assistance system. However, such situations were not uncommon, especially since the change from the old dispensatory system to the permit as of right, in 1997: foreigners who were legally resident in France would sometimes bring a relative, usually a mother or father, suffering from a chronic condition to the country to enable her or him to be examined and find appropriate treatment. Initially entering on a short-stay visa issued for the purposes of visiting family, the person would become an illegal resident when the visa expired and could then apply for leave to remain under a temporary permit, and gain access to treatment through public medical assistance. The tone of the circular on application of the measure leaves substantial scope for interpretation by officers assessing this criterion if the period spent in France has been short (less than one year, in the terms of the circular). Thus the two following cases, again from my field notes, appear administratively similar but result in opposite evaluations:

> A 44-year-old Algerian man came to France, where his sister lived, to get treatment for what he had been told was "throat cancer." When he saw the doctor in the month following his arrival, the doctor diagnosed a less serious condition—a particular form of allergic reaction that required a simple additional investigation and a medically routine treatment. Given that it was likely he would be able to return home after treatment, the criterion of residence was raised in objection to his application for a temporary residence permit and medical assistance: the social worker could not state that he "habitually" lived in France. By contrast, a 38-year-old Algerian woman came to visit her brother, who was living in France, following the death of her husband in suspicious circumstances that led her to fear for her own life, given the climate of violence that reigned in Algeria. A few weeks later she went to the doctor for depression and hormone problems, which required psychiatric treatment and biological tests. In this case, the impression that she was unlikely to return to Algeria because of the danger led

the social worker to see her as prospectively resident: a report stating that she was compelled to remain in France was written and allowed her to obtain permission to remain for treatment.

What the process produced, over and above what was presented as a simple objective evaluation of the individual's chances of staying in France, was also a judgment about the legitimacy of continued residence in the country: the claim to "habitual residence" of the man who came to get treatment for his illness was considered less legitimate than that of the woman who invoked potential threats. More generally, factors such as years spent in France in childhood or adolescence, the presence of a spouse or young children already resident, or the discovery of a serious condition requiring lengthy treatment tended to suggest long-term residence and led to the validation of the request for residence permits or for medical assistance. Medicine, as we know, always exerts a power over the ill person's time, even if only by imposing a period of waiting. But this power is exercised not only over the management of their present; it may also intervene in their future, particularly when the issue is one of deciding whether to grant a scarce commodity such as a residence permit or free health care.

Evaluation of this criterion, however, was not the outcome of a unilateral decision by the examining doctor or the social worker. Foreigners and their families might also develop tactics once they knew how the system worked. Sometimes informed of the nuances of the regulations by a lawyer or a support organization, they tended to highlight plans to settle, or restrictions on the possibility of return to their country of origin, as in the following example:

> A Senegalese man who had lived and worked in France for several years brought over his mother, who was in her 70s and suffering from age-related health problems, specifically a cataract for which he wanted her to have surgery in a French hospital. When the social worker asked him if his mother planned to stay and live with him afterward, he replied that she would, and an application for medical aid was made. However, he told the doctor who was drawing up the clinical evaluation report for the prefecture that his mother would return to Senegal once her treatment was completed.

These two assertions are actually less contradictory than they might appear, and it would be wrong to see this as simply a deliberate dissimulation. In such situations family decisions are not clear cut and can be revised, depending on the development of the condition but also on intrafamily relationships that articulate complex sets of interwoven social and moral obligations.

The second criterion of the law is "a state of health requiring treatment the lack of which could lead to exceptionally serious consequences." This is obviously the criterion that called for a medical expert opinion, from the clinicians who communicated their assessment and from the medical officers who gave their opinion as to whether the application was grounded. Here comparison between the three *départements* under study reveals major differences. Leaving aside Val-de-Marne, where the medical officer ruled favorably in 96.7% of cases, which indicates almost no differentiation of judgment, and focusing on Hauts-de-Seine and Seine-Saint-Denis, where the proportion of favorable opinions was 42.7% and 74.5% respectively, the disparity in rates relates mainly to a difference in the assessment of particular pathologies. Actually, the opinion rendered is relatively similar in cases involving conditions considered to be life threatening: 100% and 99%, respectively, in the 129 cases of cancer, 91% and 100% in the 384 cases of AIDS. The assessment rates are very different, though, in relation to chronic conditions: 28% and 84% for the 121 cases of diabetes, 24% and 92% for the 122 cases of heart disease. The positions even become diametrically opposed for psychiatric problems: 0% and 80% of favorable opinions out of the 119 applications submitted.

Three classes of condition emerge at the level of application of medical expert opinion. The first consists of life-threatening conditions, which almost systematically result in favorable opinions, with the additional remark that treatment will be of "indeterminate" duration, allowing the individuals to receive a one-year residence permit regardless of how long they have been in France. The second comprises serious conditions that require prolonged treatment or regular testing; here assessment is on a case-by-case basis, and particularly takes into account the criterion relating to the possibility of the persons receiving treatment in their own country, as we shall see. The third category is that of mental illness, with regard to which two clear-cut and contrary positions emerge: according to some medical officers, not only did these disorders require medical treatment on the same basis as any somatic condition, they also resulted at least in part from the patients' legal position, and the granting of a residence permit would therefore have a therapeutic effect; according to others, these problems related to living conditions, notably financial and legal insecurity, but for this very reason there was no point in starting a course of psychiatric treatment that could only result in chronicity of the mental health problem, whereas return of the patient to his country might provide a social and even therapeutic environment more conducive to healing. There were, however, intermediate positions, as the following case illustrates:

A 33-year-old Tunisian man applied for a residence permit for the purposes of treatment in order to complete costly additional tests he had been recommended to have for chest pain. He had come to France four years earlier to seek work as a car mechanic, in order to "help his family" in Tunisia, and in the hope of "making his life" there. But with no residence permit he was limited to "informal work" that was badly paid and only just enabled him to get by. The frustration engendered by the failure of his plan to settle and the resulting anxiety were probably responsible in large part for the symptoms he presented with, which various specialist tests already carried out suggested were physically benign. The medical expert opinion that might support his application for a one-year residence permit was thus couched in the terms of one of the medical officers: "Living in a precarious situation brings people down. It's not easy for us to make rulings about lowness, the blues, being down." While in this case his opinion recommended legalization "for the purposes of treatment," on the grounds of the additional tests to be carried out, it is likely that this residence permit would allow the man to find a job, provided it was accompanied, as the law stipulated, with the authorization to work. Therefore, at the cost of a pathologization of his condition (in which psychic and somatic aspects could not be separated) and a medicalization of his care (he was being treated more or less regularly by five doctors), his symptoms would serve to facilitate legal recognition and integration into society, perhaps even ultimately leading to the dissipation of the medical problems for which he had been granted his temporary residence permit.

One might be tempted to see this as a medically virtuous circle (legalizing the individual helps him to recover and may even avoid unnecessary medical expenses), but one has to be conscious that it institutes the body as the immigrant's site of ultimate truth.

This investment of the body is conducive to all sorts of truth tests, to which those seeking the precious residence permit are subjected, but in which they tend to develop their own tactics. Four figures of truthfulness can be distinguished, depending on the extent to which the condition and the identity of the applicant were based in reality (table 5).[13] The terms used for each relate to the way they are regarded by society, starting with health professionals themselves: thus they do not represent an objective reading, but rather an interactional typology. I present each of them and briefly evoke illustrations.

The figure that occurs most frequently—and is the one that least interests me here—is clearly that which we might describe as "conformity": the immigrant who gives his or her real name and invokes an established disease.

TABLE 5. Figures of truthfulness

	True pathology	False pathology
True identity	Conformity	Simulation
False identity	Usurpation	Imposture

Note: The terms used to describe these configurations correspond to the way each is viewed and, often, named in the social world: thus the genuinely sick person who presents herself under her true name is considered "conforming," while the person who invents or exaggerates symptoms is considered a "simulator." This is a logic of labeling, in the sense of the interactionist theory.

However, we have already seen the problems of interpretation posed by this situation, which is only superficially simple.

The second figure corresponds to what civil servants describe as "usurpation of identity": precisely because he or she is illegally resident, the sick immigrant may undertake medical tests or seek treatment under a different name, so that the cost of treatment is covered, or simply to avoid being denounced and deported.

A Moroccan man applied for a temporary residence permit on health grounds. He was suffering from arteriosclerosis, the main complication of which was a stroke suffered a few years before, which had led to surgery to replace part of the blocked carotid artery. However, he had been operated on under a different name, which appeared on the operation report. Although his true identity was indicated on the most recent additional tests, the different names aroused the suspicion of the public health nurse assessing his application at DDASS. Since she could not herself carry out a clinical examination, she asked a hospital doctor to verify that the pathology did indeed match the patient. In this case it was easy to check, as the scar from the operation on his neck testified to the reality of the surgical procedure. The person had not been lying.

The third figure is generally known as "simulation": the immigrant gives his or her real name, but with a fictitious pathology. As in any situation where pathology offers potential secondary gains, the procedure for acquiring a residence permit for the purposes of treatment engenders suspicion as to the reality of the pathology. Rather than an entirely invented condition, what is suspected is usually that the patient is overstating a real pathology, sometimes with the doctor's complicity.

A 33-year-old Malian man, who had lived in France for a number of years, applied for legalization, providing as evidence a handwritten letter from a doctor with an impressive list of X-rays, echocardio-grams, and laboratory tests concluding that more investigations were needed to "determine the cause of a hematological anomaly and a build-up of gas that was compressing the diaphragm." Doubting whether the hematological disorder and the intestinal signs were serious, the medical officer sent a request for further details to the general practitioner. This time the latter replied that the patient simply complained of "various problems as vague as they are numerous," but that "everything was clinically and biologically normal." The abnor-mal blood count and the suspect radiographies were suddenly brought within normal physiological limits. In this case the doctor himself had been party to the simulation.

The fourth figure results from a double falsification and is often termed "imposture": in this case, both disease and identity are borrowed or invented.

A West African man submitted an application for a residence permit for the purposes of medical treatment. The thick medical file that a humanitarian organization made up for the directorate indicated an advanced stage of AIDS. However, as the most recent blood examina-tions were several months old, the hospital was asked for an update. These new tests produced astonishingly different results, and led to the discovery that there was no HIV infection. The medical file submitted was a forgery using someone else's name.

The third and final criterion for granting leave to remain was "effective impossibility of receiving appropriate treatment in the country of origin," as the circular on application of the measure stated. This text also specified that the condition "depends not only on the existence of appropriate health care resources, but also on the patient's ability to access these resources." This is an important point: it indicates that the doctor must take into account not only the availability but also the accessibility of treatment, understood in terms of both diagnostic equipment and therapeutic procedures. More-over, the circular added that in this assessment of the medical situation in the country of origin, the medical officer must "take into consideration the existing structures, equipment and funding, as well as the presence of pro-fessionals competent in the condition in question," and check whether, "given that these individuals are usually among the most impoverished, social insurance exists and how far it extends, or whether the cost of treatment is covered by the collectivity." A Burkinabé man I met recalled his interview with a nongovernmental organization volunteer to whom he had turned: "I showed her my prescriptions, she said I had to have a serious illness. I can't buy medicine in Burkina Faso, it's only for rich people there. She told me to go and see my doctor and if I've got good supporting evidence, I'll get the residence permit, no problem. All I have to do is show we can't get treatment at home." Here too, however, things were not so simple.

The liberal interpretation allowed by the regulation resulted in major variations between examining doctors. Some sought to ascertain as best they could the health care situation in the home country, and even complained about the lack of centralized service providing relevant data from all countries, though the circular suggested that the "technical medical officer at the Directorate of Population and Migration" might fill this role: we may surmise how unrealistic was this suggestion, which envisaged universal knowledge of health care systems combined with a global assessment of each place. Most abandoned imagining this as a possibility and tended to match their assessment to the severity of the disease: for life-threatening pathology such as cancer and AIDS, it was assumed that conditions for access to complex and expensive treatment did not exist; in the case of chronic pathologies including diabetes and hypertension, the seriousness of the condition served empirically to distinguish patients who should be treated in France from others. Like the preceding second criterion, this criterion, which could not be objectified, proved largely redundant in practice.

There was one exception: mental health. As we have seen, two contrasting attitudes arose among clinical psychiatrists and medical officers. On the one side were those who believed that psychic problems required the same quality of treatment as other pathologies: return to the home country would be doubly damaging, because it would expose the individual to conditions he or she had sought to escape, and because it would interrupt psychiatric treatment as envisaged in the French medical context. On the other side were those for whom the patient's origin, especially if he or she was African, led to a very particular assessment: returning home would have a doubly therapeutic value, both by restoring the familiar social environment and by giving access to local treatments, be they rituals, herbs, or magic. Apparently benevolent but contrary assumptions resulted in the two sides harboring diametrically opposed opinions, one relating to the harmful context in the person's country and a universalist argument, and the other supporting the assumed beneficial nature of the home country, with a culturalist justification. This line between universalism and culturalism profoundly divides the field of mental health.[14] Here it was drawn on the basis of whether the situation that has led to emigration, or the condition prevailing in the society of immigration, was considered the more pathogenic. Once again, it was a conflict of truths.

Of the three criteria—duration of residence, nature of the disorder, and accessibility of treatment in the case of forced return—the government chose to intervene on the latter when, from 2002 onward, it deemed that the number of immigrants being granted permits on medical grounds needed to be reduced. The Ministry of the Interior, together with the Ministry of Health, made several attempts to establish lists of countries indicating for each the therapeutic resources available for each of the main pathologies, the idea being that this would make it easier to control the opinions rendered by medical officers. This position was inspired by the principle, operative in cases of asylum, that led to the identification of "safe countries," nationals of which were a priori excluded from refugee status. In contradiction with the tenet of medical confidentiality, the list would therefore allow any prefect, provided that he knew the immigrant's illness, to overrule the medical officer's opinion. Thus the government's efforts to restrict the extent of legalization on health grounds, including those that went against basic ethical rules, indirectly reveal the power of humanitarian reason.

In addition to the three criteria discussed, other factors not explicitly stated in the law often entered into the experts' deliberations. "It's not simple, but it can't be simple," explained one medical officer to me. "We try to examine each situation by taking into account the length of residence, the situation in the country of origin, including the political situation, the person's age, whether they have family support, whether they have children." In other words, data relating to health—in principle the only factor determining the opinion rendered by the directorate—represent just part of the elements taken into account by the physician in a context where affective and moral factors play an essential role. This is particularly the case when state experts are not content with examining the application, but enter into that unusual face-to-face encounter that brings together a patient who is seeking not a treatment but a residence permit, and a health professional who cannot examine the patient since he or she is supposed to deal with populations.

The following comment made to me by a medical officer evaluating several hundred applications annually offers an indication of the empathy that sometimes developed: "The more time you spend with a person, the more you tend to say yes." It was probably to reduce this interpersonal tension, and the compassion it engendered, that the regulations repeatedly instituted more neutral and distant procedural norms, with the expert increasingly being required to generate decisions on the sole basis of the application. But the fact remains that whether it is in a meeting with the patient or merely in the reading of the files, the truth of the body, as instituted by the law, acquires its legitimacy only in relation to the larger truth of the person, as evaluated by the expert. This truth includes his or her history and current situation, but also brings into play his or her rhetorical capacities (persuasiveness) and relational qualities (to arouse sympathy). For the immigrants aspiring to documents on humanitarian rationale, the assessment by the clinical expert and the medical officer effectively emerges as a test in which they are judged far beyond their health condition.

Within the course of a decade, the principle of legalization of immigrants with health problems was established and the provision, presented as a compassionate measure, was initially welcomed. But this unanimity of moral sentiments was short-lived. Ten years after the humanitarian rationale, recast as medical grounds, was inscribed in French law, its widespread application had become the subject of polemic. In the right-wing magazine *Le Point* on October 11, 2007, columnist Jacques Marseille derided immigrants legalized on health grounds: "28,797. That's how many foreigners were granted a French residence permit in 2004 for the purposes of treatment 'the lack of which could lead to exceptionally serious consequences for them, provided that they would be unable to receive appropriate treatment in their country of origin.' In 1998 there were only 1,078. More than half these serious conditions are psychiatric disorders. France —a true land of asylum for people who are a bit down."

    In fact my research points to much graver situations than his cynical statement suggests; not only were AIDS, cancer, chronic hepatitis, and kidney failure frequent among the statistics in question, but even with illness of a less serious nature, the social reality faced by those concerned was generally not an appropriate topic for sarcasm. Moreover, the figures presented in the column had been crudely manipulated: in fact, 16,164 foreigners, not 28,797, were granted a temporary permit on health grounds in 2004, so the number cited was overstated by 78%. As for the alleged proportion of psychiatric disorders, the indicated proportion suggested that the medical officers had breached medical confidentiality by disclosing the conditions on which they had made rulings, which was unlikely; despite attempts to introduce such a measure in prefectures, notably in the working version of a 2006 ministerial circular, this attack on deontology had not yet been applied when the article was written. Notwithstanding its scornful humor and inaccurate figures, this commentary is doubly significant. On the one hand, it emphasizes an undisputable fact: the rapid growth in numbers legalized for health reasons. On the other, it reveals a new phenomenon: the breakdown of the consensus around humanitarian reason.

Until the early 1990s, illness was used as grounds for seeking a residence permit only in exceptional cases. Ten years later, the health criterion had become one of the primary grounds for legalization, and the one that was increasing most rapidly. This evolution needs to be interpreted with caution. First, it corresponded not to a massive influx of new patients but rather, principally, to the recognition of a right for people who had often been living in France for several years; it should therefore strictly speaking be seen as legal regularization of a situation that the health authorities considered progressively more problematic. Second, it was greatly exaggerated by the fact that almost all the permits granted were only valid for one year and thus had to be renewed, artificially inflating the ministry's figures; in fact, new permits represented just under 40% of the total. Yet, even with these two caveats in mind, the increase in the number of people admitted on health grounds for the first time, as opposed to being renewed, from 455 in 1998 to 7,737 in 2005, cannot be denied.[15] It was in this context that the government proceeded to issue increasing numbers of measures aimed at restricting access to this right (notably, as mentioned, through the establishment of lists of treatments available, rather than accessible, in each country), exerting pressure on medical officers (by threatening them with sanctions if their decisions were deemed too accommodating), and multiplying the administrative obstacles to deter immigrants (above all by refusing to assess applications and by demanding high fees). But beyond these practices, what was taking place through the increasingly frequent challenges to the right to health care, discredited on the grounds that it was being abused— the article cited being just one among many—was the tentative delegitimization of humanitarian reason.

This delegitimization was not limited to France. When humanitarian reason was introduced into French law in order to protect sick immigrants against the risk of deportation, it was optimistically thought that, under pressure from nongovernmental organizations (the European sections of Médecins du Monde in particular were campaigning on this), and given the state of European Union legislation (especially within the framework of the European Convention on Human Rights), the provision would be extended throughout the Union. Actually, a number of countries did adopt measures of this type, although generally in a restrictive and discretionary manner (the United Kingdom, for example, merely resolved not to proceed with the deportation of terminally ill individuals), and European jurisprudence was gradually becoming established (on the basis of a broad interpretation of Article 3 of the Convention, which prohibits torture and the imposition of degrading and inhuman punishment). Even though it was of limited applicability, this extension of legal protection for sick people was still considerably reduced by a decision of the European Court of Human Rights on May 27, 2008, in a ruling in the case brought against the British government on behalf of a Ugandan woman suffering from an advanced stage of AIDS. Considering first that it was possible to get treatment in Uganda, despite the prohibitive cost of antiretroviral drugs there, and second that European countries could not be required to redress the disparities in health care between nations, the court rejected the woman's appeal and authorized her deportation.[16] The logic of state sovereignty in the control of immigration clearly prevailed over the universality of the principle of the right to life. The compassion protocol had met its limit.

4. Truth Ordeal

Attesting Violence for Asylum Seekers

> From its inception the experience of a refugee puts trust on trial.
> The refugee mistrusts and is mistrusted. In a profound sense, one
> becomes a refugee even before fleeing the society in which one
> lives and continues to be a refugee even after one receives asylum
> in a new place among a new people.
>
> VALENTINE E. DANIEL AND JOHN CHR. KNUDSEN,
> *Mistrusting Refugees*

In 2004, with 58,550 applications submitted, France became the industrialized country with the highest recorded number of requests for asylum, ahead of the United States, the United Kingdom, and Germany, which until then had been the top three countries for refugees. Yet in the same year, the rate of acceptance of applications by the Office Français de Protection des Réfugiés et des Apatrides (French Office for the Protection of Refugees and Stateless Persons, OFPRA), which had declined continuously for thirty years, reached its lowest level, at 9.3%. Thus, if we count not the applications submitted but the actually granted refugee status, France, with just over one hundred thousand refugees of the nine million in the world in 2004, was far behind not only Pakistan, Iran, Tanzania, and Chad, among others (for it should not be forgotten that it is the countries of the global South that take in the majority of refugees), but also Germany, the United States, and the United Kingdom (which then had 960,000, 450,000, and 280,000 refugees, respectively).[1] In other words, despite the government's alarmist declarations, which were echoed by media representations of refugees overwhelming the capacity for receiving them, the situation remained demographically under control and politically of no great concern. France's generosity toward victims of persecutions was indeed limited.

For some twenty-five years, this tension between a high number of applications for asylum and a low rate of granting refugee status, which was obviously problematic for a nation that continued to present itself as the "cradle of human rights," had been resolved ideologically by increasingly discrediting the word of asylum seekers so as to justify the progressive reduction in the rate of acceptance of their request. OFPRA officials were

forced into becoming stricter by the burgeoning numbers of "bogus refugees," it was claimed. Under these conditions, the asylum seekers' accounts,
long the only evidence testifying to their story and justifying their request,
were no longer sufficient to confirm the truth of the alleged persecution.
The body, which could have retained a trace of it, came to be seen as potentially providing tangible proofs.[2] Medical practice was then called on to
contribute its expert opinion on the scars left by the violence suffered, and
organizations specializing in supporting foreign migrants began to produce
medical and psychological certificates, such as the following:

> Mr. V., a 40-year-old Tamil man, asserts that he has been persecuted by
> the Sri Lankan authorities because of his alleged links with the LTTE
> [Liberation Tigers of Tamil Eelam, the armed rebel movement opposing
> the government in the Sri Lankan civil war]. He states specifically that
> he has been shot when fleeing arrest on May 5, 1998, and then left for
> dead after being stabbed twice by Sri Lankan soldiers. Clinical exami-
> nation reveals: on the right hand, a sutured scar on the back and a smaller
> puncture scar opposite it on the palm, compatible with the entry and
> exit points of a bullet; a puncture scar on the left cheek, opposite a mouth
> scar, likewise compatible with a bullet wound; a scar to the left of the
> sternum; a round scar in the right iliac fossa, 3 cm in diameter; a 1 cm
> round scar on the inner left arm; a puncture scar on the inner left leg;
> a 6 cm vertical linear scar in the middle of the chest, compatible with a
> knife wound; a 10 cm linear scar on the outer left shoulder, compatible
> with a knife wound. The observations made in the examination are
> compatible with the injuries recounted by Mr. V. Certificate drawn up
> at the request of Mr. V. and handed to him.

As in almost all cases, there is no way of knowing what action Ofpra took
with regard to this precise and expressive testimony written by a physician
working with the Comité médical pour les exilés (Medical Committee for
Exiles, Comede), which was set up in 1979 to provide health care, social
support, and legal assistance for sick, mostly undocumented immigrants
and asylum seekers. Was it taken into account or not? Was Mr. V. among
the 4.9% of Sri Lankans granted asylum by Ofpra in 2005, or among the
95.1% who were rejected? We know no more about this case than about the
563 other Sri Lankans who sought help from Comede that year, 84% of
whom asserted that they had been victims of violence and 47% of whom
claimed to have been tortured.[3] In its annual report, Ofpra noted: "Sri Lanka.
Applications, the large majority of which come from persons of Tamil origin, always cite violence and fear of persecution or maltreatment, either
from the authorities or from the LTTE. They refer to arrests, detention and
abuse on the grounds of the logistical support, food and medical care they

or their close associates provided or are wrongly accused of providing to fighters from the Tamil separatist organization." Even more than the suspicion implied in the detached tone of this passage, the gap between the content of the commentary, with its evocation of dreadful events, and the rate of acceptance of applications, which remains particularly low, reveals the lack of credence given to the word of asylum seekers. In that year, which had started with the disaster of the tsunami and where political violence was part of the everyday for many, only one in twenty Sri Lankan asylum seekers was granted refugee status by Ofpra. Of the nineteen who failed to persuade the official responsible for assessing their case, one might succeed in extracting refugee status from the Commission des Recours des Réfugiés (Commission of Appeal for Refugees, CRR), which evolved from 2008 into the Cour Nationale du Droit d'Asile (National Court for the Right to Asylum, CNDA).[4] The remaining eighteen would likely become lost among the illegal immigrants, with some being arrested and sent back to Sri Lanka, often at risk to their lives. Under these conditions, a medical or psychological certificate such as that presented by the Sri Lankan applicant just cited became a crucial element of proof.

It is this new regime of truth[5] that I focus on here, this search for a truth for which the asylum seekers' word no longer constitutes sufficient evidence, but of which their body still bears the trace, in the form of the physical consequences of torture that only medical examination is competent to state. I seek in particular to understand the conditions in which this regime of truth emerged by setting it within the context of the contemporary history of asylum. I then attempt to analyze how medical and psychological certification of persecution suffered put organizations supporting asylum seekers to the test. Finally, I examine how the shift from the narrative and the word of the refugee toward the body and the expertise of the physician or the psychologist modifies political subjectivities.[6] Through this exploration located at the core of the politics of asylum, my aim is to grasp the tensions and contradictions at work in the moral economy of Western societies when they assert generous principles of protection for victims of persecution while at the same time managing their recognition through the restrictive terms of immigration control.

THE SITE OF VERACITY

At the height of the violence in Colombia, Michael Taussig reported his visit to a young far-left activist who had been arrested, abducted, and tortured for attempting, with the other members of his small group, to denounce the abuses of human rights committed by the army.[7] Still profoundly affected by this experience, which he had miraculously escaped after being left for dead in a park, the young man "proceeded to tell me how he was tortured, how bad it was when they changed the handcuffs for rope, how he felt like drowning with the wet towel stuffed down his mouth, and what it was like being in the bag and shot but not killed. He leant his head forward almost onto my lap and guided my finger through the hair to the soft bulging wounds of irregularly dimpled flesh. 'Like the worshippers with Christ's wounds,' murmured a friend days later to whom I was telling this." In fact, virtually the same gesture is performed by two Algerian men, one showing the large scar across his neck, the other revealing a round scar on his lower back, in Olivier Pasquiers's photographs in an exhibition titled *Exile Sickness* that took place at COMEDE in 2000[8]—as if they had something to prove as their story was challenged by the French authorities in charge of asylum. Torture leaves the marks of the torturer on the body, and it was now these scars that bore witness.

The body is the primary site on which the imprint of power is stamped. In traditional societies, initiation rites have the dual function of inscribing the law of the group on the body and ensuring its inculcation, and of imprinting within bodies the codes and norms organizing the relations of power and authorizing their reproduction.[9] In contemporary wars, both imaginaries of violence and theories of extermination have made use of practices (ranging from collective rape to the branding of prisoners) derived from logics that exceed pure brutality to signal the presence of power.[10] Thus, whether it is set in the context of the order of social reproduction or the disorder of barbaric violence, the body is invested, in the sense that it is the means by which power is both expressed and demonstrated. In its extreme version, incarnated in the radical dictatorial and totalitarian regimes of the twentieth century, it was the disappearance of the body that manifested the absolute and arbitrary nature of crude power, when even the physical trace of individuals or of entire peoples was erased. The body is political in the sense that in the last resort, it is what bears witness to power.

In pacified Western societies, however, this incorporation of the political order was gradually attenuated, as physical violence lost its legitimacy in the imposition of that order, and the "trace of 'torture' " in criminal justice became "enveloped, increasingly, by the non-corporal nature of the penal system," as Michel Foucault put it.[11] The proscription of torture and the abolition of the death penalty form part of this relinquishing of physical power. But politics has not lost all relationship with the body. By a remarkable historical turn, in contemporary societies—at least those in which the state more or less exercises a monopoly on legitimate violence—the body, no longer the principal site at which the strength of power is manifested, has become the site where the truth of individuals is tested. For both the poor who must exhibit the stigmata of poverty in order to receive public aid or private charity, and the immigrants who must demonstrate their sickness or suffering in order to obtain a residence permit, as we have seen earlier, the body has become that which bears witness to a truth.

The importance ascribed to medical certificates in applications for asylum in France in recent years has to be understood in light of this new regime of truth.[12] Expected by the institutions responsible for deciding whether these requests are eligible, sought by lawyers and support organizations so they can better defend their clients, avidly hoped for by the immigrants themselves, who are aware of or imagine its authority, a certificate issued by a physician, or sometimes a psychologist, testifying to persecution endured, has become an essential component of the application submitted for evaluation by the state. The procedure for granting refugee status in France is effectively the responsibility of two national bodies created by the law of July 25, 1952: OFPRA, the office that generates the initial ruling, and the CNDA, the court that reviews appeals from rejected applicants. Candidates for asylum submit their application to OFPRA, which decides whether or not to interview them and accepts or rejects the application. In the case of refusal, the asylum seekers can appeal to the CNDA, whose judgment is normally considered final. Medical expertise may be sought at either stage, by these state bodies, the asylum seekers, or the agents involved in legal or social mediation between the two, whether lawyers or nongovernmental organizations. While it has not eliminated the need for the autobiographical account through which applicants for political refugee status strive to prove that they meet the criteria allowing them to claim the protection of the 1951 Geneva Convention, this medical expertise is increasingly required as verification of the validity of the applicant's story. Scars, mostly physical but also increasingly psychic, become the tangible sign that torture has indeed taken place, that violence has indeed been perpetrated. The body is the ultimate site of veracity. Like the doubting disciple Thomas, the French state needs to touch the wounds in order to believe the word of the asylum seekers.

For refugees, the body is therefore the site of an inscription whose significance relates to two levels of temporality. First, it represents the inscription of power, through the persecutions suffered in the country of origin.

Second, it becomes the inscription of truth, to the extent that it bears witness to these persecutions for the purposes of the institutions in the country of arrival. In other words, the case of asylum seekers places us at the articulation of two histories of the body: that through which power is manifested, and that through which a truth is stated. There is no need to point out that torture has always claimed its legitimacy from the alleged search for truth, even when its primary goal was to impose an order of power through terror. The fact that the individuals exposed to such persecutions in the country they have left are subjected to a new test through which power strives to produce a truth (naturally without physical brutality but not without a degree of psychological violence, which I have witnessed, and of which the consequences are revealed by the testimonies I collected) in the country in which they seek refuge, is not the least paradox of the contemporary politics of exile.

THE BEST OF PROOFS

The following letter is extracted from a file of lawyers' correspondence collated by the nongovernmental organization COMEDE:

Paris, [date]

Dear Sir,

I write in respect of the Commission of Appeal hearing on [date]. In order for you to obtain refugee status, you *must* send me a medical certificate testifying to the traces left on your body as a result of the torture and abuse inflicted on you, particularly with respect to your eye. Please do not hesitate to contact me if you have any difficulty.

Yours sincerely . . .

This letter reveals the extent to which the body has become the site of production of truth about asylum seekers. From the late 1990s to the early 2000s, COMEDE recorded a doubling in the number of medical certificates supplied in support of applications for political refugee status: more than one thousand per year were being drawn up, and some readily spoke of an "epidemic of requests for medical certificates."[13] The growth in the number of certificates requested from COMEDE was striking: in 1984, when medical expertise was beginning to be more widely used, 151 certificates were produced; in 1994 the figure was 584, and by 2001 it had risen to 1,171. Considering the number of consultations for treatment, the physicians working for the organization were devoting five times more of their schedule to providing medical expert opinion than fifteen years earlier. Moreover, during the recent period it was only possible to manage this increase via the forced limitation of the number of examinations made. While internal policy and expert practices varied between OFPRA and the CNDA, support organizations were all observing the same phenomenon, which they repeatedly condemned: "Is a piece of paper necessary to prove torture?" exclaimed the anonymous author of a report on medical certification in the June 2002 edition of the newsletter of the Primo Levi Association, founded in 1995 to support the victims of political violence. The article highlights a "progressive rise in requests to both physicians and psychotherapists." This increase needs to be resituated in the historical time of asylum.

As with other nations, France is more generous the less it has to bear the cost of its generosity. When requests for asylum are few, in an economic context wherein refugees easily supply needed labor, the country demonstrates its solidarity with the victims of persecution throughout the world, faithful to the spirit of the 1793 Constitution.[14] In this sense, we could say that throughout the nineteenth century there was not really an asylum problem, although a degree of demographic pressure was exerted during periods of conflict outside the country's borders. It was only during the twentieth century that the "refugee question" became an issue, particularly following the First and, especially, Second World Wars, when foreigners fleeing persecution or violence became undesirable throughout Europe.[15] The initial international response was the creation of the High Commission for Refugees in 1921, under the aegis of the League of Nations. This step was more directly related to the Bolshevik revolution in Russia and the hundreds of thousands of exiles it created than to the war itself, but the rise of totalitarianism and nationalism in Europe between the wars quickly overwhelmed the commission's modest regulatory and financial resources.[16] The signing of the Geneva Convention in 1951 heralded the official entry of refugees into contemporary policy. It is often forgotten, though, that from the first there was a powerful tension between, on the one hand, a humanist ideology that promoted the right to asylum and offered an ennobled representation of the refugee, and on the other, a pragmatic politics that mistrusted these stateless populations and reduced them to the economic status of immigrant.[17] The utopia of the former, still marked by the spirit of "never again" following the discovery of the Nazi atrocities, came face to face with the realism of the latter, already imprinted with the "liberal rationale" of a globalization accelerating through the need for labor in the reconstruction of a destroyed Europe, and soon succeeded by international economic expansion. Thus, once the enormous influx of refugees during the immediate aftermath of the First World War had been absorbed, states easily granted asylum to the exiles. Indeed, these refugees were less recognized in a spirit of justice than tolerated for their contribution to the wealth of the nation.

In the early 1970s the situation altered dramatically, against the background of the oil crisis and the rise in unemployment, but also, through the efforts of social protest movements, with the revelation of the living conditions suffered by immigrants: a comprehensive state policy combining control of flux and social integration was put in place.[18] The control was targeted first at the labor force, which was tightly restricted from 1974 onward, and later at family regrouping, particularly after 1984. Integration was focused on housing, and aimed to absorb most of those in transit centers and unfit private housing. In this new context, the number of asylum seekers rose sharply, from 2,071 in 1974 to 15,500 in 1976. The figure increased gradually during the subsequent years to reach a peak of 61,422 in 1989. Over the space of fifteen years, the number of asylum seekers swelled thirtyfold.

However self-evident the relationship between the decline in labor immigration and the increase in requests for asylum may consequently appear in OFPRA's statistics, it is nevertheless complex. There is a widespread belief that when migrants saw the possibilities for entering France diminishing, they turned to the still open avenue of asylum, given that 90% of requests were granted by the authorities in 1974, with the rate even rising as high as 95% in 1976, compared to only 28% in 1989. The interpretation may be partially correct, and it is likely that some of those seeking to immigrate learn to take the opportunity of the routes available to them. But this explanation, which clearly feeds the discourse discrediting asylum seekers, ignores the converse reality that until the 1970s, in the absence of any government policy for managing immigration and as the law of supply and demand was the only regulating factor, a contract of employment generally acted as de facto residence permit. Under these conditions, many potential asylum seekers did not need to subject themselves to OFPRA's assessment, since finding a job was a means of ensuring both financial and legal security.

In the new configuration of immigration, asylum policy was fundamentally redefined. In the mid-1970s, nineteen out of every twenty applicants were granted refugee status. By the onset of the 1990s, only three out of twenty received a positive response from the French authorities. OFPRA's rate of acceptance has fallen still further since that time, dropping to almost one out of twenty during the first decade of this century.[19] Four decades ago, asylum was the subject of a relation of trust in which the asylum seeker was assumed to be telling the truth—or more accurately, since the number of refugees was then not an issue, knowing whether the truth was being told was similarly a nonissue. By contrast, today asylum is set in a climate of suspicion where the applicants are suspected of taking advantage of French hospitality—or more precisely, the asylum seekers are systematically suspected of being economic migrants passing themselves off as victims of persecution. It is in this new context of delegitimization of the asylum seeker's word that the development of medical certification of scars and trauma acquires meaning.

"As the number of requests for certificates has increased, the number of asylum seekers being granted refugee status has decreased." In putting it this way, a doctor working for a refugee support organization sought to point out the futility of the medical certificates he was requested to produce. Their lack of efficacy seemed factual because he observed a decreasing return in terms of asylum: on the one hand, the proportion of applications granted continued to fall, while on the other, medical expertise was increasingly being sought. In fact, the relationship of cause and effect is exactly the opposite: it is because asylum was no longer legitimate, and was increasingly difficult to obtain on the basis of the applicant's account alone, that certificates acquired greater importance. In a context where the validity of asylum requests was systematically contested, not only was any evidence positive for the applicant, but those proofs in particular, from an agent credited with ideological neutrality and expert knowledge, had even greater power. As one assessing judge on the CRR indicated in an interview: "All proofs are acceptable. The judge builds up a personal opinion on the basis first of all of the applicant's account, which remains the central element—its coherence, credibility, or contradictions—and then, somewhat like in criminal trials, where a confession is considered the height of evidence, the medical certificate tends to be seen by lawyers and asylum seekers as the best of proofs."

These remarks point to a dual phenomenon: first, the imaginary invested in the medical certificate, and second, the limited efficacy it has in reality.[20] Paradoxical fetishization, given that it has little basis in empirical fact: from the person who submits to judgment to the person who metes out justice, the symbolic and practical value of the medical certificate is actually, if not inverted, at least altered. Lawyers and asylum seekers see it as an open sesame. OFPRA officers and CNDA judges view it as one piece of evidence among others. For both, however, it was a political innovation: the validation of asylum seekers' accounts via the corporal inscription of the persecution they had suffered invented a new form of transnational government.

ETHICS PUT TO THE TEST

Among refugee support organizations, a crucial question then emerged: Should they continue to issue medical certificates? Their doubts were underlined by Sibel Agrali, then director of the Primo Levi Association:[21]

> The precautionary principle suggests that someone who says she has been raped or tortured should be believed. What is the point of asking therapists to confirm the truth of what their patients have endured? When a request for medical certification breaks into the therapeutic relationship, it is rarely spontaneously. The patients, usually pressured by their lawyer, compatriots or support organizations, ask for the document as if it were an essential requirement of the asylum application procedure. This logic of proof is totally incompatible with the logic of torture—which, beyond the suffering it imposes on the body, essentially represents an attack on the individual's fundamental psychological and social structures. What purpose is served by participating in this dysfunctional system?

Reading the minutes of their meetings and their activity reports over fifteen years, and listening to veterans of nongovernmental organizations recounting their experiences, it becomes apparent that all those supporting asylum seekers and victims of torture have continually faced this question about the efficacy and meaning of the certificates. Thus in a 1991 COMEDE internal document, the secretary of the Certification Committee, attempting to give an account of sometimes stormy discussions, was already writing: "A general unease with the current formula, with which no one is happy, was identified, some expressing a wish to cease all such activity, others a feeling of saturation, a dissatisfaction with the lack of time they have to draw up these certificates." An article published at the time by COMEDE's medical director provided a more detailed description of this unease:[22]

> A growing number of individuals who suffered ill-treatment and torture in their country of origin come to see the physician in order to obtain a medical certificate supporting their application to the authorities for asylum. This increase in requests is alarming for two reasons. Firstly, the demand for proof takes on increasing significance for the applicants, and results in serious destabilization: how can they make the authorities understand that they have a reasonable fear of reprisals if they return

to their country? Secondly, OFPRA officers and CRR magistrates almost instinctively attach greater importance to the bodily conse-quences of torture, whereas in fact it forms part of a program of destructuration and depersonalization of the individual: physical violence, the most widespread image of torture, is also the most reductive evidence of it.

As we see, the problem of the certificates is nothing new.

The strongest criticism of medical certification relates to its deviation from the Geneva Convention, according to which any person who has "a well-founded fear of being persecuted for reasons of race, religion, nation-ality, membership of a particular social group or political opinion, is out-side the country of his nationality and is unable or, owing to such fear, is unwilling to avail himself of the protection of that country" is considered a refugee. The fear of persecution does not imply that the individual should actually have been tortured: it may stem from direct or indirect threats, from real or suspected links with a threatened political, religious, or ethnic group, from the murder or disappearance of people close to him or her. Even if the individual has suffered torture, it does not necessarily leave visible traces: asylum seekers often recount rape, nightstick beatings, electric shocks, prolonged immersion in water, or being hung upside down. Asking for a medical certificate that confirms the existence of scars compatible with the account considerably restricts the field of application of refugee status un-der the Geneva Convention, and, conversely, reduces the chances of those who have no scars to show.[23] No one, of course, suggests that refugee status cannot be granted in the absence of a certificate, but the added value ac-corded to bodily traces diminishes the power of the principle of the "fear of persecution," which has no physical manifestation. While the certificate may play a positive role for the individual concerned, in the long term it results in a restriction of chances and a reduction in rights for refugees in general.

But the medical certificate is not only a document that reduces the spirit of the founding text of asylum to violence inscribed on and in bodies: it is also implicated in discrediting the word of victims, because it brings in an expert who is called on to speak the truth in their place. The accounts pre-sented by asylum seekers were increasingly mistrusted as policy became more restrictive and stronger constraints were exerted on OFPRA officers and CNDA judges. The more the government pressured institutions and their agents to reduce the proportion and number of applicants granted ref-ugee status, the more those agents needed to persuade themselves that many asylum seekers were exaggerating, faking, or making things up, so that in the end they could reassure themselves that decisions to reject applications were not entirely negating the meaning of their work. As one judge from the United Nations High Commission for Refugees, serving on the CNDA, explained, they gradually internalized the rate they were encouraged to aim for, and used criteria that allowed them to accept an average of only one application in ten in the first decade of the twenty-first century, when they had been accepting proportionally nine times more in the 1970s. Under these conditions, drawing up certificates testifying that, as the standard wording put it, the observations of the medical examination were compatible with the asylum seeker's account, was to substitute an expert opinion for the applicant's word and contribute to the delegitimization of individuals' accounts. This devaluation of the asylum seeker's word is particularly poignant for facts about which the physician can say little, notably in cases of sexual violence where, fortunately, the physical aftereffects usually disappear over time. In such circumstances the psychic imprint is sometimes substituted for the missing bodily trace, cast as trauma.[24] Psychologists therefore began to work alongside physicians to explore the truth of stories, seeking nightmares and other symptoms that might testify to a state of posttraumatic stress.

With regard to these issues, two attitudes existed among support organizations. A first group was relatively unconcerned about these ambiguities and dangers of medical certification. In the view of these organizations, the main aim was to give a chance to the asylum seekers by adding credibility to their application through a medical certificate. There was no internal debate about the issue. This was the position taken by the Centre Minkowska, which specializes in mental health care for refugees and immigrants, the Association for the Victims of Repression in Exile, and the Center for the Law and Ethics of Health. A second group was torn by the contradictions between the idea the organizations had of their mission and the role they were asked to play. While they were supposed to provide care and support to victims of persecution and, going beyond individual cases, to champion their cause in the public arena, particularly in the context of increasingly restrictive asylum policies, they gradually found themselves drawn into collaborating with state authorities, helping them select among the applications for refugee status. They were stirred, and sometimes split, by recurrent impassioned debate. But despite their shared analysis, they did not all draw the same conclusions. Some, however much they disagreed with the procedure, felt they could not withdraw from giving expert opinion. According to them, applicants had the right to request a certificate, physicians had a duty to respond, and a certificate might ultimately act as evidence to obtain refugee status. Moreover, there was a fear that if organizations no longer issued certificates, they would be replaced by a body of accredited experts certainly less inclined to defend asylum seekers and definitely more expensive. COMEDE, which currently provides more than ten thousand consultations a year at a hospital located in the south of Paris, chose to continue issuing certificates. Conversely, for other organizations, the ambiguities and contradictions of the certification prevailed over the imagined benefits. Their position was to break off relations with the OFPRA officers and CNDA judges who sought their opinion, and therefore to avoid any collaboration, which they tended to see as potential complicity. The Primo Levi Association regularly announced its intention to stop issuing certificates.

It would be tempting to see the first position (criticizing but certifying) as deriving from an ethic of responsibility, and the second (refusing to collaborate) from an ethic of conviction, to use the Weberian distinction.[25] The former would privilege the potential anticipated benefits for the asylum seekers both individually and collectively, whereas the latter would defend more general principles of political autonomy. However, the theoretical distinction is not so clear, since on the one hand, the first posture includes deontological arguments (the medical doctor cannot refuse to provide certificates) while the second involves consequentialist elements (the long-term effects of participating in the discrimination of candidates to the status of refugee). Moreover, the options described correspond to the more or less stable official position of the various nongovernmental organizations, but they do not fully account for actual practices. Within each organization the attitudes and discourses of physicians and psychologists remained diverse, as is revealed by interviews, observation of their interaction with clients, and examination of certificates drawn up.

The intense reflection and discussion on these questions among members, the emotions and rifts they aroused in debate, and the doubts and difficulties they gave rise to in the daily practice of every clinician form part of the ethical world of these organizations.[26] To issue, or not to issue, medical certificates: in both conversation and action, each individual revealed an ethical passion that derives from the affective logic peculiar to the management of asylum.[27] The reason is that, beyond their disagreements, the physicians and psychologists were well aware of the gap between the meaning that violence could have for those who had suffered it and the semantic reduction operated by the clinical description of physical scars—between the deep-rooted reasons for their own commitment to the cause of refugees, which led them to work in these organizations, and the administrative actions of verification they were required to perform. Defenders of the right to asylum, they found themselves implicated in a policing of bodies.

But it can also be hypothesized that ethical tensions between and within these organizations were that much stronger because their room for maneuver was restricted. For on one level the questions of whether they should issue certificates and whether they had some efficacy were settled outside the space where they were debated. They were fundamentally determined at the level of the European Union, with the 1990 Dublin Convention, which established relations of solidarity on asylum among member states; the 1997 Treaty of Amsterdam, which instituted provision to set a common policy on immigration and asylum; the 1999 Tampere Summit, which, while affirming that the two areas are distinct, linked policy on immigration and asylum; and finally at the Paris Conference in 2008, which established the European Pact on Immigration and Asylum.[28] They were further decided via the guidelines issued by the government and the administration to their agents to reduce the number of people obtaining refugee status, but also through these agents' own acceptation of a set of common beliefs about the exponential rise in asylum requests, the invalidity of most of them, and the need to bring an end to overgenerous granting of residence permits— all considerations that were obviously not unique to the French context.[29]

Given these conditions, it is no surprise that since 1995 the cumulative rate of acceptance by OFPRA and the CRR has remained relatively stable, regardless of the variations in the international situation and the fluctuation in the number of requests. During the following ten years, the rate ranged between 15% and 20%, as if the CRR's expanding generosity compensated for OFPRA's increasing strictness to maintain an implicit statistical norm. This disquieting observation suggests that certificates had only a marginal influence, "saving" a few applications while making little difference to the general economy of granting asylum. Ultimately, changes in policy (for example, the invention of the administrative concept of the "safe country" that allows almost systematic rejection of applicants for asylum from those countries), and the individual attitudes of decision makers (OFPRA officers or CNDA judges who are more or less liberal in their interpretation of the administrative-legal structure given to them), carried much more weight than the medical certificates about which the support organizations were so concerned. Much ado about nothing, it would be tempting to suggest, if the only concern was efficacy. But the issue was different in these debates that shook the organizations supporting asylum seekers: it was the defense of moral principles in politics, particularly the recognition of the reason of victims of persecution faced with the reason of state.

WRITING TO TESTIFY

Once these organizations agreed to draw up certificates testifying to the existence of traces of the persecution endured by asylum seekers, they still had to define the best way to do it. How can one write about violence without eluding its political meaning, without betraying the experience of suffering, without substituting for the word of victims?[30] To this general question, which concerns writers as well as historians and anthropologists, there is a specific answer in the present case. In effect, for the expert tasked with testifying to the trace left by torture on a body, the problem is principally a technical one. A skill has to be applied in the service of a cause. The medical and psychological consequences of the persecution must be described in order to authenticate validity to a narrative. The following example is the conclusion to a long medical certificate written by a COMEDE physician about a man "of Zairean nationality":

> The account Mr. B. gave us of the circumstances of his arrest and the ill-treatment he received then and during his time in N. prison is very detailed, highly coherent and sometimes even tinged with emotion. However, clinical examination revealed relatively few traces. The chest pain is probably linked to posttraumatic chondrosternal arthritis, which cannot be detected by X-rays. The fact that Mr. B. has a tooth missing while the rest of his teeth are in good condition supports his case. Mr. B. was unable to ascribe his abdominal scar to a specific trauma, saying that he more or less lost consciousness. However, taken as a whole the signs point to the truth of the facts he alleges. Certificate issued to the applicant for the appropriate legal purposes.

Medical certificates follow a standard model. They begin with the words "I, the undersigned" and continue with the applicant's "declaration"; then come the "complaints," further the "examination," and finally the "conclusions," which end with the formula "Certificate issued to the applicant . . ." In this instance, the declaration, in direct style and indicative mode, is long, running over thirty-six dense lines. Reference is made to the political circumstances: "Mr. B. told us: 'I was working for S. company as a warehouseman when one of the managers asked me to let through some propaganda material transported by the airline in the name of Mr. V., a Belgian Socialist who supported the clandestine opposition party, the UDPS. I accepted and I let several shipments pass through.'" The account of the arrest is detailed: "On July 30, 1985, five BCRS (political police) agents came to my house to arrest me. They started beating me from that moment, and continued in the jeep they took me away in. I was kicked in the left cheek and felt that one of my teeth had been broken, it really hurt, I began to bleed, then I realized the tooth had fallen out." Subsequently, physical ill-treatment during the man's internment in a detention camp is described:

> In the afternoon they came for me and took me to an office to be interrogated by one of the officers. I told the truth about what happened and then one of the soldiers slapped me and because I wouldn't answer any more questions they hit me on the head and shoulders with rubber nightsticks. I couldn't take it any more, I was knocked out, they threatened to kill me. Then they handcuffed my hands behind my back and took me outside. They threw cold water over me and told me I had to stay lying there. I saw that my stomach was wounded. After an hour they stood me up again and carried on hitting me and telling me to talk. They tried to make me carry someone on my back and when I couldn't they kicked me three times in the chest. The third time, I lost consciousness.

The complaints listed in the certificate consist of "chest pain," "one missing tooth," and "an abdominal scar." The medical examination has only a small contribution in comparison with the account: "antero-posterior pressure on the thorax is painful," writes the doctor, but the X-ray "shows no bone lesion"; "the absence of the second upper left pre-molar" is noted, but there are of course many ways of losing a tooth; there is certainly a "roughly horizontal, straight-line scar" on the abdomen, but again it is difficult to determine its origin. Hence the conclusion quoted earlier, which reveals, rather than a clinical truth read from the body, a personal conviction evoked by the story told. Unable to ascribe the physical signs to torture with any degree of certainty, the physician underlines the coherence and emotion of the account, ending an undemonstrative description with a surprising expression—"point to the truth of the facts he alleges"—that has something of a profession of faith.

This medical certificate was issued in 1987. It belongs to the initial period of clinical expertise on torture, when the institutional demand for such certificates had recently emerged. Support organizations had not yet developed a doctrine about certification. Physicians approached by asylum seekers or the asylum authorities responded as best they could, mixing the canons of medical certification (standard formulas, careful description, prudence in interpretation) with the concern for accurate expression (respecting the applicant's account, highlighting probative details, revealing personal conviction in the conclusion). General rules did not get in the way of the freedom of expression of the practitioner. Moreover, analysis of a series of certificates written during this period indicates a fairly wide stylistic variation, as might be expected when the exercise was left to each individual expert.

But that time is past. As early as the beginning of the 1990s, under pressure from the social and political fronts, Comede instituted standard wording, an initial version of which appeared in an internal document in November 1991. Physicians were henceforth asked to "try to be brief and accurate." The brevity related mainly to the applicant's account. While the certificate just cited covered a page and a half, more recent ones are no more than a few lines, in indirect style and conditional mode, as in this far shorter document dating from 2002: "This patient, of Tamil origin, alleges that he was arrested in 1996 because he was involved in helping the Tigers, and imprisoned. He states that he was tortured, stabbed with a bayonet and burned with cigarettes."[31] By contrast, the guidelines on the clinical section of the certificate indicate that doctors should "provide a detailed account of the complaints or the observations from examination." Everything that relates to medical expertise is detailed, as the following extract from the same certificate suggests: "At the base of the right thumb, two scars, one longitudinal, 3 cm long, the other oval, compatible with a wound from a blade; on the left forearm, five round lesions typical of cigarette burns; on the right leg, several scars with loss of flesh due to blade wounds." Finally, the conclusion, as the recommendations go on to state, should attempt to "link the facts declared as closely as possible to the ill-treatment observed," without mentioning "negative elements in the complaints or the examination." It was therefore no longer advisable to note, as in the earlier certificate, that "clinical examination revealed relatively few traces," or that "the scar cannot be ascribed to a specific trauma," demonstrating an honesty that had been considered to be ultimately effective but was no longer seen as appropriate. In fact, the final formula was standardized in the dry wording: "As a whole the observations are compatible with the patient's statement." Although the medical certificate followed the same rhetorical structure as previously, thus redefined with more rigor and soberness, it acquired a quite different social signification.

The shortening of the account of violence, now reduced to the barest facts, has three main reasons: first, a desire not to repeat the applicant's story, which would contribute to reducing its legitimacy; second, a concern to keep to the principle of the exercise, according to which physicians should speak only about what they can attest; third, the effect of exhaustion given the number of requests, which resulted in a sort of routinization of certificates. Yet to diminish the part played by the applicant's story in the certificate to submit to the Ofpra officials or the CNDA judges is literally to participate in the dehistoricization of refugees, both in terms of the individual histories of the asylum seekers and in terms of the collective history of violence they are inscribed in.[32] Interestingly, this reductive process formed part of a broader shift within the world of nongovernmental organizations: it can be described as a differentiation of functions and a distinction of roles. The defense of asylum seekers was increasingly conducted on three main fronts: the legal cases, through which authorities were reminded of their responsibilities, including before European courts; the narrative support, which consisted in assisting people in wording their story to make it more compatible with the criteria on which they would be evaluated; and finally, as we have seen, medical expertise, based on certification of the traces of violence. The first of these fronts relates to the collective (refugees and even the principle of asylum itself), while the other two focus on individuals (through personalized intervention).

Thus, in the division of tasks between those specializing in support for the account and the experts in medical certification, there was a separation between the narrative and the corporeal. Physicians, of course, had to link what the body revealed through scars to what they had learned from the account. But they did not venture beyond their realm, the clinical sphere, leaving the reconstruction of biography to agents specialized in this activity—that is, lawyers, but also organizations such as the Service oecuménique d'entraide (Ecumenical Service for Solidarity, CIMADE), and providers of accommodation including the Centres d'accueil pour demandeurs d'asile (Reception Centers for Asylum Seekers, CADA). The validity of the physicians' expertise was based on the demarcation of their field of competence, as expressed in the certificate. Relinquishing the moral sentiment and political commitment that had inspired them to become involved in the care and support of asylum seekers was the price they paid for ensuring that their certificates were credible and might have a positive effect. They no longer spoke of the sincerity of the account, and made no mention of their believing the applicant's word. Their job was to examine and describe the "scars observed," striving to assert the likelihood of a link with the "alleged facts." They had imagined themselves as activists of the cause of asylum, but realized they were actually practicing forensic medicine to attest to the traces of persecution.

Nevertheless, expertise had another function that remained unnoticed. In fact, it was not only addressed to the OFPRA officers or the CNDA judges: it also had a role that the physicians considered therapeutic, but which I would rather view as ethical. Drawing up certificates meant recognizing that the persons concerned had indeed suffered the violence they claimed to have endured. Not only were they listened to; they knew they had been heard. While those who have faced the extremes of horror have a painful "experience of the unspeakable,"[33] they are also often confronted with an experience of the inaudible, which is no less harrowing: no one hears their account. Today, the dominant ethos of the authorities with regard to asylum is suspicion. Doubt is cast on stories, facts are disputed, evidence is dismissed. Convincing the doctor may therefore be a first, and sometimes decisive, step in the production of one's truth. The mark is no longer only on—or in—the body: it is present in a document that has legal value. The scriptural trace, whether it repeats the account or testifies to bodily traces, envelopes the fragile words and invisible wounds of the asylum seeker in its legitimacy. Thus writing does not have merely practical virtues. It also has a symbolic, and hence political, value, of which the medical certificates remind us. In a context of generalized skepticism, written testimony represents the highest form of truth telling.

However statistically modest their presence in Europe—particularly compared with the number of refugees in the countries of the global South—asylum seekers represent a major issue in the contemporary world. Like the "displaced persons" after the First and Second World Wars, the victims of violence who seek protection today put not only the regulatory structure of the Western states but also their moral sense and their political responsibility to the test. From this point of view, we could say that if, as Hannah Arendt suggests, the stateless were the supreme moral and political figures of the twentieth century in Europe,[34] asylum seekers now appear to occupy that position. Indeed we need to make an analytical distinction between refugees as a mass phenomenon on the African and Asian continents and asylum seekers as a hyperindividualized reality in Europe and North America. The former are the subject of collective management, grouped together in camps by international organizations, while the latter receive singular treatment, with state apparatuses taking a case-by-case approach. Thus the "anonymous corporeity" of the former[35] is contrasted with the detailed exploration of the body of the latter, seeking the traces that can testify to the truth of the condition.

But here we encounter a tragic paradox. The practice of torture is, as we know, condemned by international conventions—the 1949 Geneva Convention on humanitarian law, and more specifically the Convention against Torture adopted by the United Nations in 1984. There is more than enough evidence that the existence of these texts does not guarantee the elimination of physical maltreatment: we need only remember the torture routinely meted out by the French army during the Algerian war of independence, or the recently revealed degrading treatment by the U.S. military in Iraqi prisons. From the perspective of moral and political history, the point is therefore not to ask whether torture is used less frequently today, but to note that it has become illegal, and generally illegitimate (despite the fact that some positions taken in France following the revelation of the generalized practice of torture in Algeria, and even more in the United States after 9/11, demonstrate a resistance to this historical evolution). Thus torture has not disappeared, but—as far as possible—it has to remain secret.[36] The contrast here with the practice of public torture, which was deemed in earlier times to have a pedagogic virtue, is striking. Not only must torture be hidden, its traces have to be erased for the perpetrator to avoid the risk of being brought one day before an international court of justice. This means one of two things: either making the bodies disappear completely (mass graves sometimes bear retrospective testimony to this practice) or using techniques that leave no detectable marks (whether the suffering inflicted is physical or psychological). Consequently, by an ironic turn, it is at a moment when the practice of torture is developing toward increasingly invisible forms that a visibility of marks on the body is demanded, to confirm that the persecution did indeed take place. While the word of victims of political violence is being systematically cast into doubt, it is now their body that is interrogated—but a body that has often little to tell because torturers silence it.

And even when it speaks, the body of persecuted individuals is not always enough to establish the truth of their history. I noted, with regard to the case of the Sri Lankan man whose medical certificate I quoted from at the beginning of this chapter, that we usually do not know whether the medical testimony submitted to the authorities that decide whether to grant refugee status has any effect. However, in some cases we do know, and that of Elanchelvan Rajendram is such a case.[37] According to his reconstructed biography, he came to France at the age of twenty-six and submitted a request for asylum. A Sri Lankan Tamil, he had lived in a zone controlled by the rebels of the LTTE, to which his older brother, who had been killed by the national army, belonged. He himself had been arrested by the Sri Lankan military, along with his father, shortly after his brother's death. He was imprisoned and tortured for twenty days. Following his release he hid in the premises of a party that was collaborating with the government, and for which he also worked. This time he was threatened by the Tamil Tigers, who accused him of colluding with the enemy. Another of his brothers was also killed. His parents then decided that he should leave the country.

After a long journey organized by smugglers, he arrived in Strasbourg. OFPRA rejected his request on the grounds that it was too "stereotypical" and not "substantiated." He appealed to the CRR, submitting a number of documents including a death certificate for his brother, which indicated that he had been shot, and a certificate testifying to his scars, drawn up by a French medical doctor. But the CRR judges were no more convinced than the OFPRA officers, and even stated that no link had been established between the clinical observations and the reported maltreatment. Following changes to the French law on asylum, Elanchelvan Rajendram, assisted by a Strasbourg support organization, was allowed to resubmit his application to OFPRA and then to the CRR, reiterating his "fear of returning to a country where his safety is not guaranteed": the two bodies confirmed their previous decision. After a final unsuccessful appeal to the administrative court to try at least to get the deportation order rescinded, the young man was returned to Sri Lanka. A few months later, on February 28, 2007, he died after being shot sixteen times by the Sri Lankan army during a patrol. "I don't know what more I can do to make people believe me," he had written in his last appeal. It seems that neither his account nor his documents had succeeded in making his situation credible. Even a letter from the hospital doctor testifying to the existence of scars compatible with the facts of his story had not been of any use. Thus, a modest element in the politics of asylum, the medical certificate can sometimes become the fine thread on which the existence—both physical and psychic—of the asylum seeker hangs. But in the case of Elanchelvan Rajendram, the thread broke.

Frontiers

5. Ambivalent Hospitality

Governing the Unwanted

> In contrast to the *peregrinus*, who lived outside the boundaries of the territory, *hostis* is "the stranger in so far as he is recognized as enjoying equal rights to those of the Roman citizens". A bond of equality and reciprocity is established between this particular stranger and the citizens of Rome, a fact which may lead to a precise notion of hospitality. By a development of which we do not know the exact conditions, the word *hostis* assumed a "hostile" flavour and henceforward it is only applied to the "enemy".
>
> ÉMILE BENVENISTE, *Indo-European Language and Society*

On May 23, 2002, just two weeks after taking office in the French government under Prime Minister Jean-Pierre Raffarin, Nicolas Sarkozy, the new minister of the interior, made a highly publicized visit to the Sangatte transit center in the north of France. Since September 24, 1999, the giant hangar, located in a small coastal resort, had become an almost obligatory staging post for foreigners en route to the United Kingdom to seek asylum: during those two and a half years, it is estimated that fifty-five thousand people found temporary shelter there before crossing from Calais by train or boat. Run by the Red Cross under contract to the French government, the center, which had previously served as a depot for the machinery used to excavate the Channel Tunnel, was repeatedly denounced by immigrant support organizations and human rights campaigners. Pointing to the material conditions of the accommodations and the undefined legal status of the place, these activists described it not as a center but as a "camp."[1] A rather unusual camp, however, since it was not enclosed by barbed wire, and residents were free to come and go as they pleased. When it opened it had places for 200 people, but two years later the 700 beds were no longer sufficient and in fact there were 1,300 persons living in the 25,000-square-meter space; each week 400 newcomers arrived, and almost the same number left. In drawing the media spotlight to his visit, Sarkozy was symbolically demonstrating his intention to break with the policy of his left-wing predecessors: he would be tough on immigration and strict with foreigners who had no right to stay in France, but he would not tolerate breaches of democracy.[2] He would close the Sangatte center in the name of the Republic. Branding the building "sinister," he threw his opponents' argument back at them, asserting that he rejected the "undignified conditions" to which foreigners were being subjected. He and his collaborators, notably Brice Hortefeux, who would go on to become the minister of immigration several years later, went so far as to adopt the word "camp" themselves in order to condemn past policy and justify closing the center. The term had in any case become common currency in the public arena, and it was used as an almost innocuous description in press reports: newspapers deemed the center the "Red Cross camp."[3] The paradox being that the center, opened ostensibly for humanitarian purposes, was now being closed on the same grounds. In both cases, the publicly stated compassion was just a step away from hidden repression.

The prehistory of Sangatte is longer than is generally supposed.[4] In the mid-1980s most of the foreigners in the Calais area were Pakistanis and Vietnamese waiting to cross to England. In the early 1990s there were increasing numbers of East Europeans, particularly Poles, liberated by the collapse of the Communist regimes, and Sri Lankans, mainly Tamils, fleeing the civil war in their country. During this period the British began to refuse to assess some requests for asylum and to send undesirables back to France. In the mid-1990s local initiatives emerged to address the needs of the growing masses of people sleeping on the streets and in the parks of Calais and the surrounding area: the organization Belle Étoile (Under the Stars) in 1994, and the Collectif de soutien en urgence aux refoulés (Emergency Aid Collective) in 1997. The situation became more dire in 1998, with the arrival of Kosovars who had suffered persecution under the Serbian government. "Calais, a Reflection of Chaos," read the headline of the local newspaper *Nord Littoral* on August 6, 1998: "Kosovars seeking asylum in England in the worst conditions, a Romanian who has come to try his chances on the other side of the Channel, Gypsy families rejected by the British authorities—encounters that reveal Calais as a pit of misery." The following spring the prefect, the local representative of the state, who had until then been reluctant to use this solution, found himself forced by the influx of Kosovars to open up a warehouse, but only as a night shelter. "After the time of securitization, has the time of humanization come?" asked a local journalist on April 24, 1999, the day the building was opened. But by June 4 the prefecture authorities had closed the warehouse. During the summer, asylum seekers, who no longer had anywhere to go, camped in the Saint-Pierre Park in central Calais, supported by the organization C'Sur. The Kosovars were gradually replaced by Afghans and (mainly Iraqi)

Kurds who had fled the Taliban and Baathist regimes. On August 11, 1999, in an article headed "Government Seeks a Way Out," a journalist of *Nord Littoral* declared: "The prefect's aim is to reconcile humanitarian aid to refugees with the rejection of illegal immigration: he admits he is having difficulty finding a balance between the two."

The struggle to make real a watchword that looked like an oxymoron— compassionate repression—gave rise to contradictory decisions in the days that followed. On August 14, the opening of an emergency reception center was announced. On August 19, in the streets of Calais, 210 individuals were arrested. On August 24, approximately 200 refugees were installed in the hangar. Intrigued, *Nord Littoral* commented: "While the Saint-Pierre Park returned to looking a little more like a park, the deputy prefect of Calais indicated that policy was now shifting from the humanitarian approach to the security phase." The reverse, in short, of what the journalist cited earlier from the same newspaper had surmised four months prior, when "securitization" seemed to be yielding to "humanization."

It is the tension between humanity and security, between compassion and repression, as it is manifested around the issue of refugees and more broadly that of immigration, that I wish to explore here. This tension is currently a major factor in the management of aliens in France, and to some extent also more broadly throughout Europe. In his comparative Indo-European linguistics, Émile Benveniste emphasizes the curious ambiguity of the etymology of the word "hospitality."[5] The Latin term from which the word is derived is *hospes*, itself stemming from *hostis*. The first of these terms denotes the guest, while the second signifies the enemy. "To explain the connection between 'guest' and 'enemy' it is usually supposed that both derived their meaning from 'stranger', a sense which is still attested in Latin. The notion 'favorable stranger' developed to 'guest'; that of 'hostile stranger' to 'enemy'." However, *hostis* has not always held this negative connotation. Initially, as the epigraph to this chapter points out, it referred to a contractual relationship of equality and reciprocity with the stranger who lives in the city. Similarly in Greek, *xenos*, which means "stranger," assumes a pact implying obligations and exchanges. A moment arose in Roman history, though, when social changes were no longer compatible with the type of relations of equality and reciprocity that had been established with regard to strangers. "When an ancient society becomes a nation, the relations between man and man, clan and clan, are abolished. All that persists is the distinction between what is inside and outside the *civitas*." When *hostis* came to signify the enemy, another word, *hospes*, was required to refer to the guest—each of the two terms referring explicitly to the stranger. The confusion between hospitality and hostility, which thus goes back to the etymological and political origins of this figure, is central to our reflection on the contemporary condition of foreignness.

Extending this reflection, Jacques Derrida gives an almost psychological reading of it:[6] "One can become virtually xenophobic in order to protect or claim to protect one's own hospitality, the own home that makes possible one's own hospitality. I want to be master at home, to be able to receive whomever I like there. Anyone who encroaches on my 'at home', on my power of hospitality, on my sovereignty as host, I start to regard as an undesirable foreigner, and virtually as an enemy. This other becomes a hostile subject, and I risk becoming his hostage." A dialectics of hospitality and hostility, of host and hostage: we recognize the rhetoric of immigration policies that has become widespread over the past two decades. "We can only integrate legal immigrants on condition that we are more strict in turning away illegal foreigners," ran the argument in the 1990s, conveniently forgetting that a growing number of legal immigrants became illegal foreigners because their residence permit was not renewed, their request for asylum was rejected, or they had been convicted of a crime—in other words, evading the fact that the boundary between the two categories was increasingly porous and that "legal immigrants" no longer had any guarantee that they would remain so. "We have the right to be selective in our immigration policies," one would hear only ten years later, reducing hospitality to a simple issue of utility and deeming those not "chosen" unwelcome, with the risk that asylum would shrink like an evaporating puddle.[7] In other words, we have evolved in one decade from a logic of legal differentiation (separating the legals from the illegals within the country) to one of legitimate discrimination (separating the desirables from the undesirables before they enter the country).

Sangatte is testimony to this slippage: it was not a true reception center where requests for asylum would be processed, nor was it a detention camp for those rejected and about to be deported. It was a place of indeterminate status, with a humanitarian mission but set up for reasons of security, through which foreigners were supposed to pass but where they were not supposed to stay. It was a place of transit in which illegal status was not punished (though they were present, the police were exceptionally tolerant) but in which the undesirables were rendered invisible—as long as they quickly disappeared by leaving for the United Kingdom. Neither guests nor enemies, they enjoyed a furtive hospitality that conferred no rights—and in particular no right of asylum. They were pure obligees. But as the British authorities toughened their policy on accepting these refugees and the journey became more difficult and risky, the relations between humanitarian reason and security logic in the center became increasingly tense. Ultimately, the same arguments used to justify opening the Sangatte center—humanitarianism and security—served to explain its closure.

To explore this singular combination of compassion with repression, of which Sangatte represents a revealing moment,[8] I begin by returning to what took place within and around the center, and especially how the dual invocation of these contradictory logics resulted in the suspension of the law. I then resituate these issues in the context of contemporary immigration policies, focusing particularly on the humanitarianization of asylum. Finally, I propose a rereading of the processes of globalization in light of the history of this last caravansary.

INVERTING ROLES

Anyone visiting the Sangatte reception center in early 2002 could not fail to be struck by the juxtaposition of two symbols: on one side of the entrance to the huge depot a Red Cross flag fluttered in the wind, while on the other a French riot police van was permanently stationed. On entering the center, the visitor would be struck again by the area known as the "village square": this was a sort of vast hall that one had to cross in order to reach the large military-style tents and barracks where the refugees slept. The following is a paragraph from my field notes, written on March 22, 2002:

> In the village square, most of the men are standing in small groups. In the middle there is a little wooden play structure for children; a few older children are on bikes or roller skates, and others are playing hopscotch. There is also a television area with eight rows of seats, of which only the first three can see the tiny screen, and only the first row has any chance of hearing the sound. Further away, near the infirmary, a dozen or so men are waiting on a bench to see the nurse. Behind the barriers that separate the refugees from the staff, Red Cross workers talk with one another or busy themselves with work. When new arrivals come in they are welcomed by the staff, who cross the barriers to ask them a few questions and register them, a process that takes less than one minute. Personal circumstances are discussed aloud in front of everyone around. Five meters [sixteen feet] above the heads of the crowd milling about the village square, there is a metal gangway that overlooks the area like an innocuous viewing platform. Policemen, ostensibly calm, their weapons clearly exposed, watch over the bustle a few meters below them. At several points during the day, especially at mealtimes,

patrols pass through the midst of the refugees, who do not seem to be disturbed by these now familiar walkabouts.

The space of Sangatte was structured and occupied by a dual institutional presence: the Red Cross, with its offices, infirmary, and volunteers, and the French police, with its company of riot officers, overhead surveillance stations, and discreet but quite visible presence around and inside the hangar.

Yet, the two institutions had not always cohabited in this way. The Red Cross, on the one hand, had managed the center since it opened, commissioned to do so by the state, with funding from the national Department for Population and Migration. It had tendered for this role, and in addition to the close political links the organization had with the government (its president at the time, Marc Gentilini, presented himself as a friend of then French president Jacques Chirac), it could point to its experience not only of refugee camps in other parts of the world but also of spaces of exception within France (such as the waiting zone at Roissy airport, whose Red Cross manager, Michel Derr, subsequently became director at Sangatte).[9] The riot police, on the other hand, only established a presence at the center following a number of violent incidents among the refugees, since in a context of competition between different national groups for control of the holy grail of passages to England, intimidation and fighting had become more frequent, particularly between Kurds and Afghans (I was told that the rate for those wishing to cross was between US$500 and US$1,000 in this period, the Kurds charging less than the Afghans for arranging the journey). In early 2002 the police were therefore requested to provide twenty-four-hour security, which did not however prevent various disturbances, some serious (one fight resulted in one death and two serious injuries in April 2002, and a soccer match between the two groups in May 2002 degenerated into a pitched battle). Thus humanitarian care and security concern were intimately linked, because of the increasing concentration of people in poor living conditions and the growing difficulty in crossing the Channel.

In the day-to-day working of the center, the roles of the two institutions partly overlapped. The Red Cross was frequently called on to exert a controlling function or even administer punishment. I witnessed the following scene. A refugee was trying to enter the camp with three ten-pound bags of apples. The Red Cross volunteers at the entrance would not let him in, fearing that he was "trafficking goods." The reception manager was asked to back them up. The refugee explained that the apples were for a party with his friends. The manager replied that she did not believe him. Other refugees then became involved. A woman intervened to mediate. The Red Cross staff, weary of arguing, let the man with the apples through, adding that no other foodstuffs would be permitted for the party. An hour later a Red Cross volunteer reported having found the men selling the apples near the "mosque," an unenclosed space set aside for prayer. The manager decreed that the apples must be distributed for free. The refugees protested. Soon the police had to intervene to calm them. This kind of episode happened every day: not only did the aid workers find themselves "policing" the center, but the most trivial events took on enormous significance and gave rise to a permanent state of readiness to intervene. As one Red Cross volunteer noted:[10] "It was disappointing to see how a group of humanitarian workers could become so embittered. For the staff, any initial illusions that refugees are docile and grateful recipients of assistance gave way to compassion fatigue." In reality the problem was that the task the state had conferred on the humanitarian organization was primarily one of public order, a fact that the Red Cross volunteers had not appreciated when they took it on.

But conversely, the riot police showed a fairly indifferent, even almost benevolent attitude. The officers were never aggressive toward the foreigners, never checked their residence permits despite the fact that almost none of them were there legally and that everywhere else in the country identity checks were on the rise. Nor did they apparently ever take them to the nearby Coquelles detention center, where hundreds of undocumented immigrants were waiting to be deported. They often even brought individuals found wandering the streets of the town or around the port back to the center, so that they could be cared for and have lodging. Their regular patrols through the hangar occasioned no antagonism; even when they made generalized searches for weapons. They were not interested in the smuggling networks unless fights broke out. Their security task was thus essentially preventive, and it was the Red Cross who maintained order in the center. Paradoxically, Sangatte was the place where undocumented immigrants were the least harassed by the police and—if I dare say—the safest in France.

This fragile equilibrium and institutional ambiguity was able to last as long as the center functioned as a place of transit. Refugees spent no more than a few days or weeks in the hangar before leaving for Britain, and consequently, the local tensions were only transitory. The discourses and practices of the Red Cross managers themselves confirmed this situation. A document drawn up by the International Organization for Migration (IOM) was distributed to the refugees when they first entered the center.[11]

It began with these words: "You are currently a resident of the Sangatte reception center which is managed by the French Red Cross. This center was set up by the French Government in order to provide short-term humanitarian assistance to irregular migrants like you. However, this situation is and can only be a temporary and precarious one." Given this situation, the options proposed in the title of the pamphlet—"dignity or exploitation"—seemed at best an impossible choice.

On the one hand, the document emphasized the dangers run by those who attempted to reach the English coast: "The barbed wire is razor wire. It contains thousands of metal blades. These can cause you deep injuries. The railway is electrified. It carries 25,000 volts. If you get too close, you risk electrocution. Hiding under a lorry, you can be crushed or choked to death. Jumping onto a moving train, you can be maimed or killed. The windspeeds in the tunnel reach 200 mph. You can be blown off the train." The pamphlet even referred to the deaths of four undocumented immigrants who tried to cross in 2001 and of fifty-eight Chinese migrants hidden in a truck in 2000. In addition to these threats to life and limb, it stressed the risk of an application for asylum in the United Kingdom being rejected and the applicants being returned to their country. But on the other hand, it made no mention of the possibility that refugees could seek asylum in France. Nor did the Red Cross ever divulge this information, so that the center's residents were not aware of it. It was as if the United Kingdom, despite its increasing inaccessibility, was the only country where asylum was a possibility. This strategy worked well, since of the 65,000 individuals who passed through the Sangatte center in two and a half years, only 350, less than 1%, applied for asylum.[12]

In fact, only one solution was presented at the end of the document *Dignity or Exploitation:* return to one's country, for which the IOM would provide assistance. It is easy to comprehend, however, how unrealistic this hypothetical solution was, given the months the refugees had traveled to get there, the considerable amount of money they had spent, and the many perils they had faced in order to reach the gates to what some local journalists called the "British El Dorado." But it is also easy to understand why, when five hundred mainly Afghan refugees stormed the tunnel between the two countries on Christmas Day 2001, before being arrested and then released by the police, the United Kingdom held the Red Cross responsible.[13] This was just one more episode, albeit a more spectacular one, in a long history of accusations that the French government's policy encouraged the flow of refugees into England: once again, the British called for the closure of what they termed "the Sangatte refugee camp." Negotiations, which had begun under the previous government, continued from May 2002 between French minister of the interior Nicolas Sarkozy and British home secretary David Blunkett, and resulted in an agreement under which the center would be closed in return for the British authorities granting residence to the people still staying there. "Goodbye to Sangatte" was the headline in the French national daily *Libération* on December 3, 2002, above an article reporting the departure of the last refugees.

However, the history of Sangatte, from its ambiguous opening to its paradoxical closing, has a wider significance. The replacement of the right to asylum with humanitarian reason, which the politics of the Sangatte center demonstrates in exemplary fashion, forms part of a phenomenon that emerged during the 1990s: the sidelining of asylum and the advent of humanitarianism. The background to this development is the process whereby the refugee issue became subordinate to migration control policy, a process that began at the Tampere Summit in 1999 and was completed with the signing of the European Pact on Immigration and Asylum in 2008.

ASYLUM AS SUBSIDIARY

Marie is a young Haitian woman. She came to France at the age of twenty-three. She sought asylum in 2000. The story she told me is no doubt virtually the same as that she gave the Office Français de Protection des Réfugiés et des Apatrides (French Office for the Protection of Refugees and Stateless Persons, OFPRA), and later in her appeal to the Commission des Recours des Réfugiés (Commission of Appeal for Refugees, CRR). Her father, a political dissident, had been murdered a few years earlier. Her mother disappeared some time later, and everyone believed she had been abducted and killed. One day when Marie was at home with her boyfriend, a group of young men burst into the house. She was gang-raped. Terrified, she hid at an aunt's house. Several weeks later, she managed the leave the country and came with her boyfriend to France to seek asylum. OFPRA rejected her application, probably deeming that it had not been demonstrated that the gang rape was politically motivated and that this was essentially a matter of ordinary violence that did not amount to persecution on the grounds of belonging to a particular social group, as stipulated in the 1951 Geneva Convention.[14] Marie appealed to the CRR, which was no more favorable, and her case was definitively closed. There was nothing surprising in this: the decisions were in line with the practices current during that period. Not only had OFPRA's rate of acceptance of applications plummeted to 11.3% by

2000, augmented by the 5.8% approved on appeal by the CRR (in other words, overall one applicant in six was granted asylum), but Haitians were even less likely to receive a favorable response, with only 3.3% accepted by OFPRA and 3.8% on appeal by the CRR (that is, one in fourteen applicants obtained refugee status).[15] The civil war in Haiti, the military regime of terror, the political instability between Jean-Bertrand Aristide's two terms as president, were obviously not enough to meet the criteria of the Convention.

The only choice left for Marie, like most of the 80% of asylum seekers whose applications are turned down, was to become an illegal immigrant. She hid at a friend's place, not leaving the house for fear of identity checks. After two years, depressed and underweight, she submitted to the urgings of her friends and went to see a doctor who, concerned by her condition, sent her to the hospital. There she saw a psychiatrist who wrote a report describing her as suffering from depression and at risk of suicide, in the hope that this emphasis on her condition might help the application for residence that was to be made to the prefect's office on her behalf. The physician was attempting to help her stay in France on medical grounds under Article 12a11 of the 1998 immigration law. This was a risky venture since cases centering around mental health could result in contradictory assessments, depending on the views of the medical officers called on to adjudicate: some held that mental illness could be better cared for in the country of origin and therefore did not justify residence permits, while in the view of others, the applicant's precarious legal status itself was the source of the depressive symptoms and granting permission to remain could have therapeutic benefits. But the psychiatrist did not have to deliberate long over the best strategy.

On Marie's second visit to the hospital, the results of the blood tests taken at her first visit revealed that she was HIV positive. Further investigation confirmed that she was suffering from an advanced AIDS condition. It seemed clear to everyone that the infection resulted from the gang rape. The application to the prefect's office was drawn up quickly and residence was granted without problem. Here too, statistics were coherent with this favorable outcome: Haitians constituted the third-largest group seeking residence on medical grounds, and AIDS was by far the most commonly cited condition, the opinion of the examining doctors being generally favorable in these cases.[16] Thus Marie, who had initially been refused asylum, was granted residence under the so-called humanitarian rationale. Her word about the violence she had suffered was doubted, but ultimately her body spoke for her.

Marie's story is exemplary but not unusual. How many others who were refused refugee status owed their residence permit to a serious illness that allowed them to appeal on medical grounds? Often the diagnosis of AIDS "helped" to repair the injustice of a rejected application for asylum, as in the case of the Central African woman whose husband had been tortured and murdered, the Congolese priest who asserted that he had been persecuted for his ministry, or the Cameroonian trade unionist who was jailed and beaten before his house was burned down—among many asylum seekers whose stories I collected. Advised by a lawyer, a support organization, or a relative, they had consulted a doctor with the "hope" that their medical condition would fit the criteria of the humanitarian rationale. How to make sense of this development? Reasoning pragmatically, we could of course consider that the most important thing is to obtain the precious document, and simply rejoice that Marie, the Central African woman, the Congolese priest, and the Cameroonian unionist all did so. But this would be to ignore three important aspects of the issue.

First, not all asylum seekers whose applications are rejected have a serious illness they can turn to their advantage, and the doctors they consult find it extremely difficult to have to tell them that their condition is "not serious enough" to justify an appeal on medical grounds. Second, the residence permit granted to rejected asylum seekers on medical grounds does not confer the same guarantees as the status of refugee; in particular, holders of this permit have to submit to reexaminations, usually annually, which generates profound anxieties and may lead to their documents not being renewed. Third, it seems likely that the level of social recognition and the sort of subjective experience are different for those benefiting asylum than for those allowed to remain on health grounds: there is more dignity in being a refugee victim of political persecution than in being a sick immigrant receiving charitable support for one's medical condition.

Thus, in little more than two decades, as asylum gradually lost its credence, illness gained prominence and there was a shift in the award of residence rights, from the less legitimate to the more legitimate. Let us return for a moment to OFPRA's statistics. In the early 1980s there were just under 20,000 applications for asylum per year, of which nearly 15,000 were accepted, representing a 75% success rate. In the early 1990s, although the number of applications had risen substantially to more than 80,000 per year, the number granted refugee status remained roughly the same, approximately 13,000, meaning that the proportion of acceptance had effectively plummeted to 15%. During the subsequent decade, application numbers began to decrease, as a result of major efforts to deter asylum seekers at the point of entry to the country, but although it might have been expected that this selective process would result in an increase in the acceptance rate, that rate remained low, and even began to fall again in the early 2000s, dropping to below 3,000 accepted as refugees, or 7.8% of applicants. Within twenty-five years, therefore, the rate of asylum granted had plunged to a fifth of its previous value in absolute terms, and a tenth in relative terms. The net result was a swelling in the number of rejected applicants, in other words illegal immigrants: 171,000 more in the period 2003–2007 alone. Some of these turned to other means of gaining residence, primarily medical conditions when these were deemed sufficiently serious by the administration doctors.

The substitution of humanitarian rationale for the protection of asylum is not merely a mathematical phenomenon, a simple shift from one category to another, as if some rejected asylum seekers would simply choose to seek residence rights on medical grounds. It corresponds more profoundly to a government strategy, and ultimately to a political decision. This is revealed by the amnesty program of 1998.[17] The program was the third great wave of legalization since the "closure of the borders" in 1974. The first, organized in 1981, related mainly to immigrants who had contracts of work but were not legally resident: out of 150,000 applicants, 130,000 were granted documents. The second wave, launched in 1991, examined the cases of those refused asylum: of 48,000 applications, 15,000 were granted leave to remain. The third wave, implemented after the left won the parliamentary elections in 1997, was aimed at assessing the effects of increasingly restrictive immigration control legislation known as the Pasqua and Debré laws, which had resulted in a sharp rise in the number of foreigners illegally resident in France, some of whom were considered "not suitable for either legalization or deportation," according to the semiofficial lexicon. In this wave, 180,000 applications were submitted, of which 150,000 were valid; 80,000 applicants were finally granted permission to remain, 3,238 of them on medical grounds. Commenting on these figures in June 1999, a senior official in the Ministry of the Interior's Department of Public Liberty and Legal Affairs, who had been responsible for the national monitoring of this major initiative, explained to me how they had proceeded when faced with situations where "deadly danger" of a political nature was combined with a "serious illness" requiring care not available in an applicant's country of origin: "Humanitarian reason is a new, clearly identified category. We routinely considered the political risks as secondary and the serious illness as the principal issue." Thus what might appear to be an individual decision—

by rejected asylum seekers in poor health, by the lawyers working on their behalf, by the organizations supporting them, or by officers of the prefect's office willing to give them another chance—was also a choice made by state authorities. Political asylum became subsidiary to humanitarian reason. More consensual, the logic of compassion now prevailed over the right to protection.

This is a significant shift. To use Giorgio Agamben's distinction, it marks the loss of recognition of *bios*, "qualified life," and the new legitimization of *zoē*, "bare life."[18] Being in danger because of one's political activity or one's belonging to a persecuted group is secondary to the threat to one's body from pathology. The authorities are less willing to give credit to the combatant for a cause or the victim of violence than to the human being suffering from a serious condition. "This disease that is killing me is what enables me to live today," was the striking way it was put to me by a Nigerian man who, after a dozen years spent as an illegal immigrant roaming around France and Germany, through exposures and arrests, precarious jobs and makeshift shelters, had finally been granted a residence permit on humanitarian grounds when he was diagnosed with an advanced stage of Aids: he knew that returning to Nigeria meant death from lack of treatment, and that by contrast his documents finally allowed him to live almost normally.[19] Gradually, thanks to universal health insurance and welfare benefits and the care of doctors and support organizations, he had reinvented a life constructed entirely around his disease. In short, his biological life had given him the right to a social life. And for the health professionals and those working for the charities who helped him, this was the deep meaning of their action: using a physical disorder to recover social rights. More broadly, humanitarian organizations, foremost among them Médecins Sans Frontières and Médecins du Monde but also Aids organizations such as Aides and Act Up, made good use of the "bare life" argument (one cannot deprive the sick from treatment) to obtain a minimal citizenship (incorporating the right to residence and to health care).[20] In so doing, they exposed a form of governmentality whereby the claim to bare life was the ultimate way to access a political existence. Of this logic, the episode of the wrecking of the *East Sea* offers a final illustration.

HUMANITARIANIZING RIGHTS

On February 17, 2001, a Cambodian-registered cargo ship ran aground on the French Riviera, with nine hundred people—men, women, and children—on board. Media images of boats crossing the Mediterranean to reach Spain, Italy, and Greece as well as Malta had become familiar at the time. The sight of dozens of people, usually Africans, shivering on a beach under the watchful eye of police was almost routine, as were reports of dead bodies being recovered from the sea. But the circumstances surrounding the *East Sea* were unique in a number of ways: the ship—a freighter—was carrying many more passengers than was usual in these cases; it originated from the Middle East rather than Africa; and most of those on board asserted that they were Kurds fleeing persecution in Iraq; they therefore intended to request asylum, but had planned to do so either in Germany or in Britain, and France was simply a "land of exile by accident" for them, as an officer of the French border police observed. While these "illegal immigrants," as they were initially defined, were held at the Fréjus military base, where Red Cross teams hastily fitted out disused barracks to accommodate them, the media swarmed in, disseminating images of crying children, imploring pregnant women, and the aged and infirm behind fences to which men with defeated expressions clung.

These poignant scenes prompted a strong emotional reaction in France. While the initial response of François Hollande, the general secretary of the Socialist Party, was to say that the government could not "encourage trafficking of workers and give the illusion and the hope of integration in France," Patrick Devedjian, spokesperson for the Conservative Party, was paradoxically more hospitable, declaring: "We have no choice, at this moment, but to offer support to those suffering and to welcome them naturally." It seemed that in general politicians were playing against type: the left (in the government) took the strict line of insisting that "France cannot take everyone in," while the right (in the opposition) adopted a tone of generosity, speaking of these "unfortunate people."[21] For the government, the minister of the interior, Daniel Vaillant, recognized that this was a "human tragedy," but he added that "over and above emotion, there are rules," indicating that he had no intention of prejudging the refugee status of these men and women, whereas Prime Minister Lionel Jospin declared that "the first choice would be the humanitarian route," but that "such organized criminal trafficking should not be rewarded." However, faced with the wave of public sympathy (less than a week after the event, a poll indicated that 78% of French people were in favor of accepting the shipwreck victims and 58% thought they should be "granted refugee status on a case-by-case basis")[22] and above all aware of the risk that the detention in the Fréjus camp could be declared unlawful in a court (the constitution of a supposedly extraterritorial "waiting zone" ruled as a space of exception

was illegal because the foreigners had touched French soil when they dis-
embarked from the ship), the government decided to release the survivors,
giving them safe-conduct, which allowed them to seek asylum.

Surprisingly, very few took advantage of this opportunity. Two months
later, only 196, or 21% of the initial total, had remained in France; the others
had left for neighboring countries, mainly Germany. From an examination
of the 130 applications for asylum finally submitted to OFPRA, it emerged
that actually they were not Iraqis but Syrians, that they had embarked not
on a Turkish beach but on the Libyan coast, and finally that they were indeed Kurds, but from the little-known Yezidi minority.[23] Thus the maps of
their journeys, patiently reconstituted and proudly displayed in the newspapers, were pure fiction. "If you say you're Syrian," the traffickers had
told them, "you'll be sent back." At the time, from the cynical but realistic
point of view of the smuggling networks in the Middle East, the demonized Saddam Hussein's regime appeared to have a much worse reputation
in the West than the tolerated Syrian regime of Bashar al-Assad: this appreciation of the moral geography of tyranny was probably accurate. Whether
or not the traffickers were correct, it is revealing of the imaginary of
refugees and traffickers, and hence of the idea they have of the rational
and emotional bases on which their request for asylum will be assessed.
The often stereotypical character of the accounts, of which OFPRA officers and Cour Nationale du Droit d'Asile (CNDA) judges regularly complained, is testimony to this: rather than true stories, refugees need effective narratives.

A few days after the shipwreck, one columnist wrote the following moral
of the story: "A ship, a sort of smuggled, phantom *Exodus*, came knocking
at the doors of our coast. With no other destination but the intention not
to leave again, and flying only the flag of asylum seekers who had burned
their boats, the *East Sea* has come to test the humanitarian principles of
France, the home of human rights."[24] In this sense, the drama of the ship
and its passengers represented a truth test for French society, not just the
French government. But a test for which truth? At first, as we have seen,
some described the shipwreck victims as "illegal immigrants" whereas
others saw them as "unfortunate people"; commentators rushed to condemn
human trafficking while the authorities announced that these uninvited
guests would not be staying—for the best of reasons, that is, the fight against
crime. Subsequently, however, as emotion escalated, the survivors were able
to present themselves or be represented as victims of both Iraqi persecution and unscrupulous smugglers, and new attitudes had to be assumed:
"The heart has its reasons, or even simply its reflexes, that reason needs to

understand," enthused an editorial in *Le Monde*, paraphrasing Blaise Pascal's famous "thought" in an expression of approval for the prime minister's reversal now that he was willing to "take the humanitarian route" in the treatment of individual cases.[25] In a situation where reference to the Geneva Convention of 1951 would have provided sufficient grounds, moral sentiments, and even emotional "reflexes," were being invoked to justify asylum.

With reference to the post–Second World War context, Hannah Arendt writes: "The first serious attack on the United Nations following the arrival of hundreds of thousands of stateless people was that the right to asylum, the only right that has ever figured as a symbol of human rights in the domain of international relations, was abolished. The second great shock suffered by the European world as a consequence of the arrival of refugees was the awareness that they could neither be got rid of nor transformed into nationals of the country of asylum."[26] Shortly after she wrote this text, the Geneva Convention was signed. It was possible to imagine that the right to asylum had just been restored and that refugees would now find a place in the world. Half a century later, the *East Sea* episode—which is of course just one among many signs of this phenomenon—shows that matters are not that simple and that the two tensions evoked in Arendt's chapter on "the decline of the nation-state and the end of human rights" are still manifest in France (and the analysis would not be so different for other European countries). On the one hand, the right to asylum has been, if not abolished, at least considerably reduced not only quantitatively, since the proportion of applications accepted by OFPRA dropped fifteenfold over three decades, but also qualitatively, with the tarnishing of the image of the refugees, increasingly assimilated to that of illegal immigrants and submitted to the strict rules of the Schengen space that was created in 1985 as a European zone of free circulation having for counterpart a much stricter control over the border countries. On the other hand, asylum seekers have once again become the unwanted who cannot be gotten rid of; hence the policing exercised by most European governments in an attempt to pass the burden of refugees to their neighbors, an important issue in the negotiations that preceded the signing of the European Pact on Immigration and Asylum in 2008.

States have two means of resolving this tension between the discredit of asylum and the inevitability of refugees: repression, aimed at dissuading refugees (and this is definitely more effective than is generally believed), and compassion, which renders the undesirables acceptable (by showing them in the most touching light). With the *East Sea*, the French government initially tried the first solution but finally opted for the second. In her time, Hannah Arendt, who had certainly witnessed one (repression) did not see much of the other (compassion). This is probably an indication of the contemporary political shift. In order to revalorize asylum, it has to be articulated with humanitarian reason. This process may go as far as hiding it, as at the Sangatte reception center, where information on the right to asylum was not made available to immigrants.

THE LAST CARAVANSARY

It was precisely at Sangatte that theatrical director Ariane Mnouchkine sought material for her play *Le Dernier Caravansérail* (The last caravansary), created at the Cartoucherie in Vincennes in 2003 and presented at the Avignon Festival that summer. This was an ambitious and impressive artistic endeavor consisting of about sixty scenes, performed by thirty-six actors from all over the world, and lasting eight hours (in the complete version I attended). Its theme was the refugees dispersed around the globe and their journeys to get to countries where they imagined a promise of asylum. Persecution in countries of origin, human-smuggling networks, trafficking of young women, crossings of seas and deserts, detention in camps, and escapes over barbed wire: the play aimed to reconstitute contemporary "odysseys," as the eponym subtitle of the play indicated. It made no bones about playing on moral sentiments, but it mobilized the spectator's anger rather than compassion. Its intent was political as much as poetic, seeking to bear witness to lived situations, even if they were partially reinvented.[27] The creative adventure had begun two years earlier, at Sangatte, where Ariane Mnouchkine had gone to collect refugees' narratives, accompanied by a Kurdish poet and actor. Subsequently, at the request of her company, the director and her collaborators visited detention centers in Australia, New Zealand, and Bali. The play was created from the sum of these experiences and narratives. The geography of the refugees it evokes barely distinguishes between the (open) reception center at Sangatte and the (closed) Baxter detention center in Australia, or between the *East Sea*, running aground on the French coast (whose 908 Kurdish passengers were ultimately allowed to request asylum) and the *Tampa*, carrying Afghan survivors of the wreck of a fishing boat (which was refused permission to dock in Australia).[28] Ultimately, the condition of refugee becomes the paradigm of a human condition, within which the specific contexts, national realities, and political outcomes make little difference. Homelessness, danger, uncertainty, detention, rights scorned—these are the elements constitutive of the condition. And at the end of the journey—Sangatte, the last caravansary, whose borders on the stage merged with the barbed wire protecting the Eurotunnel buildings. The permanently open and constantly crowded hangar that the French authorities tried to depict as harmless tended to become, through its artistic recreation, a threatening space of detention—a camp.

The reference to the term "camp" is subject to debate in the case of Sangatte. Adding the descriptor "transit," suggested by the short stay with its focus on leaving for the United Kingdom, evokes the image of the "transit camp" at Drancy, the Second World War internment camp outside Paris where Jews were held before being deported to extermination camps. Public authorities therefore spoke of Sangatte as a reception center while nongovernmental organizations denounced it as a refugee camp, a description that Nicolas Sarkozy, as we have seen, took up in 2002 in order to condemn his predecessor's policy. The press, both in France and in Britain, seemed uncertain, playing up the dramatic effect of "camp" in headlines but using the official formula of "center" in the body of articles.[29] The issue was perhaps all the more sensitive because it recalled a little-known local memory. Sangatte had indeed been the site of a Nazi camp. As in other coastal towns, from 1942 onward, it was a camp where Jews provided forced labor to build the Atlantic wall, often before leaving for Auschwitz.[30] The fact that all physical traces of it have disappeared and there is no memorial to mark it today does not mean that the past has been completely buried.

Let us return to this question of naming. Must we choose one or the other? I have employed the terms "reception center" and "transit center" in this text; this is, so to speak, the native terminology, which is why I use it. But this does not resolve the problem. In a strict sense, Sangatte was certainly not a camp, because it was open and foreigners were free to enter and leave under the placid gaze of the police (as is also the case, however, in most refugee camps in the developing world). But Sangatte exhibits most of the structural and organizational features of a camp—from the numbers of people living there in total dependence, to the presence of staff who provide both assistance and control, to the operating procedures that resemble those of a kind of military space, and so on.[31] In his history of French concentration camps, Denis Peschanski shows that above and beyond the ostensible role of a camp (which may run from a declared aim of protection to an assumed role of persecution) and the gamut of population it brings together (which varies in relation to political needs), some traits are common to all:[32] "One thing is constant: the weight of the situation, the primacy of time over space. Governments have always attempted to take up the challenge of the constraints of the context and the voluntarism of supervising bodies. They were always trying to manage the unmanageable." The force of contingency ("the primacy of time over space") and aporia of governmentality ("managing the unmanageable") are without doubt features of what we might call the configuration of a camp, and from this point of view Sangatte does indeed conform to these logics and exhibits this configuration. But is this similarity enough for the issues to be comparable? The question is thus less one of deciding whether this is a camp than of problematizing it. To put it another way, does the form give us the content, and can the figure of the camp be taken away from its context? It seems to me that asserting this, or even suggesting it, misses the singularity of the contemporary politics of asylum.

The powerful and controversial thesis developed by Giorgio Agamben is well known:[33] "Instead of deducing the definition of camp from the events that took place there, we will ask instead: What is a camp, what is its political-juridical structure, that such events could have taken place there? This will lead us to regard the camp not as a historical fact and an anomaly belonging to the past (even if still verifiable) but in some way as the hidden matrix and *nomos* of the political space in which we are still living." Continuing his analysis, he comes to the following remarkable definition, inspired by Walter Benjamin's famous formula: "The camp is the space that opens up when the state of exception starts to become the rule." This prompts the Italian philosopher to assimilate all forms of internment where exception is manifested, although the Nazi camps are notably absent in the following comparison:

> The stadium in Bari into which the Italian police in 1991 provisionally herded all Albanian illegal immigrants before sending them back to their country, the winter cycle-racing track in which the Vichy authorities gathered the Jews before consigning them to the Germans, the *Konzentrationslager für Ausländer* in Cottbus-Sielow in which the Weimar government gathered Jewish refugees from the East, or the *zones d'attente* in French international airports in which foreigners asking for refugee status are detained will then all equally be camps. In all these cases, an apparently innocuous place actually delimits a space in which the normal order is de facto suspended and in which whether or not atrocities are committed depends not on the law but on the civility and ethical sense of the police who temporarily act as sovereign.

The unavoidable conclusion of this demonstration is therefore that "today it is not the city but rather the camp that is the fundamental biopolitical paradigm of the West."[34] Here "city" also refers to the political space of the *polis*.

Extending this thesis, some analysts have indeed linked Sangatte to the most extreme forms of exception, including the U.S. detainment facility of Guantánamo. For example, Michel Agier writes:[35] "On different levels, recent episodes concerning the Red Cross center at Sangatte, the Australian government's isolation of Afghan refugees on the island of Nauru, and the perpetuation of a legal vacuum in relation to the 600 detainees at Guantánamo Bay, have all demonstrated the establishment of a set of spaces and regimes of exception throughout the world. It seems to be open season on the world system's undesirables." There is a significant shift in register here compared with Agamben's thesis, as Agier moves from political analysis (the state of exception becomes the rule) to polemical condemnation (open season has been declared on undesirables). But the postulate of the continuity between the forms of internment—from the Sangatte open hangar where immigrants may circulate to the Guantánamo detainment facility where supposed militants are deprived of any civil rights—remains problematically unchanged.

Both moral and historical arguments have frequently been advanced against this thesis of the camp as the paradigm of modernity: the former have contested the alarmist vision of the contemporary world (the conclusion of Agamben's *Homo Sacer* predicts an "unprecedented biopolitical catastrophe"); the latter have objected to the undermining of the unique character of the Holocaust (his *State of Exception* proposes a comparison of Guantánamo with Auschwitz in terms of the disappearance of all citizenship for the detainees in the two camps).[36] But this kind of critique is somewhat external to Agamben's demonstration, and I propose rather to adopt a critical perspective that I view as internal, trying to go where I believe the core of his analysis lies.

On the one hand, if it is true that the camp is the space that opens when the state of exception begins to become the rule, we need to identify the state of exception for what it is. At Sangatte, common law holds, more or less as it would in a homeless shelter—which is to say with many exceptions. Moreover, the police are limited not by their degree of civility or their moral sense, but by the legal framework of their professional activities. Significantly, the main area where the law is suspended is the right to asylum, which is not presented as an alternative to leaving for Britain. On the other hand, if we recognize that the camp has a political-juridical structure, we need to address the political element as rigorously as we analyze the legal aspect. At Sangatte, this politics is conditioned by the double imperative of security and humanitarianism, and is not concerned with persecution or eradication, as has been the case historically in many other camps. To maintain public order, immigrants must be withheld from the view of the local residents, but equally to protect the refugees they must be given food and shelter. Indeed, for the center to fulfill this dual function—order and protection—it had to be maintained in an extremely precarious position: this was not an accidental condition resulting from lack of means, but resulted from political reasons.

In essence, positing degrees (of exception) and differentiations (of function), as I attempt to do here, means resisting the pathos that the perennial existence of camps understandably generates.[37] More precisely, it means rejecting the principles of equivalence (everything is equal) and the logics of the indivisible (there is only one logic), and reiterating what Jacques Rancière calls the "democratic scandal."[38] And it means quite simply reminding ourselves of the complexity and ambiguity of reality: paraphrasing Stéphane Mallarmé, one could say that a paradigm never will abolish the real. This is the least that the social sciences can do when they contribute their studies to philosophical analysis. Moreover, in order to refine the analysis of camps further and test the thesis that they are all the same, it is worth drawing a last distinction among undesirable populations, between those who are assessed as suitable to be deported, whom the authorities attempt to turn back, as at Roissy airport in Paris, or at least to keep out of sight, as at Sangatte, and those consigned to extermination, whether their disappearance is physical, as at Auschwitz, or social, as at Guantánamo. This distinction is the basis for different forms of exception and politics.

So was this caravansary the ultimate haven or the last camp? In answer to this question we can say that the Sangatte center may have been the last camp in contemporary France, but that it was also an ultimate haven where the minimalist hospitality related more to humanitarianism than to asylum—ironically, a refugee camp whose residents were not considered refugees.

The closure of the Sangatte center did not resolve the humanitarian problems any more than it did the security issues posed by the presence of refugees waiting to cross into England. Actually it deteriorated both. In the days that followed this event, immigrants took up residence on beaches and near the port, in makeshift shelters and tents, in warehouses and abandoned Second World War blockhouses. The police returned to their mode of operation from before the center was opened, but using new methods: local organizations accused them of "hunting" refugees, of "gassing" them (by using tear gas inside shelters), and "smoking them out" (by setting fire in blockhouses). An organization called Collectif After Sangatte was set up to bear witness to a situation very different from the preceding period, in two ways: on the one hand, the situation of the hundreds of refugees making their way to the beaches on a daily basis was much more precarious, but on the other it had become almost invisible in the public arena. A name was given to this novel reality: "the jungle."[39] Thus the history of the center, right up to its closure and the aftermath, offers precious insights into the moral and political attitude toward asylum in the contemporary world.

Seen from Europe, the contemporary world has become ever more polarized between North and South, with the gap between the two continuing to deepen. Even in the present context of economic crisis, the European Union remains a political space that is privileged in terms of civil peace, human rights, and social security (whatever one's views on the evolution of European policy). The linguistic and legal distinction between "residents of the European Union" and "foreigners" is becoming increasingly significant in the political imaginary of Europe, with the understanding that "foreigners" are those out of the European Union, but that the only "foreigners" who pose a problem are those from non-Western countries: the requirements for entry to and residence in European territory are different for Canadian citizens than for nationals of African states.

In this context, Europeans' privileged situation is perceived to be threatened by three types of insecurity. The first centers on public security, both external and internal. On one side, there is the external danger of terrorism that the attacks in Madrid and London in 2004 and 2005, respectively, concretized and that has been used to justify heightened border control, although less so than in North America. On the other, there is the internal threat represented by the children of immigrants who have often become citizens of European countries, and the riots in France during the fall of 2005 illustrated how explaining the disturbances in terms of immigration was used to justify still more restrictive immigration policies. The second dimension is social security. Immigration is seen as a threat to hard-won rights to jobs and education, unemployment benefits and pensions, medical insurance and family welfare benefits, regardless of experts' demonstrations of the often beneficial effects of demographic and financial contributions made by foreigners. The third concern has to do with identity security. Given little prominence until recently, it has crystallized around mistrust and even hostility toward Islam as a religion and Muslims as a group, and is manifested in the desire, most marked in Italy, the Netherlands, and France, to assert the continuity of a white, Christian Europe, even going as far as proposing it as foundational in the preamble of the European constitution. The debate over Turkey's entry into the European Union has been largely underpinned by this question of identity. This triple threat to the security of Europe results in asylum policy being made subordinate to immigration policies, which are themselves conceived on this background of anxieties that has been consistently maintained by the far right and often the right, without much resistance from the left, for at least three decades. In this respect, France offers the example both of the high electoral capital held by the theme of the immigrant threat and of the porosity of party boundaries around these issues. The creation in 2007 by the newly elected president, Nicolas Sarkozy, of a ministry associating for the first time the words "immigration" and "national identity"[40] may be seen as a logical outcome of this process.

Given these conditions, the aim of policy makers is to restrict the coming of migrants as much as possible, even if they are in fact seeking asylum. For if globalization allows some people to free themselves of territorial restraint, and hence of borders, others conversely are confined to their territory or, when they seek to escape it, held back by impassable frontiers. In the area of Europe subject to the Schengen Agreement—that is, to a treaty authorizing free circulation within twenty-five countries—and to a lesser degree in the rest of the European Union, a series of legislative measures has made circulation of individuals increasingly easier.[41] But at the gates of Europe the difficulty of entering and the ease with which one can be expelled have continually augmented. Thus border control has been reinforced, particularly at airports, with always more sophisticated technologies of biometric identification, going as far as the requirement to produce genetic evidence of relationship (DNA tests), and data coordination, with the establishment of the European Agency for the Management of Operational Co-operation at the External Borders of the Member States of the European Union (known as Frontex). At the same time, repressive measures aimed at more efficient deportation of immigrants have been strengthened, notably with the passing in June 2008 of the "Return" directive, which allows individuals to be held in detention centers for up to eighteen months (rather than the thirty-two days until then permitted in France, which already represented a recent tripling of the legal maximum) and imposes a mandatory sanction of a five-year ban on residence (which did not previously exist in France except where explicitly decreed in a court judgment following conviction for a crime). This regulation is paradoxically all the more strict because the European space is also a space of the rule of law—and hence of rights, notably human rights. Should they forget, European institutions are reminded of it by nongovernmental organizations, law-yers' associations, and magistrates' unions, who defend the rights of those who are on European territory. Hence the efforts of European govern-ments to reduce as much as possible the numbers of individuals entitled to claim these rights by keeping the borders closed. In order that the ideal of a land of human rights can be maintained, those applying to benefit from it must be as few as possible.

This limitation of the recourse to the law has resulted in a proliferation of extralegal structures. Waiting zones, which increasingly perform a fil-tering function upstream of asylum, are one example: picked up as they leave the plane, a growing number of foreigners are held in detention within airport premises while their case and, where appropriate, their request for asylum are examined. In France, they can claim the legal assistance of the Association nationale d'assistance aux frontières pour les étrangers (Na-tional Association for Border Assistance for Foreigners, ANAFÉ), the only support organization permitted to be present in the waiting zones, provided they access it before being deported. Thus France currently has sixty-five of these waiting zones, with an extraterritorial status that means applicants can be refused the possibility of asylum. In the Roissy zone alone, an area known as ZAPI 3, which is by far the largest, the yearly number of immi-grants held rose from an average of five thousand in the mid-1990s to an average of more than twenty thousand since 2001; the rate of acceptance of applications for asylum plummeted over the same period from 60% in 1995 to 3% in 2003, before rising again.[42] But these mechanisms can only be a last resort, from the point of view of states, since they are costly and have a relative degree of public visibility because of the presence of orga-nizations such as ANAFÉ. This explains why European governments develop convergent initiatives that aim to complete this filtering even further up-stream, by establishing camps at Europe's borders—on the outermost fringes (as in Poland), in the most isolated regions (for example, some Greek islands) or the most enclosed zones (like the Spanish North African territories of Ceuta and Melilla), or even on the other side of the borders (in the east, in Albania and Croatia, and in the south, in Libya and Morocco).[43] At the Thes-saloniki Summit in 2003, Britain presented a plan for externalizing control and detention, which involved establishing "transit processing centers" ef-fectively designed on the model of the camp but concealed under a bureau-cratic term.

Two strands to the overall logic of these structures may therefore be identified. Governments are, of course, concerned with preventing migrants from arriving and dissuading potential migrants, but the structures are also aimed at making this thankless task invisible, or even having it performed by others. This is indeed the problem facing European nations. As long as places like the Sangatte center exist, there is always the possibility of protest from nongovernmental organizations or even the risk that citizens of the host country will feel compassion toward the undesirables, seen as unfortunate rather than criminals. It is therefore essential to obscure the activity of mass rejection and selection as much as possible, either rather imperfectly in waiting zones or more efficiently in camps outside of European territory where the security operations can be performed. There are always of course some who will manage to surmount all these obstacles. These escapees will be recognized through humanitarian reason rather than right to asylum. In this regard, Sangatte provides precious evidence of a time when security and humanitarianism were still entangled.

However, the evidence is viewed as such essentially by us, Western spectators of the odyssey, for, in the journey of migrants seeking asylum, Sangatte represented no more than a parenthesis, as Michael Winterbottom's 2002 film *In This World* reminds us. When the young Afghan hero, who lives with his family in a refugee camp in Pakistan, embarks on a trip to Europe at his parents' instigation, he does so for economic reasons, because they believe that the youngest have to flee the situation they are in. His epic journey with his cousin through central Asia and the Middle East leads him from one danger to another and one smuggler to the next until he reaches Istanbul, where he boards a cargo ship, hidden in a container in which his cousin dies of suffocation, along with several companions. After traveling through Italy and France, he arrives in Sangatte where he stays briefly at the center before crossing to Britain. The film thus depicts a time when it was still possible to do so: seven years later, Philippe Lioret's 2009 film *Welcome* revealed a different reality—that of the jungle which has replaced the center and of a crossing that has become impossible.[44] But let us return to the young Afghan man. As a minor, he is granted a subsidiary protected status in Britain, which he knows he will lose when he reaches the age of eighteen, and he finds work illegally, as a kitchen porter, in a place he has little chance to leave before long because of his precarious juridical situation. Thus, in addition to reminding us, in the prologue filmed in Pakistan, how many more refugees there are in the developing world than in Western countries and how difficult the distinction between economic and political refugees remains, the film shows that ultimately, with or without asylum, the hospitality offered by the "British El Dorado" is merely the integration into the clandestine underclass. Sangatte was the last password to enter it.

PART II

Worlds

6. Massacre of the Innocents

Representing Childhood in the Age of AIDS

> In the eye of nature, it would seem, a child is a more important
> object than an old man, and excites a much more lively, as well as
> a much more universal sympathy. It ought to do so. Every thing
> may be expected, or at least hoped, from the child. The weakness
> of childhood interests the affections of the most brutal and
> hard-hearted.
>
> ADAM SMITH, The Theory of Moral Sentiments

When the Thirteenth International AIDS Conference opened in Durban on July 9, 2000, South Africa was already seen as the nation most seriously affected by the epidemic. By a remarkable, but until now little-understood, phenomenon this country, which in the early 1990s had appeared so spared by the virus that it became the subject of studies seeking to explain this relative immunity (at that time less than 1% of the population was infected), a decade later had become the world epicenter of the pandemic (HIV seroprevalence was estimated at 24% among adults).[1] In a tragic coincidence with this unprecedentedly rapid development, the devastating progression of the disease, which mainly affected the African population (the local designation of black people), came precisely at the moment when the South African nation was emerging from a long period of oppression and segregation that had culminated in the forty-six years of apartheid. The bright future heralded by the long-awaited liberation was heavily overshadowed by the biological threat of a condition that, by 2000, had already infected 4.5 million people, and which, it was predicted, would within two decades reduce life expectancy among the African population of the country by twenty years. Chris Hani, a hero of the antiapartheid struggle, who was assassinated by a white extremist not long after this statement, had foreseen the new peril South African society would face: as early as 1990 he declared that after having overcome white supremacy, the next fight would be against AIDS.[2] But ten years later the political commitment of the leaders of the "new South Africa" seemed less firm. Nelson Mandela was criticized for his lack of urgency with regard to this issue. Thabo Mbeki, his successor as president, was accused of outright obstruction of the struggle against the epidemic. The scandal arose when his links with Western heterodox scientific circles, most notably in California, which denied the viral origin of AIDS and blamed the deaths of patients on antiretroviral treatments, came to light. Giving credence to these theories, Mbeki convened a panel of scientists to assess the state of current knowledge, and claiming that the scientific truth had not yet been established, he appointed equal numbers of leading researchers and marginalized dissidents. To add to the provocation, he organized this meeting just a few days before the international conference, which many participants threatened to boycott. It was therefore no surprise that half the conference delegates left the auditorium in protest during his welcoming speech.

If the villain of the event was the president, its hero was a child. Nkosi Johnson, who mounted the podium after Thabo Mbeki in front of thousands of participants, had in effect become an icon of the disease.[3] He had been born eleven years earlier, of an unknown father, in a township near Johannesburg. When his mother, who was suffering from AIDS, abandoned him, he was adopted by Gail Johnson, a white woman who specialized in public relations and was the general manager of a health clinic. At the age of eight he made headlines in the South African press when a school in his white district refused to admit him because he was HIV positive. The ensuing protests forced the school to reverse its decision, and the little boy became a symbol of the struggle against AIDS discrimination. When his biological mother died, his attendance at the funeral was highlighted in the media. Later, he was present at the opening of the first of Gail Johnson's "Nkosi's Havens," which cared for HIV-positive mothers and their children. It was therefore obvious to many that he should be invited as keynote speaker at the International AIDS Conference. Intimidated by the crowd, he began: "Hi, my name is Nkosi Johnson. I live in Melville, Johannesburg, South Africa. I am eleven years old and I have full-blown AIDS. I was born HIV positive." He went on to give an account of his life, his two mothers, the discrimination at the school, the funeral for his biological mother, and the refuge opened by his adoptive mother, and movingly concluded:

> When I grow up, I want to lecture to more and more people about AIDS—and if mommy Gail will let me, around the whole country. I want people to understand about AIDS—to be careful and respect AIDS—you can't get AIDS if you touch, hug, kiss, hold hands with someone who is infected. Care for us and accept us—we are all human beings. We are normal. We have hands. We have feet. We can walk, we

can talk, we have needs just like everyone else—don't be afraid of us—we are all the same!

This was, at least, the speech that Nkosi had prepared with his mother, and that he was supposed to give that night.[4] Overwhelmed by the stage, the lights, and the audience, moved by the standing ovation he received, and also perhaps struggling with technical problems, he stumbled over his words and did not manage to make his text audible. What remained of him for posterity were his smiling presence in a suit too big for him and the written version of his speech. A few months later his health deteriorated. He appealed to the South African president, asking him to make antiretroviral drugs available to all those with HIV/AIDS, and above all to work for the prevention of transmission from mother to child that was his own fate. A morbid media watch began, and each day, as his condition worsened, journalists published messages from him inviting the head of state to visit him and pleading for access to drugs. When Nkosi died on June 1, 2001, without having seen Thabo Mbeki (whose wife, however, did visit him in a private capacity), many expressed anger at his lack of sensitivity to the child's suffering. But a controversy emerged during the days following his death when it was revealed in the press that the young boy had been in a coma for several weeks and that the poignant messages attributed to him and widely commented on in the media had in fact been written by his adoptive mother, a campaigner for treatment.

AN ICON OF AFFLICTION

Nkosi Johnson's tragic demise indecently exposed in the media marked a turning point in the epidemic: it signaled the entry of the theme of childhood into the public arena. Until then children had been virtually absent from issues and discussions about AIDS. When the first cases were diagnosed in the 1980s, the disease was thought to be restricted to homosexuals. At this time African teenagers were in the streets, demonstrating for an end to apartheid and provoking the white police. As the situation became more worrying in the townships and some of the former homelands in the 1990s, people asserted that it was a condition that affected sexually active adults. During this period, even though increasingly dire rates of HIV infection were being detected through antenatal screening, suggesting that newborns might be infected, childhood seemed removed from the epidemic: in the context of the reconstruction of society, children symbolized the future of the nation, which could not be altered by such grim perspectives. With

Nkosi Johnson, not only did South Africans become aware of the epidemiological reality of an infection that affected tens of thousands of children, but his suffering made it possible for them to conceive a different moral representation of AIDS. Whereas mainly white homosexuals, and later African men and women, were blamed for their infection on the grounds of what were imagined to be their sexual practices (with prevention messages continuing to focus on the theme of promiscuity and the issue of responsibility), children bore the mark of innocence: they were born infected. Guilt had no reason for being in the misfortune they suffered. On the contrary, they were the victims of both the reckless behavior of their parents, as health care workers readily reminded HIV-positive pregnant women when they arrived at the maternity ward to give birth, and the inappropriate decisions of the government, which was too slow to introduce programs for reducing the rate of transmission from mother to child.

But with Nkosi Johnson, the child was not only a victim, he became a hero.[5] He had been an icon, thanks to his adoptive mother, when the issue of discrimination against children with AIDS in schools was raised publicly, and had become one, again through his mother's intervention, when he championed access to treatment. This new status was affirmed by the poster produced in 2001 by the Treatment Action Campaign, the leading AIDS activist organization, in collaboration with the Congress of South African Trade Unions (COSATU). That year marked the twenty-fifth anniversary of the Soweto uprising, which began on June 16, 1976, with the death of a young demonstrator, Hector Petersen: the image of his body, carried by a weeping friend, became a worldwide symbol of the struggle against apartheid. It was this representation that the Treatment Action Campaign had chosen for their poster calling for access to antiretroviral drugs. It featured two black-and-white photos, each with a simple caption: "16 June 1976 Hector Petersen age 13" and "1 June 2001 Nkosi Johnson age 12." For those who saw these images pasted on walls, the juxtaposition of the two heroic figures was almost natural. It was customary by that time in South Africa to think of the fight against AIDS as the contemporary equivalent of the struggle against apartheid in the past: this comparison between the two causes had become a commonplace that no one thought to question any longer.

On closer examination, though, one wonders if the two deaths did signify the same thing. Hector Petersen was shot by police charged with quelling a protest against the imposition of the Afrikaans language in schools in the townships. Nkosi Johnson died of a disease for which no preventive treatment existed when he contracted it at birth. Even though both tragic events prompted a nationwide surge of compassion, the political death, so to speak, of the former did not have the same meaning as the biological death of the latter. More broadly, the battle against AIDS can only be likened to the struggle against the racist regime if we ignore the historical context of the two campaigns. By assimilating the two causes, today's activists seem to tar the previous enemy (the white supremacist government) and the current adversary (the multiracial democratic government) with the same brush. Many have reproached the movement for this, particularly when the campaign of civil disobedience against Thabo Mbeki and his government was launched, because this was precisely the weapon used by the townships in their struggle against the apartheid regime a few decades earlier.

Whatever the case, with Nkosi Johnson, childhood entered onto the South African AIDS scene—and, more specifically, into its moral realm. Arguably it did not so much initiate as reveal a phenomenon that continued to mushroom in the following months and years: the presence of children as a central issue in the epidemic. But this presence subsumed different realities. In fact, three figures emerged one after the other. The first was that of the suffering child: it crystallized essentially around the risk of transmission of the virus from mother to child. The second was that of the abused child: it related especially to girls, sometimes infants. The third was that of the orphan: it put the future of South African society at stake. The common element in these three figures is that they combined a moral and a social representation, innocence with vulnerability. However, these images were not stable: they could even be inverted, with victims being seen as dangerous in certain circumstances. What I want to analyze in this chapter, taking each of the three figures in turn, is therefore the "cultural politics of childhood,"[6] particularly their moral dimension. To do so, I analyze the way in which questions were debated, comparing it to my own observations during studies conducted in the townships of Soweto and Alexandra, in Johannesburg, and in the former homelands of the north, in Limpopo Province[7]—in other words, confronting the moral simplification of public discourse with the inevitable complexity of social realities.

THE ECONOMY OF SUFFERING

"Suffer, the Little Children" ran the headline of the editorial in the *Saturday Star* of January 30, 1999. "The cost of saving the life of the most pathetic, vulnerable human being, a baby, from a grim AIDS death is surprisingly small: just 400 rand [around US$60 at the time]. Yet Health Minister Nkosazana Zuma doesn't seem to be prepared to pay it," the columnist wrote. Comparing the sum in question with the military expenditure then under negotiation, and demonstrating the economic benefits of prevention given the predicted expense of treating young patients with HIV, he concluded: "Well beyond the financial implications, there are moral issues. Do we have the right to condemn these children to death when we could save them? And do we have the right to deprive future generations of potential leaders, artists, peacemakers? As a nation, we will be judged on what is in our hearts and what we do for one another, not on what is in our arsenals or our budget deficit."

For several years the press regularly featured articles and editorials with similarly dramatic headlines: "Babies Too Poor to Live," "The High Cost of Living Babies," "Babies' Lives in Balance," "How Many More Babies Must Die?" A few days before the opening of the Durban conference, three highly regarded South African researchers had exhorted Thabo Mbeki to "leave science to the scientists" in an article illustrated by a photograph of a sleeping baby over the caption: "An eight-month old abandoned girl with AIDS in a hospice; the unintended consequences of the president's doubts about the causes of AIDS could lead to unimaginable suffering and many avoidable deaths." The day the international conference started, another newspaper ran the same photo under the headline: "Innocent Victim: This infant has AIDS and when old enough to understand, will have to be prepared to accept the terrible truth about the future." And as the scientists' meeting was drawing to a close, the same newspaper blazoned its front page with the pictures of forty-four babies' faces under the headline: "Each Day We Could Save All These Little Children from HIV." During this period accusations of "genocide" and references to a "holocaust" featured almost routinely in public debate, articulated by the highest scientific and moral authorities in the country, and sometimes repeated in conversations among the general population.[8]

These challenges to the government centered on the issue of transmission from mother to child. At that time, new protocols, first developed in Western countries and then tested in the Third World, were beginning to be introduced. They consisted of giving antiretroviral drugs to the mother during the final weeks of pregnancy then to the child at birth. Clinical trials conducted in Thailand and Uganda respectively had demonstrated the efficacy of AZT, and subsequently the still greater efficacy of nevirapine, in producing a significant reduction in the transmission of the virus to the newborn at low cost. These promising experiments were followed by further trials in a number of locations, including South African hospitals.

However, the trials generated controversy. On one side, some in the medical community were highly enthusiastic about this simple, effective, innocuous, and inexpensive method, and they were easily able to win over the media: the "magic bullet"[9] had been found, and this treatment should immediately be made available to all. On the other side, the government temporized, expressed reservations, withheld therapeutic trials, and delayed the introduction of the treatment at national level: the official reason was that the principle of precaution was being followed, but members of the government, the president among them, were sensitive to the "heresy"[10] of Californian dissidents which suggested that antiretroviral drugs were killing patients.

The resulting accusation of lack of action passed quickly from the press to the courts. The nongovernmental organization AIDS Law Project brought a case against the local government of Mpumalanga Province, in the name of "baby Tinashe." This little girl, then aged six months, had been infected at birth, and the lawyer therefore charged the public authorities for not having informed her mother of the existence of a means to reduce the risk of transmission.[11] The case was followed by a number of others, which after several appeals eventually resulted in April 2002 in a judgment against the South African government and an order compelling it to introduce prevention programs. It was, however, several more years before drugs actually became accessible in hospitals, mainly because of the serious organizational problems inherited from the apartheid era, but also because of the indifference manifested by many health professionals toward patients.

Seen in retrospect, the representation of children as victims of both the disease and power emerges as a central element of the social mobilization and the media campaign during the profound crisis that traversed South African society around the issue of AIDS. It furnished activists with a powerful argument, and journalists with a useful resource. Who would oppose the principle of saving the lives of newborns? And how could one not condemn a government that was endangering the most vulnerable of its population? The moral obviousness of the argument of saving lives is at the very heart of humanitarianism. It overcomes any competing argument—for instance, in terms of social justice or simply practical feasibility. But using the pathos of the threatened babies had two consequences that were never discussed.

First, it set the responsibility of adults in stark relief. A sort of scale of innocence and vulnerability was implicitly established among the three categories of individuals with the virus. Men were generally seen as bearing the greatest burden of guilt: they were not only charged with conjugal infidelity and paternal irresponsibility, but also accused of violence; the stereotype of the "rapist" was routinely invoked, partly supported by epidemiological and sociological surveys that revealed the frequency of sexual violence. Women seemed to occupy an ambiguous intermediate position: on the one hand, they were deemed guilty of "sexual promiscuity," which was represented as a cultural trait among the African population; on the other, they were seen as "vulnerable" to the brutality of men and in particular to the imposition of unprotected sex. Finally, children were both innocent and vulnerable: if they were infected it could only be the fault of their parents, one would think. But studies of life among families in the townships and former homelands, while they did not question the reality of matrimonial instability and male domination, showed that this reality itself was set in the context of extreme insecurity and routine violence, both past and present.[12] A political economy of AIDS is more illuminating in this respect than a moral version of rational choice theories: by failing to understand these broader determining factors one is reduced to psychological interpretations that essentialize behaviors and blame the victims.

Second, while highlighting the innocence and vulnerability of children makes it possible to justify the introduction of programs to prevent mother-to-child transmission of the virus, it also leads to silence about the treatment of mothers. The new regimens, at least initially, were concerned only with reducing the chances of infection of the child: antiretrovirals were given to a woman not for her own benefit, but simply to decrease the risk for the baby, and were therefore interrupted after the birth. Furthermore, such short-lived treatments at the end of pregnancy risked leading to subsequent resistance to these drugs, which were precisely the most commonly used for treatment. This was effectively confirmed by studies conducted during the subsequent years: when they were treated later, women who had been in this protocol presented high levels of inefficacy for a whole class of first-line treatments because of viral resistance. Ultimately, saving babies meant unintentionally putting their mothers' lives in danger. The priority given to children and indifference toward women are in fact common to a number of so-called maternal infant programs implemented in the Third World in the past few decades.[13] Presenting children as victims comes at a cost that is both symbolic (the contrasting damning representation of other categories of AIDS sufferers) and practical (the implicit justification of the relative neglect of mothers, at the risk of compromising their future health).

Yet my aim here is certainly not to contest the validity of programs for reducing mother-to-child transmission, nor to question the commitment of AIDS activists on this front, but simply to reveal the unforeseen consequences of the moral construction of childhood. Moralization of a cause effectively tends to give rise to moral discrimination between what can be more or less legitimately defended, and often to support moral judgments already at work in the social world. Thus testimonies gathered from women with AIDS and observations of hospital practice suggested that compassion for children had the corollary of a lack of interest or even cruelty toward the mothers. One woman told me how the midwife at the rural maternity hospital where she was informed she was infected denigrated her in public, accusing her of importing the virus from Johannesburg. Another, who was in very poor medical condition, nevertheless refused to be admitted to the hospital where I had taken her, recalling the discrimination she had suffered there because of her HIV infection. The delivery process could be a harsh ordeal for these women, who were sometimes abused, insulted, and accused of being responsible for their baby's misfortune.[14] Of course, the representation of newborns as innocent in the public arena was not the cause of this ill-treatment, but it shored up prejudices that suggested the mothers were guilty, just as the representation of women as vulnerable supported accusations of violence leveled against men. The only difference was that the men had to justify themselves not in a hospital but—sometimes—to the police and the courts.

THE SCANDAL OF RAPE

"Things Fall Apart": the special report that was published under this headline borrowed from Chinua Achebe's novel by the *Weekly Mail and Guardian* on November 9, 2001, was damning. The article began in literally apocalyptic tone: " 'The coming of the Lord is nigh, I'm telling you,' asserts Jan Pietersen, his gaze fixed on the sunset. 'They have rejected the name of the Lord'. He falls silent. Standing in front of his humble house in Louisvale, a township on the dusty margins of the town of Upington in Northern Cape Province, his dark eyes reflect the last glimmers of dusk. Pietersen smiles sadly, shaking his head. 'It's frightening, beyond my imagination.' " The event that prompted these remarks was a drama that rocked South African society. A nine-month-old girl had been raped in this "colored" township. The penetration had caused major injury. The suspects were six men from the neighborhood, including the little girl's great-grandfather. They were drunk at the time of the incident. The father, aged twenty-four, and the sixteen-year-old mother, who had left the child alone, were themselves drunk when the rape occurred. The article described the scene in detail, citing the clinical account supplied by the doctor, reporting the dismayed or vengeful responses of neighbors, and quoting local residents' comments about the trauma for the neighborhood and the curse it would bring on the township. The reporter took particular care with the writing, mixing realism with a poetic tone. The full front-page photo showed the grandmother and a neighbor: the two women were covering their faces with one hand, to allow their tears to flow, it was suggested, but in fact more probably to conceal themselves; one sister of the victim stood at their side looking at the camera. The caption spared nothing: "In the weak light of the lounge, the women discovered a bleeding, gaping wound as they parted the infant's legs." In spite of its reputation as a serious and even intellectual publication, the *Weekly Mail and Guardian* yielded to the temptation of rendering the intolerable sensational.

While this terrible abuse has a particular resonance in the recent moral history of South Africa, it emerges in a broader context of the chronicling of horror. On a daily basis the press intones a litany of brutality and crime, not only the publications that specialize in sensationalism, but also the major national newspapers. There is something remarkable about the media's readiness to propagate this striking and even repulsive image of South African society. Without wishing to underestimate the reality of the violence, it is difficult to elude wondering about the meaning of this national representation of self in the register of abjection. The imaginary of South Africa is thus less that of fear of violence—however real this is in individuals' experience—than of its obscenity. In this respect reports about children are the most distressing—especially the stories about the rape of very young children, the case of the little girl in Louisvale obviously representing an extreme example.

Although they are fortunately rare, these incidents are particularly visible, partly of course because they are so appalling, but above all because of their extensive media coverage. "Picture of Child Rape Too Horrific to Publish" ran the headline in one daily. Despite this putative warning, the author of the article spared no sordid anatomical detail, and readily substituted the image with a description beginning with these words: "The photograph of the six-year old rape victim's injuries tells a story of inconceivable pain and savagery." A proliferation of articles recounted that "child sex abuse case shocked the court," that "thousands of children are raped every day," or that "HIV threat adds to tragedy of child rape," even stigmatizing "the increasing bestiality in South Africa."[15] Thus the press offers a media gallery of horrors, in which crimes against children are portrayed as the most intolerable, all the more when committed by family members. This display is set in the context of a global phenomenon of the increasing visibility of sexual abuse of children, particularly incest, which was little recognized until recently. But the radicalization of the exposure of these crimes, and the transformation of it into a spectacle of monstrosity, call for reflection on its significance: Why is South African society presenting itself in this way to the world, and above all to itself? Two hypotheses, which are not mutually exclusive, can be suggested.

First, the treatment of child rape as a crime of extremes, in terms of both the age of the victims and the physical injuries caused, tends to conceal the fact that sexual violence is a routine phenomenon, both in frequency and in practices. The focus on the most horrific incidents has a paradoxically reassuring effect. The men who perpetrate these barbaric acts of pedophilia would be dangerous psychopaths, against whom society must be protected. There would be a sort of externality of evil. But levels of sexual abuse are very high in South Africa. With all the usual caveats about the methodological problems of studies of sexual violence, it is estimated that 7% of women have experienced nonconsensual sex; the figure is, unexpectedly, higher among younger women (suggesting either a recent increase in sexual abuse or a greater propensity to report it) and, even more remarkably, twice as high among white women as among black women (possibly due to self-censorship among the latter). In surveys of men, 15% admit to having raped or attempted to rape their wife or partner within the past ten years. With regard to children and teenagers, in the two main general population studies, 1.2% of the women interviewed in one study and 1.6% in the other stated that they had been subjected to nonconsensual sex before the age of fifteen, and almost always after the age of ten.[16] The abusers were often teachers who took advantage of their power—for example, by threatening to give the girls bad marks.

By contrast, the rape of very young children is fortunately quite exceptional, with only a handful of particularly dismaying incidents each year versus the 221,000 sexual assaults reported to the police by girls under the age of seventeen in 1999—certainly a large underestimation. In general, although the media portray child rape as "the scourge of the new South Africa,"[17] all the studies confirm that this is a statistically insignificant phenomenon and that there is a much more serious problem with the ordinary sexual violence perpetrated against adolescents or young and mature women, often within the context of their relationship with a regular partner or family member. This was what I found in my own studies; for example, in the cases of two young women from Alexandra township: Sophia, who since the age of fourteen had lived with a boyfriend little older than she who abused her out of jealousy, and Astrid, whose father, until then very tender and attentive, had raped her one day when he came home drunk from a party, just after her sixteenth birthday. In other words, the sensationalist coverage of crimes such as child rape masks common abuses against girls and young women. It highlights the barbarity of exceptional practices, to the detriment of reflection on male domination, domestic violence, sexual harassment, and incest, all of which take place everywhere from schools to work, from home to the street.

The second hypothesis is that the hyperbolic treatment of child rape derives from a form of racialist exoticism that is fairly widespread in South African society. This process consists in representing social facts as cultural traits. Making a spectacle of atrocities committed contributes to a picture of the country as "a world apart," as suggested by the title of Chris Menges's well-known antiapartheid movie. And this singularization is implicitly—but transparently for South Africans—applied to the African population, or rather, to African men. This was at the core of the controversy aroused by a series of articles written by journalist Charlene Smith after she was raped. She first wrote an account of her traumatic experience, and then proceeded to denounce this "society of rapists" in both the national and the international media: while she never described the problem in racial terms, she gave her readers all the clues they needed to understand that her words related to African men, referring in particular to "tradition," "culture," "sexual promiscuity," "sugar daddies," and the "virgin cleansing myth" (the alleged belief that men could be purified by raping virgin girls).[18] While recognizing Smith's courage in speaking out, Thabo Mbeki accused her of "racism," sparking protests from the white liberal opposition, which returned the criticism, condemning the instrumentalization of the race issue. A few months later, Smith repeated her accusation in an article provocatively headlined: "Should We Put Chastity Belts on Our Children?" In this article she described a range of supposedly exotic sexual practices observed throughout Africa.

The representation of black men as sexual predators was, of course, nothing new. The Western imaginary of African sexuality has a long precolonial and colonial history fed by a fantasy representation of the other, which was taken to an extreme in human zoos. In South Africa, the proximity of whites and blacks in the cities and industrial centers from the late nineteenth century onward gave rise to a common discourse on "African sexuality" that stigmatized "sexual impulses," describing African women as licentious and men as dangerous; the "black peril" became a standard trope, and it has in fact never completely disappeared from the mental world of white society. With AIDS it reemerged in caricature form under apartheid, and euphemized in the years following the dismantling of the apartheid regime.[19] Thus what is operating here is clearly a social construction developed over time that tends to culturalize violence—that is, to essentialize it in cultural terms, making it a feature specific to African societies, in other words to the black population. However, apart from the fact that studies indicate that sexual violence, including incest and marital rape, is at least as common among the white population, it is important to understand that it emerges within the context of a social and historical reality of violence. The brutality of relations between men and women or boys and girls cannot be separated from the brutalization of social relations over recent decades, whether through apartheid or in the struggle against the regime. Many of the black men of today were teenagers during the years of virtual civil war when the use of force was generalized not only in political activities but also in daily life, within local neighborhoods and families. The culturalist essentialization of violence ignores the historical conditions of its social reproduction.

This basic truth is revealed in a shift that has recently taken place in the debate on sexual violence in South Africa. When the issue first became the focus of public attention in the late 1990s, the victims were always children. By contrast, a few years later, children were frequently portrayed as perpetrators. A series of studies expresses a new anxiety about rapes of girls and boys by barely older teenagers, either individually or in gangs, in schools or local neighborhoods, and also in juvenile detention centers. Social workers and children's judges assert that the abusers are increasingly young. They explain this phenomenon in terms of the ready availability of pornographic materials, or more mundanely, watching TV soap operas.[20] The moral panic around child sexual violence that has developed over the past ten years is now being reconfigured in a way that partially undermines the foundations of the moral sociology of childhood. Once innocent, children are now guilty. Adults are no longer the only perpetrators of sexual abuse: teenagers themselves can somehow become predators on their own kind. Nevertheless, it is still their vulnerability that is highlighted in these cases, with calls for protection from adults. Conversely, the economic and social realities within which these violent practices are set—the breakdown of families as the parents migrate for work and the abandonment of children to the extent that some become de facto heads of households—have been little explored. The discovery of the rape of children by other children mainly reinforces the common representation of a society in which barbarity, a supposedly innate cultural trait, spreads gradually to all ages and classes.

THE TRAGEDY OF ORPHANS

"Why should AIDS orphans be given special treatment when other parentless children go hungry?" asked then president Thabo Mbeki in a speech to traditional chiefs on April 3, 2007. Responding to one who complained about positive discrimination in favor of this one category of orphans in some programs, and criticizing the well-meaning activities of international donors focused solely on the consequences of AIDS, he continued: "An orphan is an orphan. You cannot say these orphans are special because their parents died from AIDS and they therefore require special treatment. An orphan whose parents died in a car accident is an orphan. We can't have a situation where there are five hungry children, and you take two and go and feed them and leave the other three."[21] This polemic may seem surprising. Yet it is illuminating.

In effect, during the past decade, the question of "AIDS orphans" became a concern of international aid policy throughout Africa. Alarmist statistics and projections were widely circulated: according to calculations made by the United Nations Children's Fund (UNICEF) and UNAIDS at that time, the number of children orphaned by AIDS was supposed to reach twenty-five million worldwide in 2010, 82% of them in Africa; this figure concerns children who have lost one or other of their parents, but some authors assert that it is much underestimated with regard to the social reality of families.[22] Significantly, at a time when USAID was reducing its programs promoting prevention through condom use in favor of abstinence and fidelity, considerable resources were being targeted specifically toward orphans; the compassionate conservatism championed by the Bush administration found an ideal expression for the application of its differentiated moral choices here.[23] In South Africa the situation was clearly worrying, even if figures in that period were still relatively low: on the one hand, rates of HIV infection among young adults indicated that a rapid increase in the number of orphans was likely; on the other, the recent explosion of the epidemic suggested a time lag, because the peak of mortality had yet to be reached. The general tone of the discourse was nevertheless one of anxiety. The minister for social development warned of the worst possible consequences of the epidemic, with one million orphans in the short term, and nongovernmental organizations raised the stakes by publishing even more dire statistics. On October 20, 2000, the *Weekly Mail and Guardian* published a "survival guide for AIDS orphans." Pathos was culminating.

There were two key elements in the dramatization of the issue of AIDS orphans: statistics and compassion. Statistics established the seriousness of the problem, while compassion appealed to the public's emotions. Both seemed obvious—but the apparently self-evident truths on which they lie merit further examination.

Let us begin with the figures. A close look is crucial here. Demographic projections for South Africa indicated that by 2015 there would be 2 million children who had lost their mothers, and between 3.6 and 4.8 million who had lost one parent or other (representing 9%–12% of the total population). However, studies within the population suggest a more cautious approach to observations and their interpretation.[24] In the early 1990s, before the beginning of the spread of the epidemic, 2.0% of children had lost their mothers, 7.6% had lost their fathers, and 0.6% had lost both parents. Statistics were even more tragic when considering how children were actually brought up: 12.9% of them were not living with their mother, 35.3% were not living with their father, and 9.7% were not living with either parent. Only 31.9% of South African children were being raised by both parents. Ten years later, when the disease had become the first cause of mortality among adults, a survey revealed that 3.2% of children had lost their mother, 8.9% their father, and 1.1% both parents. Children being brought up without their parents comprised 12.8% not living with their mother, 39.0% not living with their father, and 7.2% not living with either parent. Finally, just 27.8% of South African children were living in a family where both parents were present.

These rarely discussed figures call for remark on several important points. First, the number of children living without at least one of their parents is around six times the number who have lost one parent, and this ratio decreases only slightly with the onset of the epidemic; in terms of children living without either parent, the first study found there were fifteen times more who were living apart from their parents than who had lost them, and the second study found there were still seven times more. This first observation signifies, on the one hand, that children living apart from their parents represent a much more serious demographic issue than that of orphan children, and on the other, that both these problems existed before the AIDS epidemic, which merely amplified an already grim reality. Second, many more had lost their father than their mother—four times more before the epidemic, three times more ten years later—which might seem surprising given that in the epidemiology of AIDS young women are affected in greater numbers than men, therefore implying a higher mortality rate among mothers. Similarly, absent fathers are three times more common than absent mothers. This second observation implies, on one side, that AIDS is responsible for a limited proportion of children whose mother has died, and a small proportion of those whose father has died, and on the other side, that the number of children whose father has died or is absent is much higher than the number of children whose mother has died or is absent, although it seems likely that over the next few years AIDS will have a stronger impact on female mortality.

To sum up, we can therefore say that the problem of children raised in the absence of one or other parent, or both, existed before the AIDS epidemic, but that previously it was not seen as a matter of interest, even though two-thirds of children were affected; and also that the focus on AIDS even today neglects both the majority of orphans, who have lost their parents through other causes, and the total number of children living without their parents because the latter have left the family home. The two conclusions are linked: it is the social conditions in which families live, the breakdown of households that has been ongoing for a century owing to migration for work and male mortality due to murder and violence more generally that need to be taken into consideration, not just the epidemiological phenomenon of AIDS. Most of the men and women in Soweto and Alexandra who told me their stories had been raised by grandparents, because their parents were working several hundred miles away, and sometimes even created a second family far from their home. Even today, many of the children I met in these families were living with a grandmother or an aunt, sometimes following the death of their parents but much more often because of forced exile in search of work. Therefore, contrary to what international aid programs lead us to believe, the issue of orphans and more generally of children separated from their parents is not primarily the sad consequence of a biological misfortune, but above all the result of historically constituted structural inequalities.[25] Rather than just the moral economy of orphans, we need to focus on the political economy. But clearly, this would risk the compassionate consensus losing its edge through the effect of social criticism.

Returning to the mobilization of emotion about orphans, we observe that most of the reports produced by international development agencies and nongovernmental organizations focus the spotlight on the tragedy of motherless children (fathers are rarely mentioned), the psychological and emotional consequences (rather than the historical precedents and social causes), and the vulnerability and suffering of orphans. Considering recent trends, however, it is noteworthy that other themes have gradually emerged in official documents, depicting a catastrophic situation on the African continent, where orphans left to look after themselves become street children who threaten public order, or even child soldiers recruited by rebel movements. In the case of South Africa, the rise in crime, already a concern, was anticipated with warnings of a "time bomb," as in a paper published by a researcher at the Institute for Security Studies and quoted by most subsequent international reports:

> Age and AIDS will be significant contributors to an increase in the rate of crime in South Africa over the next ten to twenty years. In a decade's time, every fourth South African will be aged between 15 and 24. It is at this age group where people's propensity to commit crime is at its highest. At about the same time, there will be a boom in South Africa's orphan population as the AIDS epidemic takes its toll. Growing up without parents, and badly supervised by relatives and welfare organizations, this growing pool of orphans will be at greater than average risk to engage in criminal activity.

In a second article the author reiterates his analysis, introducing a psychological dimension:[26] "The loss of parents to HIV/AIDS may increase the emotional vulnerability of children. Children who lose a parent to AIDS suffer loss and grief like any other orphan. However, their loss may be exacerbated by prejudice and social exclusion. That is, the shame, fear and rejection that often surrounds people affected by HIV/AIDS can create additional stress and isolation for children—both before and after the death of their parent or parents. In addition to stigma, children may suffer additional trauma. Such factors may have a number of implications for levels of crime and victimisation." Here humanitarian concern for unfortunate children is combined with an increasing anxiety about security in relation to dangerous children.

The boundary between the two is thin and porous: the victim can easily become a criminal. Although such analyses, founded on a mixture of prejudice, intuition, and unquestioned statistics, are not based on any sociological study and have even been contradicted by ethnographic observations in countries that have been affected by the epidemic for longer, they provide a sort of lingua franca for international agencies and nongovernmental organizations, which are less inclined to criticize them because they support calls for resources to fund orphan aid programs. Yet there is no evidence that children brought up without their parents do not find relatives to raise them. They may be separated from their parents because their parents are dead or have left, but live in their family rather than in the street. Fostering, or informal adoption, usually by a grandmother or aunt, is a tried and tested practice in South African society, which, as mentioned earlier, has several generations' experience of separation of children from their parents owing to labor migration—neither miners' hostels and farms (in the case of men) nor the kitchens of large houses (where women toil as servants) have been conceived to accommodate children. In my own observations, orphans were always taken in by relatives, and these arrangements frequently resulted in conflicts between the father's and mother's families. Indeed, the presence of these orphans was not without problems, but not always the expected ones. In an apparent paradox, which would have surprised many aid organizations' members, families often fought for custody of the children. Since the government had instituted "foster child grants" for adoptive parents,[27] paying a sum higher than the average worker's wage, the anticipated financial resources inspired vocations for looking after orphans, and even led to conflict between family members for the right to take care of them and receive the corresponding grant.

Without my endorsing them, the reservations expressed by Thabo Mbeki, who was always highly sensitive about issues of sovereignty (children as the generation of the future are at the heart of issues of sovereignty throughout the Third World) and suspicious of the West (since the beginning of the epidemic, initiatives regarding AIDS having been driven from Europe and North America), become more intelligible in this light. The outpouring of international generosity toward AIDS orphans and its justification in terms of a discourse of catastrophe derive from an understandable but problematic pathos. It often reflects a failure to apprehend both the past (and therefore how far back the orphan problem goes) and the present (notably the family and institutional resources mobilized in South Africa). The exaggeration of both compassion for current suffering and anxiety about future disorder adds to the confusion of emotions surrounding a tragedy of which neither the historical nor the political aspects are being taken into consideration. This confusion can be noted not only at the international level, but also locally. In South Africa as elsewhere, the middle and wealthier classes seem more ready to help far-off orphans than to tolerate their presence within their own environment. For example, the residents of affluent districts in Durban campaigned for the closure of an orphanage that had been built in their neighborhood. "We believe this center should be positioned with the community it supports and where the children are predominantly from. They are from the underprivileged communities and they should go back there," wrote the residents in a letter to the town council. One of them complained that "the mere sight of a black child in this neighborhood devalues my property," while others insulted children, "telling them to go back to the townships."[28] Compassion has its limits, which are territorial, but above all social and racial.

Childhood as a social category is a phenomenon of modern history, as we know from historian Philippe Ariès and others after him.[29] As a moral and political category, or more precisely as a moral category in politics, it is however more recent. It emerged in western Europe and North America at the end of the nineteenth century, with legislation against ill-treatment of children and the institution of social work focused mainly on working-class contexts, and more broadly with the gradual spread of child protection policies. It advanced progressively through the world after the Second World War, notably with the creation of UNICEF in 1946, the adoption by the United Nations of a Declaration on the Rights of the Child in 1959, and a Convention on the Rights of the Child held in 1989. This development paralleled a growing mobilization of nongovernmental organizations on the issues of child abuse from 1970 onward, then child labor during the 1980s, and finally pedophilia and incest in the 1990s. The representation of childhood that underlies this policy highlights the moral quality of innocence and the social quality of vulnerability. The former refers to original purity, to which adults must bear witness; the latter suggests a need for protection, for which adults must be responsible.

AIDS, with the moral connotations of sin and deviance that have been associated with it since the beginning of the epidemic, and the social dimensions of inequality and violence that mark it in the South African context in particular, is revealing of the stakes that crystallize around childhood. Previously absent and invisible, children became omnipresent in the past decade, at the very moment when scientific and political controversies around the disease were proliferating. In a radicalized public arena where opposing sides accused one another of the most heinous crimes including genocide, where opponents were demonized in racial terms, and where the memory of the tragic past of apartheid was constantly reanimated, children became an issue. Their innocence was contrasted with the behavior of adults, who were portrayed as irresponsible. The three figures analyzed here thus emerged. The sick child, whose only responsibility for his or her misfortune was to have been born, appeared as an innocent victim of adults and the incompetence of the authorities. The abused child, often raped by a family member, presented the most obscene and intolerable image of this status of expiatory victim of men's madness. The orphan child, enduring both grief and isolation, became the iconic image of the present, but also the future victim.

Of course, these figures relate to concrete situations. And of course, the children concerned deserve the attention paid to them. The way in which these figures were exposed in public nevertheless calls for a critical analysis. We need to take the measure of this exaltation of misfortune, the exaggeration of the figures, the exhibition of horror, the staging of suffering, the catastrophization of the social world. The end justifies the means, one might think, and compassion spurs action. Parading sick children forces the government to introduce preventive treatments. Telling the story of raped children makes society aware of sexual abuse. Publicizing the plight of orphans stimulates national and international aid. But this emotional mobilization is fragile and ambiguous. The sick child becomes a burden on society, the abused is revealed as a future perpetrator of sexual violence, the orphan is transformed into a potential criminal. Above all, the affective emphasis reifies children as victims in a way that removes them far from the social reality in which they live. The weight of poverty and the role of exploitation in the spread of HIV/AIDS among disadvantaged communities, the ordinary violence in social relations, the permanence of traditional forms of family solidarity—all these things that constitute the life context of these children—disappear. By eluding this complex reality, which makes moral judgments less certain and solutions less univocal, compassion may paradoxically prove to be an emotion that spares those feeling it from having to take more demanding action.

7. Desire for Exception

Managing Disaster Victims

> The tradition of the oppressed teaches us that the "state of
> emergency" in which we live is not the exception but the rule.
> We must attain to a conception of history that is in keeping
> with this insight.
>
> WALTER BENJAMIN, "Theses on the Philosophy of History"

The tsunami that hit South Asia on December 26, 2004, causing the death of more than 285,000 people and sparking a campaign that resulted in donations estimated at more than 5 billion euros, dramatically highlighted the historical fact that natural disasters, insofar as they represent both the most massive (in terms of numbers of victims) and the purest (being putatively beyond human control) of collective misfortune, belong to the modern moral universe. As Theodor Adorno's well-known argument put it: "The Lisbon earthquake sufficed to cure Voltaire of the theodicy of Leibniz."[1] For European societies, and particularly for the intellectual elites of the Enlightenment, the disaster operated on two registers: on the one hand, moral theory, notably the principle of the best of all possible worlds, which the tragedy brutally overturned, and on the other, moral sentiments, first and foremost the compassion aroused throughout Europe by this misfortune that was so unexpected, and so close.

Although today explanation of these events is no longer sought in terms of the wrath of God as it was in earlier times—sociodicies have tended to replace theodicies, though the latter have not completely disappeared as one could ascertain in the comments about the 2010 earthquake in Haiti—the capacity of disasters to mobilize sympathy for the victims has lost nothing of its power; rather the opposite, in fact, since the media transmit their distress home to us through the immediacy and proximity of images and emotions and via moving descriptions and harrowing personal accounts. In this sense, the earthquakes in Turkey and Pakistan, Hurricanes Mitch and Katrina, the eruption of the Nevado del Ruiz volcano in Colombia, and the floods in Bangladesh form part of our everyday affective landscape, with the pathos of its terrible disasters, and presuppose unconditional empathetic engagement, even if it is at a distance in the form of a check sent to a humanitarian organization. In short, natural disasters[2] represent consensual parentheses in the flow of history, privileged moments in which solidarity is displayed, inequality is erased, and conflict suspended. For example, it was widely—although not quite convincingly—asserted that the tsunami seemed to obliterate the disparities of condition between Western tourists and local people in Phuket, Thailand, as well as the violence of the civil war in Banda Aceh, Indonesia. All that counted were the dead and the survivors—all, apparently, objects of the same solicitude.[3] The fact that these are fleeting moments, and that the reality of inequality and conflict quickly reasserts itself, only underlines the moral and political exception that these events represent. In this regard, the disaster known in Venezuela as the *Tragedia* offers a stark demonstration since the humanitarian response to it was paradoxically the declaration of a state of exception.

On December 15, 1999, following torrential rain in the capital Caracas and the neighboring region of Vargas, mud torrents and landslides resulted in a disaster unprecedented in recent Venezuelan history: over the following days, several thousand were reported dead, and tens of thousands lost their homes.[4] Faced with this exceptional ordeal, the National Constituent Assembly declared a state of emergency and gave full power to president Hugo Chávez: "Considering that extraordinary weather conditions prevail over the entire country, the executive is authorized to take all decisions and measures necessary to prevent further damage, to care for those affected and to coordinate joint action by national, regional and municipal bodies. The Venezuelan people are called on to mobilize in solidarity and to collaborate with the aid operations, and must therefore obey the authorities' instructions."

What was remarkable was the national consensus—beyond the Constituent Assembly, which consisted largely of the president's supporters and therefore followed his lead—around the principle of this state of emergency: the tragedy justified exception. Indeed, the elected representatives acted with a degree of moderation in their proclamation and did not suspend basic freedoms. Similarly, the president, an army colonel who had attempted a military coup a few years before but was now democratically elected, avoided an excessive display of power. Militarization was limited to the worst-hit area, where the army took full control, officially in order to bring aid to victims. In fact, rather than the dialectics of law and anomie, this historical moment was marked by the tension between empathy and order. What makes the *Tragedia* a singular event is that it produced a humanitarian state of exception, if I can venture that oxymoron. The state of emergency was universally perceived as the obvious response, not because of the danger to public security that would traditionally be represented by a declaration of war or currently by the threat of a terrorist attack, but in the name of the emotion aroused by the disaster and its human consequences. It was not the fear of peril that legitimized the exceptional measures, but sympathy for the victims that called for and sanctioned them. For this is the unique feature of the situation: far from being the unilateral decision of the sovereign, the state of exception was desired by broad sectors of society, prompted to some degree by a wave of generosity toward the victims, but also by a feeling of trust in the person of the president. Usually dreaded and condemned, here the state of exception was desired.

It might be tempting to view this situation of exception as exceptional in itself, given both the circumstances of the declaration of the state of emergency and the sentiments that legitimized it. Venezuela might then appear to be a unique case—and this was indeed the image that was constructed in the national public sphere. If, however, we analyze the place now occupied by humanitarian government on a global scale, particularly in war zones, the way in which military intervention is justified in the moral register of humanitarianism (for instance in Somalia or Kosovo), and the way humanitarian organizations accompany military operations (such as in Afghanistan and Iraq), the Venezuelan case should perhaps be considered exemplary rather than exceptional.[5] The fact that exception can be declared in the name of humanitarianism is perhaps ultimately a manifestation of a remarkable and ironic feature of the contemporary world: the routinization of exception and its justification on humanitarian grounds. To explore this process,[6] I first question from an anthropological perspective the idea that exception has become the rule, then depict the mobilization of emotions and the production of an illusory equality of conditions in the aftermath of the disaster, and eventually describe the space of violence opened by the humanitarian exception.

THE ROUTINIZATION OF EMERGENCY

Walter Benjamin's illumination[7] that the state of exception had become the rule is historically situated: it appeared, like a bolt of lightning, in a text written during the early months of 1940, a few weeks before his suicide, and published posthumously two years later. The philosopher was deeply and intimately affected by the violence of this tragic era, which had caused the precipitate conditions of his exile, his wanderings through a Europe indifferent to the rise of fascism, his internment in a French camp following the declaration of the Second World War, his flight from Paris when the German army arrived, and the confiscation of his apartment and his library by the Gestapo. But above and beyond his personal tragedy, his work is entirely in tune with a more collective reality:[8] the irremediable loss of a world in which he was both witness and victim; the coming of a new age he saw beginning with the First World War, and whose advent was heralded by the suspension of the Weimar Constitution in Germany; and the entry into a cycle of humanity in which, he wrote, "the art of storytelling is reaching its end." Exception has become the rule: this expression was therefore a biographical as much as a historical truth, marked by the culmination of a process redefining the meaning of politics in the first half of the twentieth century.

The entire reconstruction of the world after 1945 proceeded, under the consensual litany of "never again," from a global attempt to end even the possibility of a state of exception because it could instigate a return to what had been experienced and what no one wanted to experience again; this attempt was manifested on the rhetorical, but also on the legal and institutional levels. Of course, many situations ran counter to this effort, from the totalitarian regimes of the East to the dictatorships of the South, from colonialism to postcolonialism, but it was still possible until recently, with the announcement of the "end of history,"[9] for the utopia of a global democracy, constructed on a reinvented Western model, to prevail.

But in recent years this supposed "law of history" predicting the universal advent of democracy has been called into question, and the idea that we live again in an age of exception become the rule seems increasingly accepted. In this new consciousness, many have seen the aftermath of 9/11 and the extralegal conditions of the fight against terrorism, rapidly transformed into a war against the "axis of evil," as a historical turning point.[10] Given these conditions, the surprising return to favor of the work of Carl Schmitt, a theoretician of the state of exception who influenced Walter Benjamin, among others, but was discredited because of his justification of the Nazi state and his personal compromises with its representatives, seems especially significant.[11] However, in its most radical form the theory of exception as the rule goes beyond the particular context of the destruction of the twin towers and of imperialist politics of the United States. For

Giorgio Agamben[12] in particular, "the voluntary creation of a permanent state of emergency (though perhaps not declared in the technical sense) has become one of the essential practices of contemporary states, including so-called democratic ones." The shift is thus not new, having continued uninterrupted throughout the twentieth century: "Faced with the unstoppable progression of what has been called a 'global civil war,' the state of exception tends increasingly to appear as the dominant paradigm of government in contemporary politics." From Hitler's promulgation of a "Decree for the protection of the people and the state" in 1933, which suspended the freedoms instituted by the Weimar Constitution, to George W. Bush's issuing of a "Military Order" that allowed for the indefinite detention of terror suspects in an extension of the Patriot Act, he suggests a continuity, if not obviously historical, at least genealogical.

Yet from a social sciences perspective, we cannot take the terms of the discussion thus posed at face value. We must problematize it, examining both the alleged normalization of the state of exception and the generalization of the discourse on exception. Today one is always accompanied by the other, and the facts are indissociable from the articulation of them. It is in this sense that we can—paradoxically—speak of the routinization of exception: routinization of the practical use and of the theoretical framework. There is a rhetorical inflation that corresponds to the political inflation—and vice versa.[13] But in order to transcend what risks becoming a play of mirrors between reality and its construction, we need to set our reflection within an empirical test. Beyond the assertion of a generalization of exception, what is its concrete manifestation in contemporary societies? To what observable realities does the state of emergency correspond today? How can we grasp the issue of sovereignty in the full complexity of its meanings and its consequences? In studying the political management of a natural disaster in Venezuela, my concern is first to account for a specific historical moment, the neo-Bolivarian "moment," and second to inscribe it in the ethnography of contemporary Venezuela, to break down the apparent unity of the category of exception.[14] A political anthropology of exception rests on this dual requirement to make sense of individual situations both historically and ethnographically.

As Carl Schmitt famously argued, "Sovereign is he who decides on the exception."[15] Exception is therefore what defines sovereignty, and it proceeds from decision: the three terms are inextricably linked. Rather than a merely legal notion, it is a theoretical concept for which Schmitt uses various words, referring to it almost indiscriminately as *Ausnahmezustand,*

Ausnahmefall, Notstand, and *Notfall;* these terms can be translated respectively as "exceptional situation," "exceptional case," "emergency situation," and "case of emergency." Schmitt's hesitation underlines the fact that the issue is not the definition of exception in law, of which it constitutes the negation, but more pragmatically the identification of it as a situation "that makes relevant the subject of sovereignty"—the subject being the individual who "decides whether there is an extreme emergency as well as what must be done to eliminate it." In its clearest form the state of exception is instituted in response to a danger to public order (particularly war), and is characterized by the suspension of constitutional guarantees and the ceding of full power to the sovereign (often a military). The contemporary state of emergency, in the forms in which it is most frequently encountered, has two features that distinguish it from this traditional model: first, it does not necessarily respond to war per se, but rather to the presence of a threat (the aftermath of 9/11 might constitute the paradigmatic example); second, it does not involve the abolition of the law, but rather a challenge to certain freedoms (as in the case of Guantánamo). In other words, the contemporary state of exception needs to be seen as a modulated, and therefore euphemized, condition, in terms of both its causes and its effects—a paradox few commentators have noted.

It is within this changing reality of the exception that Hugo Chávez's response to the *Tragedia* becomes meaningful. The fact that humanitarianism—the convergence of moral sentiments for the victims of the disaster—served as a justification for the state of emergency in this particular case illustrates the more general feature that characterizes humanitarian intervention: its sense of urgency.

THE COMMUNITY OF AFFECTS

"Y el Ávila bajó al mar" (and the Ávila slid into the sea). Through this expressive image, a special report in the newspaper *El Nacional* attempted to describe the disaster caused by torrential rain in the coastal region of Venezuela: almost five hundred inches of rainfall—four times the level considered potentially dangerous—had fallen on the Cordillera running along the coast, particularly on the slopes of the Ávila, a mountain that overlooks the city of Caracas on one side and slopes down to the state of Vargas on the other. This led to two compounding phenomena. The swollen soil was destabilized, resulting in landslides (*derrumbes*) that carried entire neighborhoods with them: the poorest parts of the city, built on what were deemed unbuildable slopes and also often made up of illegal constructions (*ranchos*) were the main zones affected by this kind of risk. In addition, the rain swelled the rivers, which poured torrents down the valleys, carrying blocks of stone and massive mud deposits (*deslaves*), overflowing their beds, and carving new routes through streets and between houses: although luxury hotels and holiday complexes (*urbanizaciones*) in the resort areas at the foot of the mountain did not escape the deluge, it was the houses in the marginal and illegally constructed zones that were the most vulnerable to destruction. As in many Latin American cities, land and environment policies produced the objective conditions for disasters that, while they might appear to be beyond human control, are highly predictable given the exposure to risk, particularly in the zones of unregulated construction on the fringes of major conurbations. Disasters of a small scale thus occur annually during periods of heavy rain, but the victims, too few and with too little legal status, remain invisible.

But in December 1999 two features made this event a national tragedy: the first was the spectacular destructiveness of the cataclysm and the number of dead, injured, and homeless, which moreover was initially overestimated; the second was the apparently indiscriminate nature of this natural violence, which affected not only the poor but also the wealthy. A nun working as a nurse in a Catholic hospital in the state of Vargas recalls:

> Within the community we felt terrified, so much that some of the sisters said we shouldn't go to sleep. We knew something dreadful was happening. There was a huge crash and then the electricity went off. From that point on we could hear the shouts of people in the streets running to escape the fury of the river and trying to save their families from being submerged in the flood. It was a torrent of water, earth, sand, rocks, trees, houses, people, animals, cars, all sorts of detritus all mixed together, fifteen meters [fifty feet] high and running at an incredible speed. We felt destruction and death very close to us.

Besides, the entire population, regardless of status, seemed to be affected, as the same nun described when she spoke of those gathered in her hospital the day after the disaster: "There were all kinds among them: rich and poor, educated and uneducated, good and bad, white and black, priests and criminals." The magnitude of the catastrophe and the sharing of misfortune combined to create a feeling of solidarity and compassion, at least during the first few days after the event.

December 15, 1999, is the date retained in the chronicle of the disaster as the fateful moment. While warning signs were present in the preceding days, with localized collapses of housing and several accidental deaths reported, there is no question that the torrential rainfall and the surge of the river waters made that day the turning point. But this date held a powerful political symbolism because of another event of major significance, this one entirely predictable. December 15 was the day of the national referendum on the constitution that was to lay the foundations for the new "Bolivarian republic," called as promised by the president. After his failed coup on February 4, 1992, Hugo Chávez had been democratically elected on December 6, 1998, following a campaign in which he had called for refounding the nation inspired by the epic journey of the great *Libertador* Simon Bolívar, who died in Colombia in 1830 but whose ashes were repatriated to Venezuela in 1842.[16] The Constituent Assembly, which the president had formed a few months after taking office, had developed a text with 350 articles, which was to be voted on by the people. The results of the vote—88% in favor of the new constitution—clearly demonstrated the very broad consensus Chávez enjoyed at the time (despite the abstention rate of 63%). The new president literally embodied the regeneration of a Venezuela that observers, politicians, and ordinary citizens saw as a country in terminal decline. Oil money was flooding in, but a clientelist elite was profiting from it while the majority of the population sank ever deeper into poverty.[17] In this context Chávez, a charismatic leader with a reputation for integrity, represented both the revival of a glorious past and the institution of a novel ethics. Making liberal use of mystical language and messianic symbolism, sprinkling his interminable speeches with religious elements, he offered the bruised and divided nation the perspective of redemption. When the disaster occurred, the conditions were gathered for the neo-Bolivarian hero to become a Schmittian sovereign.

The climactic date of December 15 thus combined, in a single event and within a single day, both communion in misfortune, which affected all social categories indiscriminately and brought the entire country together, with redemption via a democratic process that, under the auspices of a new constitution, held the promise of national regeneration. Appeal was made to the "sacred union" of all sides in confronting adversity. The rhetoric employed was indeed one of a political theology. The figure of the leader who decides to arrogate all power in order to save the endangered nation was rendered legitimate in this context. It recalled a time when the "king's two bodies"[18] manifested both the immanence and the transcendence of power. But on that fateful day, the sovereign also had to demonstrate the extent of his sympathy for the victims. In other words, he had to present himself as both authoritarian and compassionate.

THE ILLUSION OF EQUALITY

Over the past two decades, humanitarian intervention has increasingly become part of the management of world affairs. Far from the traditional model of the Red Cross, which was both intimately bound with scenes of war and in principle neutral with regard to the protagonists, contemporary forms of humanitarian action, however diverse, have in common a certain degree of difficulty in situating themselves in relation to military actors. Indeed, from Bosnia to Afghanistan, from Rwanda to Iraq, the very notion of "military-humanitarian" intervention has become a commonplace of the political rhetoric used to justify what were previously known as "just wars." In the global development of the "new humanitarian order,"[19] social scientists have mostly been interested in nongovernmental organizations and United Nations institutions; less attention has been paid until recently to nation-states in their capacity as agents of humanitarian policy, often closely tied to military practices. The Venezuelan case offers an illustration all the more remarkable because it is not a Western country.

But what is "humanitarianism"? Empirically, it is a notion with variable morphology, a sort of ethical object with high added value, to which many agents lay claim in order to define or justify their actions. Beyond this self-proclamation, three objective features can be identified. The first relates to the temporality of humanitarian intervention, which is that of emergency: the violence of the event, either disaster or conflict, calls for immediate action, in contrast to other modalities such as development that are inscribed in the long term. The second element has to do with the object of the humanitarian mobilization, which primarily consists in saving lives: the powerful legitimacy with which it is invested derives precisely from the fact that it can point to those rescued from death due to famine, epidemic, or injury. The third aspect concerns the spirit that drives humanitarian action, which derives from moral sentiments: it operates in both the emotional registers and the register of values, what people feel and what they believe. Let us depict each of the three dimensions at work in the *Tragedia.*

"Emergencia nacional" (National emergency) read the headlines in the daily newspapers in the days following the disaster. Emergency was simultaneously an empirical evidence and a political gesture. Remarkably, a state of emergency had been decreed in Vargas as early as December 6, and an army battalion had been dispatched there on December 11 to bring assistance to five hundred people made homeless. But on December 16 there were tens of thousands of victims, and it was even impossible to count the human cost of the events because communication was virtually nonexistent. While the president called for national unity and the Council of Ministers declared an emergency in five states, the first rescuers began their work, but without any coordination. One volunteer reported: "During the mass evacuation there was total disorganization, and whole families of victims were lost. There was chaos at the airport because instead of closing it, as emergency protocol requires, victims from nearby neighborhoods were allowed in." It was the Ministry of the Interior's civilian-staffed crisis unit that was responsible for intervening in such cases and thus for coordinating operations from the airport, where helicopters and planes were shuttling back and forth as they evacuated victims. However, the lack of resources and the absence of organization made rescue missions difficult: as the head of the crisis unit confided in an interview, "The management of the disaster was a disaster." On December 17, noting the inability of the civil defense structure to deal with the situation, the Constituent Assembly met and, "exercising its inherent constituent power, decreed a state of emergency over the whole of the Republic for the duration of the disaster." It "authorized the President to adopt any measures necessary to avoid major damage." That evening the disaster zone was completely militarized. The "emergency" phase, which lasted until December 27, involved the mobilization of 13,200 members of the three armed forces and the police, together with planes, helicopters, and ships. Their mission was to transfer those made homeless to shelters, to respond to urgent needs, to collect and distribute humanitarian aid, to administer medical care and recover bodies, to clean the water pipes and sewers, and to clear the streets. Emergency as temporal condition and legal procedure became a justification in and of itself for all action taken in the name of rescue: "We are in a state of emergency and we can do whatever we like," declared a security official.

"Many people despaired of saving lives," recounts "disaster expert" Enrique Alberto Martín Cuervo[20] in the report he drew up for the Humboldt aid organization. During the first days the main priority was to evacuate those who had managed to climb onto roofs, terraces, and balconies, and were rescued by helicopters or even by planes, and those who had been able to reach the mud-covered beaches, where lifeboats were sent to pick them up. A young woman related how she thought she was going to die until she was finally saved by rescuers: "I was in water up to my waist. It was flowing very fast. My skin was almost rotting away." Dramatic accounts offering vivid images of the conditions of survival amid the disaster piled up. A twelve-year-old boy, discovered by chance in a poor neighborhood, was saved by firemen: "He was buried in debris from the old Caracas-La Guaira road," explained a nurse in *El Nacional* on December 18. This account, like many others gathered by journalists, illustrates how close those evacuated came to dying. The precariousness of existence and the bareness of life were the very matter of humanitarian intervention, both in these individual rescues and in the later counts of the number of persons saved. Victims were first and foremost physical bodies in the naturalness of their needs and their vulnerability.

In this situation, the illusion of equality between human beings confronted by calamity, but also encountering compassion, was a powerful driver for the collective action. As a doctor explained it: "All social levels were mixed, rich and poor, we treated everyone the same way." But the reality was more complicated. While initially the rescuers appeared to draw no distinction between victims, and despite the fact that wealthy men did not hesitate to offer their personal helicopters to help in the evacuation, as soon as the period of emergency had passed the sense of hierarchical values reasserted itself as if it were the natural order. Overwhelmed by the numbers sheltering in refuges in the capital, the military quickly organized mass transfers to the interior of the country, hundreds of miles from the site of the disaster. Two women evacuated by the armed forces to Barquisimeto recounted their arrival at the airport of this town in the Cordillera east of Caracas. The first, a working-class woman who came from the poor neighborhoods of Vargas, was put up in the garrison, where she was able to wash and get warm straight away. Since she had nowhere to go, she and her children were subsequently housed and fed for several months, in return for cleaning duties. The second, a middle-class woman from the resort areas on the coast, met an engineer at the garrison who was involved in the rescue operation; he invited her and her daughter to come and shower at his office. She then called friends who lent her a house, and her daughter, who had immediately flown home from the United States where she was living, secured a lift back to Caracas in two cars that her company chartered for her. This anecdote exemplifies how quickly the bare life of the victims was "resocialized" along the customary lines of inequality, as soon as the brief period of rescue was over.

"We suffered like the poor, we gave them everything we had without expecting anything in return. . . . We were with them and felt all of their pain and need." Thus the Little Sisters of the Poor expressed their experience of the disaster.[21] The most widely shared moral sentiment in that time of calamity was certainly compassion, understood as a communion of suffering. There was no doubt with regard to the rescuers on the ground: all indicated that they felt personally affected by what was happening to their fellow citizens and how they spared no effort to save those who could be saved. But in order for "this fine lesson in solidarity that Venezuelans are giving to their leaders" (as an editorial in *El Nacional* put it on December 21) to take form, the entire nation needed to be able to share in this empathy. Here the media played an essential role, transforming the abstract reality of the numbers of dead or homeless into dramatic personal stories. The one that touched Venezuelan society most deeply was without a doubt that of little Maria Eugenia, whose riveting rescue, broadcast live on television, corresponded to a form of "mediatization" of disaster that had become well established since the 1985 Armero tragedy in Colombia.[22] On the morning of December 16, a cameraman filming mudflows in the parking lot of a residential block zoomed in on the arm of a child waving from beneath a pile of debris. He called for help and residents rushed to free her under the watchful eye of the camera. This sequence, which was repeatedly rebroadcast over the following days, ended with the image of the little girl huddled in the arms of her rescuer. Updates on Maria Eugenia's story proved no less poignant: while her mother was never located, her brother was found alive in a tree, and her little dog, identified from a family photo shown on television, was returned to her a few weeks later.

The issue of the gaze, and the material support provided for it by the media, especially television, is key to understanding the emotional impulse that brought the country together and transfigured the nation: the gaze brought people closer, and it was through it that they felt compassion. This was the impulse that drove humanitarian aid. After the 7 million bolivars of donations collected during the first five days, which according to the Venezuelan press testified to the generosity of the Venezuelan people, international contributions were seen as so many "gestures of friendship." The U.S. and French governments were the first to offer aid, quickly followed by the United Nations Development Programme, the Inter-American Development Bank, and nongovernmental organizations, first among them the Catholic aid charity Caritas. This fine display of international solidarity was barely affected by Hugo Chávez's decision to refuse permission for U.S. vessels to dock, in defense of national sovereignty. The Venezuelan president himself missed no opportunity to appear on the ground among rescuers or alongside victims, bringing the comfort of his charismatic presence and displaying the compassion of a leader for his people.

Humanitarianism, independently of the goodwill of the rescuers, constructs an unequal relationship between the one giving aid and the one being aided. The fact is attested in any number of places where the urgency of a disaster reduces the condition of victims to their bare physical existence and prompts ambiguous impulses of pity and solidarity. The recipients are not blind to the way they are being treated, particularly when they are from disadvantaged backgrounds, as the stigma of poverty intensifies the stigma of misfortune.[23] Credit should be given to Hugo Chávez for recognizing how this social injustice inherent in the humanitarian gesture added to the shared misfortune of natural disaster. In a remarkable symbolic gesture, he proposed, in fact, to reverse the stigma by renaming the victims. The Spanish word for them, *damnificados*, while it is common usage, still bears the etymological reference to religious connotations of damnation, however removed it might be here from the idea of sin. To break with this negative connotation, Chávez suggested in his weekly radio broadcast *Alo Presidente* that the term be replaced by *dignificados*—those whose dignity was recognized. In other words, misfortune should not humble people, but elevate them. From being damned, the survivors became the redeemed. Of course, this new designation had little effect on the material conditions of their confinement in military camps. More would be required to change the attitudes of society toward its poor, and the practices of the army during a state of emergency. But the inversion of the term reveals the force of symbolism in the management of the humanitarian crisis. The word *dignificados* links power and redemption. It brings together the grace of misfortune and the justification of exception.

COLLATERAL DAMAGE

Philosophers from Thomas Hobbes to John Rawls have argued that violence is at the heart of the modern social contract. The exchange is played out between a society that agrees to delegate its power and the state that assumes that power, thus ensuring greater well-being for its citizens.[24] This is indeed the core of the contract implicitly concluded in the state of exception in general, and the state of exception defined as humanitarian in particular. In declaring a state of emergency, the Constituent National Assembly, which at that tragic moment embodied popular sovereignty, gave the president not full powers, which would have suggested a suspension of constitutional guarantees, but a completely free hand to define what was to be decided for the common good. The moral sentiment uniting the nation behind its leader, and the higher need represented by the duty of saving lives, justified the state of emergency. Yet even in situations where military intervention for humanitarian purposes is most justified, violence lies at the heart of the exception, buried beneath the ethical justifications, but ready to emerge where circumstances dictate.[25] The intervention of the army in Vargas did not escape this rule.

The violence instituted in the political order by the retreat of the rule of law was, of course, seen as the price to be paid for avoiding the greater violence that would involve not only the fury of natural elements but also the breakdown of social order. The first signs of anomie appeared as soon as the second day after the disaster: looting and vandalism in the affluent neighborhoods began as early as December 17. "During that night, the devil entered the body of criminals who, instead of thanking God for allowing them to survive, took the life of innocent Venezuelans," reported the representative of the Humboldt Association. The feeling of insecurity grew among survivors, who tried to take refuge in public places in order to escape being attacked. "There were numerous acts of vandalism and confrontations between rival gangs who were killing each other, violence and destruction of all kinds. It was a second tragedy, perhaps even more serious than the one we have just lived through. . . . We did all we could to get military protection, until on Tuesday our pleas were finally met with the arrival of a battalion of the Inteligencia Militar [Military Intelligence Corps]," recalls the nun from the Little Sisters of the Poor quoted earlier. The army was pressed just as much to maintain public order under threat from anomie as to organize aid for those who could still be saved from the disaster. For many Venezuelans, the army represented a guarantee of both efficient aid and security in the face of disorder. In reality, however, the roles were shared between the three forces (air force, navy, and army), which organized rescues and evacuations, and the National Guard, Military Police, the Directorate of Military Intelligence, and also members of the Interior Ministry's much-feared Dirección del Servicio de Inteligencia y Prevención (Disip), the secret police, which took on crime-prevention duties.

Under these conditions, the declaration of a state of emergency appeared almost a technicality, a practical way of managing the crisis, a common-sense necessity in order to avoid the worst. Great care was taken to maintain all the appearance of democratic process. The Constituent Assembly issued a decree that spoke of a "state of alert," but still gave the president all prerogatives he might judge useful to address the seriousness of the situation. Constitutional guarantees were maintained, although no practi-

cal provision was made for monitoring the action of "special comman-
does" in the disaster zones. The government avoided any authoritarian
action, but it allowed the army to issue a text calling on residents of the
region not to leave their homes between nine in the evening and seven in
the morning, thereby instituting a curfew that was translated as a command to soldiers to "open fire" on anyone on the streets at night who
failed to comply with the order to show their papers. In other words, the
state of emergency, although never officially declared, was effectively in
force. The minister of the interior seemed to recognize it as he used the
expression "declaration of emergency." Thus for several weeks the military and civilian forces of law enforcement exerted wide powers over the
devastated territory of one Venezuelan state. Society not only saw nothing to question in this, but on the contrary viewed it as a desirable and
necessary demonstration of authority. Security and humanitarianism
went hand in hand, it appeared.

But beyond and above this pragmatic justification, it is necessary to
consider the longer political history of the state of emergency in Venezuela. As Chancellor José Vicente Rangel stated as a sort of excuse for the
abuses perpetrated by the military, in an interview reported in *El Nacional* on January 11, 2000: "In Venezuela we live in a culture of arbitrary
power which we cannot end overnight by changing the government or the
constitution." Since its independence, Venezuela has been governed almost
permanently, at least up until 1959, by generals and military juntas. The
very construction of the nation is tightly bound up with this singular experience of the army's power. The evident continuity in the *longue durée*
should nevertheless not lead us to underestimate the profound change introduced by Hugo Chávez. First, he came to power democratically, and it is
not the least of paradoxes that this failed putschist appeared to the very
large majority of Venezuelans who elected him in 1998, and reelected him
in 2000, as the redeemer of democracy. Second, he referred not to the traditional caudillismo of his predecessors but to revolutionary Bolivarian-
ism, the product of an ideological reconstruction that, by a chronological
leap of more than a century and a half, reconnected with the mythic origin of Venezuela.[26] Once more, we are in the register of faith that draws
from the timeless sources of religion and nation.

The test of the facts was nevertheless formidable for this mystique of
power. Having come as saviors, the military and police quickly emerged as
criminals in the eyes of a large part of public opinion. In a report titled *Emergencia en la emergencia* (Emergency amid the emergency), PROVEA, the
Venezuelan Program for Human Rights Education and Action, condemned

the abuses committed by the forces of order in Vargas province:[27] summary executions, abductions, and attacks were documented in an uncompromising assessment. A witness overheard members of these military and paramilitary groups present locally commenting on how they executed those they identified as "looters, rapists or thieves," using sticks and baseball bats in order to produce marks on the body similar to those that "might be caused by a death resulting from the disaster," and, since it was better to be safe than sorry, burying them in "mass graves": a number of accounts testify to this summary justice, with its organized suppression of evidence. In this context of arbitrary power mistakes can happen, if I dare say, as in the case of the young man who returned to fetch belongings from his apartment and, being taken for a burglar, was killed without warning. Beyond these tragic errors, those subjected to this treatment were not only criminals caught in the act of, for example, looting a supermarket or an apartment, but also those previously known to the police or the judicial system, who were sought out at their homes, taken away, and made to disappear. Moreover, the armed forces and special forces did not limit themselves to this violent repression; they also participated themselves in looting and destruction. Several testimonies report them descending on residential neighborhoods to levy a sort of war booty. In one case, officers of the secret police, called to an army captain's house that was being looted, found two dozen paratroopers raiding the premises, on the pretext of searching for weapons. As one of the civilian rescuers reported:

> During the night, there was constant shooting—hours of gun battles. The secret police against the *malandros*. The army against the *malandros*. And everyone was looting. . . . I've got photos of soldiers looting. I made the first report on violations of human rights, but I didn't go to testify. I was scared the military would find me and kill me, because there were only three of us, I was the only one with a camera and the soldiers knew it. One morning we heard noise, banging on doors. It was soldiers accompanied by a major. They were trying to force a chest open. My colleague was armed, he told them to leave and then I saw a line of soldiers with red berets moving along. I photographed them while my friend held them at gunpoint.

Colonel Manuel Carpio, the head of operations for the maritime customs authority, admitted officially, in *El Nacional* on December 23, that, of the sixty-four individuals arrested during the sack of the harbor zone, most were "wearing the uniform of police and firefighting units, and even of the National Guard." Because there was no space in the local prisons, the looters were merely sent back to their respective units.

The government had little room to maneuver between the concern for maintaining military order in the devastated region and the recognition of the abuses committed by security forces, between support for the powerful bodies of the army and the police and the response to be made to the accusations issued by human rights organizations, between the application of the state of emergency and the preservation of the rule of law. Furthermore, the situation of the president and his allies was all the more delicate because the events occurred at the very moment when the new constitution was supposed to guarantee the functioning of democracy better than in the past, and also because the disaster was the focus of major media attention in the international public arena, where the country was supposed to serve as a model. Chávez himself spoke on the subject on January 16, 2000, in his weekly radio dialogue with listeners: "There is not the slightest evidence of human rights violations, only speculation." Placing himself in the spotlight, he added, as a sign of his skepticism as much as his good faith: "Take me there with my hands tied behind my back and my eyes blindfolded to talk with the witnesses."

In fact, although inquiry commissions were appointed, the authorities preferred to present the military's successes, particularly through the public tributes paid to them. For instance, General Gerardo Briceño Garcia decorated a group of members of the National Guard for their courage in bringing aid to the victims, while simultaneously inviting citizens to report any abuses they had suffered "in order to preserve the image of our institution." At the same time, alongside testimony to the depredation and violence committed by the security forces, the press published documents attesting to the spirit of solidarity that had prevailed in the management of the disaster. Alfredo Infante, a Jesuit member of the refugee assistance team set up by his congregation, described the general mobilization in the parish of Jesús Obrero in the following way:[28] "The members of the military, coordinated by Sergeant Pacheco, who is a member of our Christian community, proved themselves up to the task, offering their valiant collaboration and demonstrating their human qualities." Leaving the last word to this worthy soldier, the churchman remembers: "This is how Sergeant Pacheco summed up his experience after the Christmas mass and meal: 'What great deeds we are able to accomplish when we work hand in hand with those who are in need! That gives me a feeling of peace.'" Collective redemption supposes this dual movement, which consists both in bringing into the open the signs of the grace that touched the entire nation through this painful ordeal and in constructing the misdeeds committed under cover of the emergency in the margins, as an inevitable and reprehensible reality. The exception was necessary, and the crimes merely an exception within the exception.

Exception is always grasped through categories of law, of which it marks not so much the negation as the boundary, since it is often included and even prescribed in the texts of constitutions.[29] But I am considering exception from a different perspective—not only as a juridical act, in this case by the assembly, nor even as a state of fact, instituted by the army, but as a political gesture that involves and cuts through the whole of society. Exception is not only the state of exception declared (and as we have seen, it was not fully declared in the Venezuelan case), it is also the exceptional situation (collectively lived as such). It is here that the *Tragedia* acquires its full significance. Faced with the greatest and most inevitable misfortune (this is at least what was asserted, highlighting nature's fury), the population united and the nation was redeemed. There is no better indication of this than the leitmotif of media articles and interviews, in which reference was constantly made to the indiscriminate exposure to misfortune and to the universal communion in assistance: there was no distinction as to class or race either in the suffering of the victims or the aid given by rescuers, it was repeated. Residents of the affluent neighborhoods spoke of sharing the misfortune of the poorest, doctors in private clinics found themselves treating working-class patients they had never previously encountered, gourmet restaurants set up temporary canteens for the survivors. Of course, this mobilization is an illusion of equality that supposedly compensates the weight of inequality in Venezuelan society, a blessing of generosity that counterbalances the routine nature of corruption. But it is also a common humanitarian impulse: the exception perhaps emerges less in the decree that instituted it than in the sentiment that justified it. Analyzing one without understanding the other would mean missing the genuinely theological dimension of this politics.

"Dios existe" (God exists), wrote Yelitza Linares, a university professor and journalist, in her account of her conversion to Christianity at the moment when, sheltering on the roof of her house, which had been destroyed by the torrents of mud and rubble, convinced she was going to die, she joined her neighbors in praying aloud, begging tearfully for divine assistance, until the waters receded and finally allowed her to be saved. The significance of what she perceived as a miracle does not only correspond to an individual truth. It can only be understood in the broader context of a national history in which the *Tragedia* was presented as an ordeal from which the nation had to emerge strengthened. In the process of regeneration of the state, articulated in a rhetoric that was ultimately less revolutionary than mystical, and which drew on a symbolism that was as much religious as it was political, the disaster was lived as a test that made it possible to reconstruct national unity, and exception appeared as the concrete modality of collective redemption gained at the cost of symbolic and even physical violence. The unanimous humanitarian impulse prompted by the disaster was admittedly short lived, and it is noteworthy that the unity forged in misfortune also formed the point of departure for future divisions that have since taken the form of profound splits and left the country on the brink of civil war on several occasions, bringing the threat of another state of emergency, this time for reasons of internal security. When the state of grace dissipated, society appeared for what it is—hierarchized, divided, and conflicted.

The events in Venezuela can be read as a sort of parable articulating the paradoxical truth of contemporary societies faced with natural disasters. Because earthquakes, hurricanes, floods, volcanic eruptions, and landslides, unlike wars, do not seem to involve human responsibility and therefore appear to represent a pure form of misfortune, they give rise, at least initially, to forms of universal communion among all those who are, whether directly in their lives or indirectly through images, affected by the destruction, mourning, and suffering: an imaginary of shared humanity emerges, prompting the illusion that ethnic and racial, economic and political boundaries are erased in the unanimous wave of solidarity. But because this illusion cannot withstand the test of reality, the harsh rules of the everyday social play quickly reassert themselves: looting by survivors, misappropriation of donations, abuses by the military, and settling of accounts become the rule of exception, while more surreptitiously the preexisting inequalities of conditions are exposed and the complacent indifference of the privileged classes toward the victims is revealed. This ambiguity is better expressed in Spanish than any other language: the *damnificados* are not merely the wretched, but also the damned of the earth; stigma is added to their misfortune. Hugo Chávez's renaming of them as *dignificados* was a laudable intent, and may even have had performative effects. But once emotions were exhausted and generosity had run dry, this symbolic gesture did not spare them either injustice or violence.

8. Subjectivity without Subjects

Reinventing the Figure of the Witness

> If *testis* designates the witness insofar as he intervenes as a third
> in a suit between two subjects, and if *superstes* indicates the one
> who has fully lived through an experience and can therefore relate
> it to others, *auctor* signifies the witness insofar as his testimony
> always presupposes something that pre-exists him and whose
> reality and force must be validated or certified. Testimony is thus
> always an act of "author".
>
> GIORGIO AGAMBEN, *Remnants of Auschwitz*

The official history of Médecins Sans Frontières highlights one moment—the Biafran war at the end of 1968 with the urgent new imperative to bear witness, no longer simply to offer assistance—as the moment when the idea of the organization and more broadly of a new form of humanitarianism was born.[1] Whereas silence had long been seen as the condition for gaining authorization from all parties to the conflict to bring aid to military and civilian groups, to the extent that it had become virtually synonymous with neutrality, nongovernmental organizations were now on the contrary asserting not only their right but also their duty to speak publicly about abuses, crimes, and more broadly the breaches of the laws of war they were observing. With the founding of Médecins Sans Frontières in 1971, testimony became an integral part of humanitarian intervention, on an equal footing with aid.[2] It was no longer enough simply to save the victims of war; one must also plead their cause.

But how was this to be done without the organizations becoming confused with the institutions and political groups that also claimed to defend them? And how could one maintain impartiality at the very moment when one chose to speak in the name of some protagonists and condemn others? These two interrogations were crucial, because they put the very legitimacy of humanitarian organizations, and the credence that was to be given to their testimony, at stake. Their response to the first question was to assert that they limited their testimony to their area of competence—that is, medical action and humanitarian law. Their answer to the second question was that they always took the side of the victims.[3] However, in practice, both delineating the boundary of their sphere of competence and identifying who were the victims proved much more complex than anticipated: thus each concrete situation of humanitarian intervention became a test in which the organizations found themselves facing other actors, other logics, and other strategies, and discovered the difficulty of maintaining their role of moral witness.

The early 1990s saw a major shift, with the deployment of psychiatrists and psychologists in humanitarian missions, in which, until then, only physicians, surgeons, nurses, and logisticians had their place. Within little more than ten years, mental health specialists, despite being improbable actors in emergency operations, became established as indispensable to such initiatives. Treating the "wounds of the soul" that, according to them, had previously gone unnoticed, they could henceforth expose "silent pain" in the international public arena, as this extract from an article justifying their involvement in the Palestinian territories during the Second Intifada suggests:[4]

> Volunteers give care and bear witness, using the media as a resource to tell the world of the suffering of the people they help. The distress these testimonies produce among those who hear them arouses the desire to construct a response that is no longer simply material and medical, but located on the psychic level. People have an enormous need for the account of their traumatic experiences to be heard. In order for trauma not to be repeated from generation to generation, and for the vicious cycle of repetition to be broken, we need to repair suffering, even the suffering that is unspoken, even the suffering that is not seen on bodies; we must therefore start by speaking of them.

"What does a psychologist report?—What does he observe?" asks Wittgenstein.[5] In other words, to what do the experts of the psyche really have access? Is it people's experience, or simply their utterances and sometimes behaviors? This query becomes central once the psychologist—or psychiatrist—decides to testify to what victims of violence experience, speaking in their place and in their name. As Veena Das and Arthur Kleinman observe:[6] "Psychologists and psychiatrists are engaged in documenting, describing and diagnosing post-traumatic stress disorder and other distressing consequences of murder, rape, torture, molestation, and other forms of brutality." However, from an anthropological or historical point of view, mental health specialists do more than just identify clinical pictures and establish diagnostic frameworks that make it possible to discover and testify to a hitherto neglected reality—that of the suffering of victims of violence.

Through their categories and via their testimonies, they also formulate a new reading of contemporary conflicts: they tell of violence in the language of subjectivity. From this point of view, trauma—or its clinical qualification as posttraumatic stress disorder—is not only the clinical description of a state of the psyche, it is also the political depiction of a state of the world. In other words, it produces a new vocabulary of war, and brings suffering into existence by naming it.

My intent here is to analyze the transformation of the status of the witness in light of the emergence of humanitarianism.[7] I first question our anthropological understanding of political subjectivation, then discuss the two forms of bearing witness, borrowing philological clues from Émile Benveniste, and finally address the contradictions and aporia of humanitarian testimonies via ethnographical examples in the context of the Second Intifada.

THE SUBJECTIVATION OF THE POLITICAL

What political work of subjectivation does humanitarian testimony produce?[8] This is the general question I am interested in. It needs some clarification. The subjectivation I am speaking of neither presupposes subjects as rational and autonomous actors, a position sometimes celebrated by sociologists, nor refers to the subjectivities buried in the unconscious, which psychoanalysts explore. My interest is in the figures used to describe individuals, and with which they are identified, whether or not they recognize themselves through them. In Palestine the bold youth throwing stones and the distressed victim of trauma—who may potentially be the same person—are two of these possible figures. Thus speaking of political subjectivation assumes neither a Cartesian "I" nor a Freudian "Ego," neither a consciousness nor an unconscious to which the social sciences might strive to gain access, as if it were an ultimate truth. Political subjectivation, in my understanding, is the production of subjects and subjectivities possessed of political meanings within social interactions. I shall therefore not ask whether the Palestinian teenager is actually a combatant or a neurotic, but observe that he is presented and may even present himself alternately as one and the other. Nor shall I seek to ascertain his true experience of violence, but rather what are the various truth tests to which he is subjected by political authorities and humanitarian organizations, by religious leaders and psychiatrists: What truth are they trying to make him tell, or to tell through him?

Thus defined, political subjectivation recalls the figure of interpellation put forward by Louis Althusser,[9] when he gives the example of the person hearing a policeman call, "Hey you there!" who, by turning round, shows that he has recognized himself in this address, even though he was not called by name. This proposition can be generalized: any socially relevant—and therefore culturally constructed—designation constitutes both a subject who is called to identify himself, sometimes against his will, with the way he is designated, and a subjectivity that conforms, at least in part, to this injunction. In this sense, trauma produces the traumatized person just as humanitarianism produces the victim. In Palestine, the presence of psychiatrists and psychologists makes possible and necessary a particular form of subjectivation.

This way of thinking about subjectivation therefore contrasts both with the essentialist conception that reduces the experience of trauma to a "condition of the traumatized person" (always the likely outcome of psychological accounts) and with the moralist critique that condemns the "victimization of victims" (to use a cliché that has become popular in some intellectual circles, particularly in France). In fact, by refusing any reifying reading, I recognize that there are other ways of interpreting violence (not just through trauma but for instance in terms of domination and resistance); moreover, by rejecting all univocal interpretation, I affirm that individuals have multiple sites of identification (not only as victims but also as combatants or martyrs). The issue is therefore both theoretical and ethical, because the task is simultaneously to understand a reality in all its complexity and to restore the degree of freedom that individuals possess. The production of political subjects is inscribed in an irreducible tension between subjectivation and subjection, as Judith Butler[10] asserts, arguing that it "consists precisely in this fundamental dependency on a discourse we never chose but that, paradoxically, initiates and sustains our agency," and "signifies the process of becoming subordinated by power as well as the process of becoming a subject." From this point of view, humanitarian psychiatry is itself also a power that, in war zones especially, prescribes a certain form of legitimate discourse: compassion toward psychic suffering thus produces a particular modality of subjectivation that is imposed on individuals but through which it is also possible for them to make their cause heard.

It is therefore important to make no mistake when we speak of affects: with the tools available to social science, we have access only to the culturally significant expressions of these affects (and we know how much these expressions may vary from one site to another, one group to another, one period to another). Psychiatry itself forms part of this culture that allows us to interpret these affects in situations of violence (and we recall that it has evolved from suspecting trauma victims to legitimizing them). Furthermore, it should be noted that in this domain, psychology has shifted from the causes of violence (when victimology, which emerged in the 1950s as a branch of criminology, sought to understand the crime-generating factors in the victim, thus making it suspect) to its consequences (with victimology as a subdiscipline of psychiatry that has since the 1990s accorded full recognition to the victim, therefore definitively innocent). This inversion of the chain of events (from causes to consequences), and of the evaluation of subjects (suspects becoming innocent), is evidence of the profoundly moral dimension of this political subjectivation. In the conflict zone, psychiatrists and psychologists not only issue diagnoses but also produce value judgments.

What does it mean to bear witness to violence using the language of trauma, then? How does the introduction of humanitarian psychiatry, with its actors and its concepts, alter the experience of oppression and war? How do the affects of the protagonists in the conflict become political objects? What is gained in terms of meaning, and what is lost, in this discursive operation? What is a politics of testimony that substitutes its own truth for the truth of those in whose name it is deployed? These are the questions I want to address, on the basis of a series of interviews conducted with members of Médecins Sans Frontières and Médecins du Monde, and of observations over four years on the Administration Board of the former. Before discussing this material, I explore the polysemy of the notion of the witness, and its recent metamorphoses.

THE DUALITY OF THE WITNESS

Latin has two words for "witness."[11] *Testis* is the "third party" who observes an event that brings two sides into conflict, and who can help resolve the dispute for having seen what happened. *Superstes* is the person who "exists beyond" the event—in other words, who experienced it and survived it. In the first case, the witness was external to the scene but observed it: to be more precise, he has no vested interest, and it is this supposed neutrality that forms the grounds for hearing and believing him, including in legal proceedings. In the second case, the witness lived through the ordeal: it is therefore because he was present, but as a victim of the event and hence a survivor, that his word is listened to. One testifies on the basis of his observation, the other on the basis of his experience. The truth of the *testis*, expressed in the third person, is assumed to be objective. The truth of the *superstes*, expressed in the first person, is deemed subjective. The validity of the latter is based on the affects it engages, that of the former on the affects from which it distances itself. However, in current usage the boundary between these two figures is tending to become blurred.

The witness, in the sense of the *superstes*, has become a figure of our time.[12] Through his writing, Primo Levi is the archetypal witness, and also one of the first. As a survivor, he can testify to something having happened because he lived through it. Having experienced the camps, he can tell the truth about them. His intellectual engagement with his own subjectivity is the highest guarantee of the objectivity of his testimony. However, he recognizes the absolute limit of this testimony, which resides precisely in the fact that, as a survivor, he cannot report the truth of those who died:[13] "We, the survivors, are not the true witnesses. When the destruction was terminated, the work accomplished was not told by anyone, just as no one ever returned to recount his own death. Even if they had paper and pen, the submerged would not have testified because their death had begun before that of their body. We speak in their stead, by proxy." The survivor, even if he has passed through the same ordeals, cannot speak for those who did not survive. He bears witness to what cannot be witnessed.

In this extreme situation, the *superstes* thus blurs the boundary with the *testis* on two levels: because he is the only one who can speak and has no interest to hide, he makes a statement on the basis of his experience; and because he survived, he cannot speak of what he did not experience— death. Remarkably, although he lived beyond the camps, he can only bear witness as a third party. By sublimating his affects in a coldly clinical description, he becomes the privileged witness through whom the truth of inhumanity can be made present.

In parallel with this shift, the more recent humanitarian notion of the witness in the sense of *testis* has been twisted in a diametrically opposed direction. The International Committee of the Red Cross was founded in the 1870s on the principle of neutrality, and the corollary of the authorization for it to intervene in conflict situations was an implicit secrecy clause. To bring aid, the Red Cross had to remain silent. Thus the witness undertook not to bear witness. Although present as a third party, the humanitarian organization did not testify. The inherent contradiction in this situation became evident after the Second World War, when it was revealed that aid workers had worked in the camps without denouncing their existence. However, it was not until the early 1970s that this contradiction led to a split in the humanitarian movement, resulting in the formation first of Médecins Sans Frontières and later of Médecins du Monde. The former was born in 1971 out of the refusal to remain silent during the war in Biafra. The latter was created in 1980 in order to protest against the oppression exerted by the Communist regime in Vietnam.[14] The second age of humanitarianism therefore corresponds to the emergence of the witness—not the witness who has experienced the tragedy, but the one who has brought aid to its victims.

Amid this constant tension between the imperative of providing assistance and the imperative of speaking out, the careful accommodations required are sometimes subject to an abrupt breakdown, as in the Ethiopian famine of 1985, when Médecins Sans Frontières was expelled from the country after accusing the government of being responsible for the food crisis. Testimony, which is embedded in a globalized media space, is thus as essential an element of humanitarian activity as is providing assistance. Humanitarian agents testify not on the basis of what they have lived through, but on the basis of what they have seen. They have not endured the ordeal, since their intervention presupposes that safe spaces termed "humanitarian corridors," in which they are protected from hostilities, have been set up, but they render themselves the spokespeople for the victims. Even if they attempt to analyze the political issues involved in the situations they face, the register in which they set their public testimony corresponds logically to the way in which their legitimacy is constructed in the public arena: it is that of compassion. They speak of bodies, of wounds, of suffering. Through a sort of reversal of the traditional roles, they occupy the structural place of the *testis* but employ the reasoning of the *superstes*. In other words, they privilege experience over observation, but this experience is the experience of others.

This paradoxical configuration of testimony deserves consideration. On the one hand, the survivors, on the basis of a sort of ethical radicalism, state that they cannot bear witness for those who are no longer present; despite all that they have lived through, they do not take upon themselves the authority to act as spokespersons, except in order to question their own status as representatives who could speak on behalf of those who have disappeared. On the other hand, humanitarian workers, on the basis of a moral imperative, take on the role of witness for those they assist; although they are rarely explicitly mandated to do so, they set themselves up as spokespeople for the oppressed in order to make their suffering public. In the contemporary era, the prolixity of humanitarian workers thus stands against the silence of survivors. The voice of the former is substituted for the voice of the latter. Or to be more precise, wherever victims of violence and injustice are seen as deprived of the power of expressing themselves, humanitarian organizations speak in their place: they have established themselves as spokespeople for the voiceless.

But there is more. In this new configuration of testimony, in which it is not the survivors who testify to what they have experienced but the aid workers who attest what they have heard, the specific feature of the humanitarian discourse is that it deals increasingly with affects. The survivors, because they need the facts to be established and because they are aware of the risk of not being believed, distance themselves from affect. The aid workers, conversely, because they seek primarily to move their audience and know that they have a stock of credibility, engage affects. We could offer many illustrations of this process, via comparisons between the written, recorded, filmed, and exhibited testimonies of these two classes of witness. For example, we could contrast the striving to eliminate all affect in the walls of names of the dead in the Holocaust memorials with the attempt to sensitize the public to the violence of the world at Médecins Sans Frontières' traveling exhibits, where visitors are invited to learn what it is like to pass through a checkpoint or enter a refugee camp, thereby provoking "a moment of emotion and awareness." Thus the two archetypal figures of the *testis* and the *superstes* are operating in reverse: while the latter becomes resolutely objective, the former uses the subjective register. The *superstes* who has lived through the tragedy keeps strictly to the facts. The *testis*, who has only heard its account or seen its consequences, communicates the experience of it.

With psychiatry, this process of humanitarian subjectivation has found a key tool for giving form to the experience of victims of war, disaster, and famine. However, this field of operation is of recent invention. Although military psychiatry has been addressing trauma neuroses at least since the First World War, and developed novel tools with the identification of post-traumatic stress disorder for the veterans of the Vietnam War,[15] humanitarian psychiatry emerged only in the aftermath of the Armenian earthquake in 1989, born out of simultaneous initiatives by Médecins Sans Frontières and Médecins du Monde, whose members began discovering the psychic consequences a few months after the disaster.[16] Before this there was no place for mental health specialists on emergency aid missions. From that point on they have become indispensable, in Romania and the Caucasus, in Bosnia and Kosovo. After the 2004 earthquake in Iran, more psychiatrists and psychologists went there to assist than did surgeons and physicians, the traditional agents of emergency intervention.

However, contrary to what the chronology might suggest, the rapid development of humanitarian psychiatry did not result from the international dissemination of new nosographic categories originated in the United States, notably posttraumatic stress disorder, which was first described in the classification of mental diseases (DSM-III).[17] It is clear from my interviews with those who intervened in the international situations in which humanitarian psychiatry was developed that they had received no training and had no particular expertise in the field of trauma. It was only after encountering situations and symptoms related to traumatic events that they discovered, often by chance, that the clinical pictures they were observing could fit into the new classification. This sequence of events is important, because it shows that humanitarian concern preceded medical analysis. These agents focused on the suffering of victims of disaster or conflict before they recognized it as trauma. Even today, in the view of many, psychologists' and psychiatrists' presence in the field is justified not on the grounds of establishing diagnoses, which are rarely sought, or providing treatment, which remains difficult, but rather of producing testimony from the experience of victims of violence.

This testimony is constituted not on the basis of what these humanitarian agents have seen, but what they have heard. That it probably has more impact in the construction of political causes today than the testimony of survivors who have lived through the events or observers who witnessed them clearly demonstrates the evolution in the nature of what is being communicated. What counts is not that the event took place, but that it was felt. It is not the fact in itself that constitutes the proof, but the trace it leaves in the psyche or the mark it makes in the telling. In the testimony that is brought to the world's awareness, affect is present both as that which bears witness (people's suffering) and as that which is produced by the testimony (the compassion of the public). The truth sought is not the objective truth of the events that occurred, but the subjective truth of the experience of them. Thus psychologists and psychiatrists, because they supposedly have access to this subjectivity, become legitimate witnesses who speak for those who have undergone these tragic events. Alongside their role as *testis*, and in the name of those who have the status of *superstes*, they base their testimony on a third figure, that of the *auctor*, the one whose word has authority.[18] Nowhere is this subjectivation of testimony as evident as in Palestine, particularly since the start of the Second Intifada, which saw French humanitarian organizations deploy an unprecedented number of mental health teams.

Médecins Sans Frontières has had a presence in the Palestinian Occupied Territories since 1988 and set up its first psychological care program, a clinic in the Jenin refugee camp, in 1994. Médecins du Monde, whose activity in the Territories dates back to 1995, developed a small program offering psychological support to drug users in East Jerusalem in 1998. It was, however, only with the start of the Second Intifada in late 2000 that psychiatry became dominant in the work of both organizations. There were two reasons for the mobilization of mental health specialists at this particular moment: exploratory visits during the first weeks of the uprising pointed out that Palestinian society had no need of the resources traditionally provided by humanitarian organizations, in terms of medicine and surgery, since there were fully trained doctors and a well-equipped health care infrastructure already in place; and the emotional tone of the extensive media coverage of the conflict suggested that the presence of mental health specialists was essential in exposing the consequences of what was portrayed as a humanitarian crisis. In other words, they had to "be there," as they would often say, but perhaps less for the purpose of practicing medicine than that of manifesting a presence and, in this way, being able to bear witness.

Psychiatry offered an alternative here: it was reasonable to suppose that the violence, destruction, and humiliation inflicted on the Palestinian people by the Israeli army must have serious psychic consequences. Yet it was evident that conditions were not conducive to the delivery of psychological or psychiatric care. Palestinian teams were already engaged within the health services, while in local neighborhoods, particularly those most at risk, the situation was so unstable and dangerous that psychotherapeutic work was virtually impossible. Thus it was in bearing witness, rather than via the provision of treatment, which was only hypothetically possible and efficacious, that the aid missions were able to find a meaning for their work: adopting a new role, psychiatrists and psychologists began to piece together personal observations and clinical anecdotes in order to condemn what they were witnessing. Fragments of narratives about aid workers in the Palestinian Occupied Territories proliferated on websites and in journals aimed at donors, in the media and in reports to the senior echelons of international institutions. Through a reconfiguration of the roles of witness, the *testis* now spoke in the first person, taking the role of *auctor* in place of the *superstes*.

THE EVIDENCE OF THE MARTYR

But there is another etymology of the witness, for in Greek the word used is *martus*, and with the first Fathers of the Church the term acquired the more precise meaning of martyr.[19] According to Christian doctrine, witnesses attest to the existence of God by choosing to die rather than betray their faith. The sacrifice of their life bears witness. Similarly, the Arabic word *shahid*, which signifies "witness," also designates a martyr—one who dies while performing his duty as a Muslim or in a holy war. The witness is therefore the sacrificed, the one who has chosen to give up his life in order to affirm his religious—and by extension, political—truth. Unlike the survivor or the third party, who speaks in the first or third person, the martyr bears witness without speaking: he testifies through the sacrifice of his life, and after death via his image, multiply reproduced in paintings or photographs that become venerated icons for those who can testify to what he was.

In the Palestinian Occupied Territories, both those who die in suicide attacks and those who perish under enemy fire are described as *shahid*. Thus the Palestinian canon of martyrs merges at least two distinct figures—he who chooses death voluntarily, in the course of killing Israeli soldiers or civilians, and he who succumbs to Israeli army fire. While in terms of both dramatic visibility and polemic the figure of the suicide bomber dominates representations in the international public arena, it accounts for only a small proportion of the dead who are considered martyrs. During the first four years of the Second Intifada, 112 suicide attacks were committed, while 3,275 Palestinians were killed by the Israelis, including 173 women and 139 children under the age of twelve.[20] Only one Palestinian death in thirty therefore occurred in a suicide attack; the other twenty-nine resulted from Israeli fire. This demonstrates how, by conflating the person who sacrifices himself and the person who is killed, the term "martyr" links to a militant rhetoric that seeks to produce a single condition of heroic victims whose death, whether deliberately chosen or not, bears witness to their resistance to oppression. Moreover, such a shift has indeed taken place in recent years.

The massive overrepresentation of young men among the Palestinians who died during the Second Intifada is directly linked to the emergence and spread of the figure of the stone thrower, both victim and hero, who sacrifices himself and is killed: he exposes his body to Israeli gunfire.[21] What is operated through this figure is a shift in political subjectivation: where the balance of power is profoundly unequal, where negotiation has become impossible, where the path to the nation's future appears blocked, staking one's life becomes the ultimate possible mode of subjectivation in the political realm. The young boy—combatants were increasingly young and most of them were boys—who exposes his body to enemy bullets offers a dramatic representation of the powerlessness of Palestinian society.

Established figure of male adolescence, he becomes the political subject who bears witness to resistance.

However, the testimony of humanitarian psychiatry produces a very different image. A few months after the start of the revolt in the Territories, when there had already been 102 deaths among those younger than eighteen, 101 of them Palestinian and 1 Israeli, a French newspaper introduced its description of the conflict in Hebron as follows:[22] "The medical term for it is enuresis; in lay terms, wetting the bed. It is one of the most common conditions affecting young Palestinians since the beginning of the Intifada. The adolescents who throw stones at Israeli soldiers during the day, showing themselves more aggressive than their elders, often wet the bed at night, in an expression of the fear they repressed a few hours earlier. The symptom was revealed by mothers who confided in psychologists sent out by aid organizations."

This medical phenomenon is confirmed by one of these psychologists: "They have no other way of showing their fear," she explains. "In front of the soldiers, in front of their friends and even within their family, they have to present themselves as strong, almost adults. Wetting the bed is their way of showing that they are still children." Bed-wetting has become a commonplace of the discourse on the consequences of violence. Psychiatrists and psychologists have placed it alongside anxiety, stress, and nightmares as the most common expression of the climate of fear to which children are subjected, and the clearest manifestation of the regression it causes. The juxtaposition of the figure of the stone thrower and of the enuresis sufferer reveals the fragility of the young combatants: tragic heroes during the day, vulnerable patients at night. Given the importance of the appearance of virility in Palestinian youth culture,[23] this public revelation of intimate wounds that lead to shameful release of the sphincter shatters the image these youths are attempting to present. The discourse of mental health—which is based on an everyday experience—does indeed expose a reality that makes the condition of the adolescents more accessible to a Western audience: a vulnerable teenager generates a more consensual empathy than a provocative or violent youth. At the same time, it replaces the martyr subject with a neurotic subject, substituting the politics of justice proclaimed by the martyr with a politics of compassion, which has the sufferer as its object. It privileges the affect of the latter over the gesture of the former—an affect that links the victim and his audience, unlike the gesture that often divides them. Humanitarian subjectivation blurs the image of violence—or rather, through the offices of psychiatrists and psychologists, it requalifies it as trauma.

This is just one of the multiple figures produced around teenage males. The situation in Palestine is the object of discourses that are not merely politically contradictory but radically heterogeneous. It is this "discursive field," in which concurrent interpretations, especially those relating to children, meet, that needs to be engaged, rather than seeking to "distill an authentic Palestinian narrative of events."[24] In this battle of truths—the truth of the Israeli politician who condemns the hold of terrorist groups over teenagers and that of the Palestinian poet who sings the praises of the young combatants' resistance, the truth of the development worker who highlights their capacity to act for a better future and that of the lawyer who emphasizes violations of their human rights—we need to add a new voice: that of humanitarian psychiatrists and psychologists, which describes them as victims of trauma.

But this voice is not new in Palestine. As early as 1979, the Gaza Community Mental Health Program was established by a Palestinian psychiatrist trained at Oxford University who set up clinics and conducted surveys on posttraumatic stress disorder. A series of articles published in international journals, and studies made available online on the program's website, publicized statistics relating to the psychic consequences of the conflict on the Palestinian people. One of the studies established that, in a random sample of adolescents aged between ten and nineteen, 83% had witnessed shootings and 62% had seen a neighbor or relative injured or killed, 33% were suffering from posttraumatic stress serious enough to require treatment, and 65% showed moderate or minor psychological disturbance.[25] The testimony of Médecins Sans Frontières is quite distinct, however, preferring fragments of narrative to statistics, and the experience of trauma reported in everyday language to posttraumatic stress disorder as a diagnostic category; the aim is to move people via stories in which aid workers place themselves center stage as privileged witnesses of the suffering of an oppressed people. The field observations of psychiatrists and psychologists over several months were compiled in the *Palestinian Chronicles*,[26] a document that was translated into several languages and distributed in many countries, including Israel and Palestine.

These chronicles are a testimony of undefined status. Straddling a line between diagnosis and protest, pathology and experience, the narratives mix the clinical with the political. They do, of course, make reference to anxiety, depression, stress, trauma—and to enuresis among children. Very quickly, however, attention turns to the local situation, the family history, the biographical details, daily life, as if psychological disorders could not express clearly enough what Palestinians are enduring. Take the example of Ibrahim, who had been arrested, beaten, and released by Israeli soldiers some time earlier: he is described as "suffering from posttraumatic stress," but immediately after this description comes the following:

> He no longer does anything during the day. He stays in bed, smokes and ponders revenge. He is still recovering physically from the beating he received, but also presents symptoms of psychological trauma. He feels weak, complains of headaches. He says he will never forget those who beat him. He talks of how his application to join the police force was rejected, forcing him to work in the colonies, and hence for the Israelis. He believes his friends think he is a traitor. His sense of injustice is further fed by a love affair, which ended badly. In the evening he talks with his group of friends, from whom he feels excluded.

The diagnosis is therefore simply a pretext for a description of suffering that mixes sociohistorical conditions with personal events, idleness and work, love and friends—almost an ethnographic account.

Moreover, on close reading of these narratives it becomes clear that often the trauma does not bear witness to what it is intended to—the violence of war. We learn that the "distress related to posttraumatic stress" suffered by a little boy results from a serious fall from the terrace of his house. Another who, we are told, stammers "following a traumatic event" turns out to have been frightened by a dog when he was younger. In many of the adults, the posttraumatic stress disorders observed actually derive from earlier events, often unrelated to the conflict, and are hence less probative than the authors would like. They consequently fall back on conjecture, as with this visit to a family shut up in a house that had come under Israeli fire: "Despite the lull, many people seem to have difficulty relaxing and returning to normal life. We could be seeing the first signs of trauma here. If this is the case, we expect to see symptoms of this type in the near future." Similarly, following a demolition operation in which approximately forty homes were destroyed and their inhabitants prevented from returning to collect their belongings: "Winding our way through the narrow streets, we consider the psychological injuries which have been inflicted. How many will escape without too much psychological damage? And will it be this cold tomorrow? Will it rain again?" In an unwitting imitation of Baudelaire's correspondence, the authors attempt to marry psychological landscape and weather conditions to engender a sort of depressive mood.

Rather than offering evidence to back up diagnoses, the chronicles therefore communicate impressions and affects that go beyond the tragic scenes they report and are felt equally by local people and by aid workers. The reaction of a teenager after an attack on his school in Hebron is described: "He has not yet got over the shock of seeing seven of his schoolmates burned when soldiers threw a bomb into the playground. He hardly speaks of the event, gazing vacantly towards the hillside of Abousina which he sees being bombed." A psychologist expresses his feelings at seeing a bulldozer destroy greenhouses, gardens, wells, and homes in Gaza: "It's enormous. It moves forwards and backwards, tearing out trees. I'm scared. Everyone is scared. A plane breaks the sound barrier and terror prevails. All the people who have been working this land for decades are seeing their work destroyed. A father tells us how, when he comes home this evening and tells his children there is nothing left, they will cry. We leave sick at heart. When we return, the landscape will be very different." Emotion may also be conveyed through more muted description. Following the bombing of a home in Rafah: "In the destruction, a man who didn't have time to flee was thrown into his neighbor's house. It is a traumatic sight for the latter, who is the first to discover him. The body is so mutilated that only the clothes identify him." Clearly, the adjective "traumatic" here describes an affect rather than a diagnosis. The aim of the testimony of humanitarian psychiatry is first and foremost to evoke, in ordinary language, the experience of state brutality.

Through a striking reorientation, what thus emerges repeatedly in the notes of the mental health professionals is a political account of violence rather than a clinical account of trauma. The tone shifts from suffering to anger. Despair reverses anxiety: whereas anxiety is expressed via the inability to act, despair is manifested in the gesture of rebellion. One sign of this shift is that many of the fragments of life recounted in these narratives end with the same suggestion: the only future lies in death—a death that is chosen. A fourteen-year-old girl who still has a bullet lodged in her stomach from when she was shot at her home tells of her plans: "She would have liked to be a martyr, she says, but maybe she'll end being a doctor." Little girls of ten chat with a member of the aid team: "We talk about what they want to do when they grow up: 'Kill myself,' says one of them." In the narratives, all the children's drawings depict "martyrs," and most of the adolescents' accounts also refer to them. "The doctrine of martyrdom justifies the scandal of a meaningless death, of an execution that could only appear as absurd," writes Giorgio Agamben of the early Christians.[27] Beyond the psychological disorders they diagnosed to provide an account of the effects of the conflict, psychiatrists and psychologists were rediscovering this truth in the Palestinian Occupied Territories, but with a shift in focus: for children with no schooling, parents with no jobs, families with no home, it was life that was meaningless, and death that gave it back some meaning. A decidedly tragic reading, in which testimony meets the canon of martyrs in the etymological confusion of the *martus*, the witness becoming a martyr.

This almost unconscious return to the profound sources of the violence probably explains the virulence of the reactions to these chronicles among Israelis and pro-Israeli donors to Médecins Sans Frontières.[28] But for the members of this organization confronted with the experience of the Second Intifada, to testify in the name of the Palestinians was to tell that truth whereby death gives back meaning to a life that has become unlivable. Here we end up far from trauma, where subjectivation is located in the arena of violence. Noticeably, the use that Médecins du Monde made of testimony, in the same region, with the same tools and the same specialists, was yet very different.

THE END OF HISTORY

Philology offers one final witness figure—that of the Greek *histor*.[29] This witness has not necessarily observed the event that has led to him being summoned (he testifies on the basis of what he has heard, not what he has seen), nor is he required to decide between the two conflicting versions (he acts as guarantor for what is agreed between the two parties). Herodotus views the work of the historian as an extension of this role, being both an inquiry based on oral testimony gathered from the accounts of others and an attempt to maintain equal distance from the two sides of the event narrated. This witness must consequently reveal his sources and strive for impartiality.

The escalation and radicalization of the Israeli-Palestinian conflict render this position particularly delicate. Historians—and analysts in general—are easily identified as being on one side or the other. Humanitarian organizations are obviously not in the business of writing history: in principle their role is not to make statements about the past, but to intervene in the present. Nevertheless, once they decide to testify publicly to what they know, the issues they come up against are not so far removed from those encountered by historians. Like the latter, aid workers do not observe what they report, but rather communicate what they are told (and not without converting it into a form suited to the cause they seek to defend); their role is not to take sides, and they profess neutrality (a condition of their very intervention in conflict situations, as defined in their charters). However, aid workers differ from historians in two respects.

First, when they bear witness it is in the register of emotion: they seek to persuade rather than explain, aiming to stimulate action rather than interpret facts. Second, while they attempt to remain impartial, they add that their role is to take the side of the victims: in their way they are creating a history of the vanquished. The two elements that make up the (relatively) unique role of aid workers are bound together: it is because they speak of (and for) victims that they can (and feel entitled to) make use of the emotional register. The suffering of the victims justifies the appeal to affects.

In the recent history of humanitarian intervention, there has frequently been an implicit choice of victims on only one side of the conflict: Biafrans but not Nigerians, Misquitos but not Nicaraguans, Afghans rather than Soviet soldiers, Kosovars rather than Serbs, Timorese but not Indonesians, Chechens but not Russians, Iraqi civilians rather than U.S. troops. The origin of the conflict, the balance of power between the parties involved, and above all the representation of the situation in the Western public arena imply that it generally appears self-evident who the victims are. However, this is not always the case. We know, for example, that in 1979 internal ideological battles were fought within the humanitarian movement before the Vietnamese boat people fleeing the Communist regime were recognized by Médecins Sans Frontières as victims, and therefore, more specifically, worthy of aid. It was this crucial moment, and the watchword that arose from it, that formed the basis for Médecins du Monde's work in Palestine: "There are no good or bad victims," reads the cover of the report *Israeli and Palestinian Civilian Victims of an Unending Conflict*.[30] The report's introduction returns to this leitmotif, recalling its origin in the tragedy of the boat people, and goes on to list the conflicts in which Médecins du Monde has refused to take sides, concluding: "There are no good or bad victims. These principles also apply to the civilian populations in the Israeli-Palestinian conflict." The conclusion seems to go without saying: like the Greek *histor*, the humanitarian witness must do justice to both parties. However, the statement implies a real change in direction in the work of these international organizations, which until that point had intervened solely in the Palestinian Territories, on the grounds that their inhabitants were subject to occupation and oppression. Never had anyone pleaded, for instance, in favor of the Serbs bombed by NATO aircraft or the Russians killed in Chechen attacks. Within Médecins du Monde, the reorientation did not come without clashes, and what is portrayed as self-evident in the published report was not seen as such by all its members.

Indeed, this report followed an earlier one, published the previous year. The outcome of a joint investigative mission by Médecins du Monde and the International Federation for Human Rights, this first report focused on violations of international humanitarian law and human rights by the Israeli army in Palestine. It described "obstacles to provision of assistance to the sick," "ill-treatment of the wounded," "deaths and injuries resulting from the indiscriminate and disproportionate use of force," "humiliating and degrading treatment amounting to an attack on human dignity," the "use of human shields," "arbitrary and mass arrests," the "conditions of detention and treatment of detainees," the "destruction of buildings and property, both private and public," and other abuses. The report included many testimonies as evidence to support its analysis. These were extremely detailed and sought to attest to the factual truth: eyewitnesses were called, written documents were produced, material evidence such as bullets and X-rays was sought. For example, this account of events that occurred in the Askar refugee camp illustrates the "deliberate assaults on life and bodily integrity":

> The story has been reported in a newspaper article. The three witnesses were interviewed by the team and their injuries examined. On April 8, at 11.00 in the morning, Shaninaz, six months pregnant, was cleaning the stairs. Her husband Samer heard shots. He ran into the living room and saw his four children and his wife run in. Alha, aged four, had been hit. Blood was coming out of his mouth. His mother picked him up and held him out in front of her, trying to come out of the house to alert the Israeli soldiers posted 50 meters [160 feet] from the house. A soldier shot at her. A bullet hit her in the left groin area. She fell, the child falling with her. Samer was just behind her.

Records from the hospital, where the mother and child were operated on and where the mother underwent an emergency Caesarian section, are also presented. The report concludes by insisting on the responsibility of the Israeli state and its army and calling for "a just and immediate peace in the Middle East," adding that this cannot be achieved "without an end to the Israeli occupation and without the guarantee of security for Israel and the Israelis." Facts take precedence over affects; juridical qualification is preferred to invocation of emotion. This testimony produces a subject in law.

However, tensions arose within the organization following the publication of this document, which some believed was excessively harsh toward Israel. At a meeting of the Administration Board, several current and former presidents spoke of the need to "rebalance" its approach. They were immediately regarded as adopting this position for reasons of religious affinity. For the first time in its history, Médecins du Monde, in spite of its universalistic principles, found itself divided along what were imagined to be sectarian lines. In this respect it did not escape the general polarization of the debate in French society, and the suspicion that fell on anyone who took a stand with regard to the Israeli-Palestinian conflict, particularly during the Second Intifada.

The report published the following year was in two parts: the first reprinted the report on Israeli violations of humanitarian law, while the second presented a new document on Palestinian attacks. Although the International Federation for Human Rights refused to collaborate on this mission, Médecins du Monde imagined a juridical neologism: to avoid using the term "suicide bombing," which places the emphasis on the attackers rather than the victims, or "kamikaze operation," which suggests military objectives, they proposed to speak of "democidal" attacks in order to indicate that the targets were civilians, and extended the term by describing various kinds of violence against civilians as "democidal" acts. Yet, unlike the first report, most of the second was concerned not with acts but with their victims. And the focus was on the psychological rather than physical consequences of the attacks, particularly in terms of posttraumatic stress disorder, many examples of which are described in detail. One illustration is the case of David, a nurse who treated the wounded after attacks: "He presents a total and profound reorganization of his personality polarized around the traumatic event and hardened into a chronic trauma neurosis. During the interview he showed neurovegetative symptoms, extreme emotional sensitivity and psychomotor reactions. He devoted much of his account to his call for a status of attack victim, which he sees as insufficiently recognized by the medical committee for sickness benefit."

The recourse to the concept of trauma made it possible to expand the range of victims considerably: in addition to the wounded and immediate witnesses to attacks, they included those "involved"—family, friends, neighbors, school classmates, work colleagues, and even "society in general," starting with health professionals and social workers but also including bus drivers and police officers. Potentially the entire Israeli population was susceptible to suffering from posttraumatic symptoms. But the further removed an individual was from the attack, the less clinical the description: the focus is on recounting an experience rather than confirming a diagnosis. A woman living in Jerusalem described the effects of attacks she had seen on television: "My heart is bleeding, I'm flayed alive. I try to protect myself, I don't look at the pictures and I don't want to see the exact details." The narrative is in the first person: it is the victim who is expressing herself, and the focus is on affects rather than facts. In contrast to the previous document, this testimony produces a subject of suffering.

An inversion has therefore occurred between the two reports published in this single volume. Political subjectivation has shifted from a demand for justice to the exhibition of pain. Between the two, trauma has been introduced both as psychiatric category and as shared experience. Absent from the first report, it is ubiquitous in the second. But the combined claim of consistency and balance made by Médecins du Monde's senior management actually convinced few within the organization. To begin with, the second part of the document was devised only after the event, to correct the impression of strong criticism of Israel created in the first part. Furthermore, the juridical qualification presented in the first report had no equivalent in the medical-psychological analysis of the second report. Certainly the final evaluation seems to portray the crimes on the same level: war crimes on the part of Israelis who were guilty of violations of international humanitarian and human rights law against the Palestinian population; war crime and crimes against humanity on the part of the Palestinians who committed attacks against Israeli soldiers and civilians. But in the eyes of many within Médecins du Monde, desperate attacks perpetrated by individuals in a context of resistance to oppression could not carry the same juridical and even political significance as the abuses coldly committed by the army of an occupying power.

Considering the situation as symmetrical meant suspending all political perspective—which is precisely what the cartographic representation of the conflict in the two reports suggested. In the 2002 document on Israeli actions, the map uses contrasting colors to show the scattered plots of territory administered by the Palestinian Authority and their borders under the 1994 and 1995 agreements. In the 2003 report on Palestinian attacks, the map, entirely blank, shows only the names of places where these events took place, marked by little lightning flashes. The political geography of the first map is therefore replaced by the naked violence of the second. Paradoxically, many interpreted the authors' attempt to treat all crimes and victims equally as a bias, given the factual asymmetry of the respective situations, and it resulted in harsh criticism, especially from the teams in the field. At the point when the aim was to proclaim the neutrality of the *histor*, the polemical figure of the *martus* therefore reappeared. In the process the witness, the *auctor*, had lost some of his authority.

This symmetrical approach was made possible only by positing equivalence between victims: on one side, Palestinian victims of the Israeli army, and on the other, Israeli victims of Palestinian bombs. This principle of equivalence holds only if the debate is restricted to counting the dead and wounded, effectively reducing the individuals to their physical body, or if the focus is placed on hardship and suffering, through a limitless extension of the persons into their narrated experience. The Palestinian mother weeping for a son who has been shot dead by the Israelis can in this way share her pain with the Israeli mother mourning her child killed in a Palestinian attack. Some of the peace initiatives in the Israeli-Palestinian conflict have in fact been built exactly on this basis by drawing together these tragic ordeals: in other words, the equivalence of victims is not an artificial device created by aid workers but a principle that local actors work to make operative. From the point of view of the publicly disseminated testimony, however, it is clear that attention focused exclusively on experiences determines and limits political subjectivities, and that such expressions erase individual and collective histories. Both the biographical and the nationalist narratives tend to focus on the trauma, understood well beyond its psychiatric definition. The singularity of trajectories and situations as well as the specificity of processes and issues are erased: camp and kibbutz, refugee and citizen, occupied and occupier become identical in a "lived experience" of pain that is supposed to be shared by all.

One cannot underestimate the performative—and potentially positive—effect of this way of speaking of violence, in the Israeli-Palestinian conflict as elsewhere.[31] Images have real-world implications: to this extent, the subjectivation is political. But one needs also to consider the restriction imposed by a testimony that reduces violence to trauma and the subject to victim.[32] What is not said about the historical situations in which deaths and sufferings are set when the focus is placed entirely on the simple fact of dying or suffering? And how much of the intelligibility of the conflict is obscured at the moment when one speaks of the trauma and the victim? These are questions one must ask about humanitarian testimony on violence in the conflict. And the answer may be that what is lost in this translation—through which the humanitarian witness claims the position of the ancient *histor*—is, precisely, history.

The witness has become a key political figure of our time. From the survivors of the Nazi camps relating the horror of the exterminating machine to guests on television talk shows recounting intimate experiences, the burgeoning importance of testimony in the portrayal of violence in the contemporary public arena has been widely noted. However, this witness figure is much less homogeneous than is often suggested. Many have raced to conclusions about the subjectivation of pure victims that this witness figure was deemed univocally to produce. The philological detour has operated as a heuristic here, returning to the genealogies of the witness: from

testis to *superstes*, from *martus* to *histor*, what we have in fact is a configuration of testimony constituted through multiple witness figures, from
observer to survivor, from involved party to guarantor of truth. What is
more, ethnographic study of the production of humanitarian testimony in
a particular context, the Israeli-Palestinian conflict, has allowed us to understand the relationships and shifts between the different witness figures,
as well as the polysemy and instability of the configuration of testimony:
the stone thrower turned trauma victim, or the sufferer becoming a candidate for martyrdom; third-person testimony gives way to first-person
narrative while the *auctor* imposes his authority.

Humanitarian testimony occupies a unique position in the space thus
described. The witness becomes a spokesperson for the victim. In contrast
to the traditional arrangement, where witnesses speak for themselves or
those close to them, in a court of law or before a microphone or camera,
humanitarian workers speak in the name of those who are assumed not to
have access to the public arena. In so doing they illuminate, transform,
simplify, and dramatize the words of those they represent, in line with
their ultimate objective, which is not so much to reconstitute an experience as to construct a cause. This construction is based on the legitimate
principles of humanitarian intervention: the defense of victims and the
appeal to emotions. Of course, aid organizations are not the only actors
who speak in the name of the humiliated and the insulted, but on a global
scale they are now probably seen as the most legitimate for this purpose,
alongside the legal institutions such as international tribunals. It would
be interesting to contrast these new actors and their unprecedented reper-
toires of action with the religious or revolutionary movements that—in
other times—also spoke in the name of those vanquished by history.

In the case of humanitarianism, the defense of victims combined with
the appeal to emotion has long resulted in the body being used as the pre-
eminent site of manifestation of violence and the object best placed to demonstrate suffering. The recent introduction of psychiatry and psychology,
both as languages and as professions, has paved the way for the establishment of other ways of considering victims and pleading their cause. It might
have been imagined that trauma, as the psychic trace of violence, and posttraumatic stress disorder, as the diagnostic translation of violence, would
provide a new dimension for humanitarian testimony. My study of Médecins Sans Frontières and Médecins du Monde throws this assumption into
question. Admittedly, reference is made to these categories, but the often precarious conditions in which observations are gathered, the diversity of experiences encountered in the field, the resistance to an imported model seen as

too rigid, and above all the ethos of actors who are much more committed to the cause of victims than to the production of diagnoses imply that the testimony of humanitarian psychiatrists and psychologists derives less from clinical evaluation than from moral judgment. It is because they see people as victims of a violent situation that they wish to bear witness to its psychic consequences, and even when they do speak of trauma, it is often in the generic sense. The discourse produced articulates affects rather than symptoms and, via a mechanism of projection that is always aroused in championing a cause, says as much about the speaker as about the victim in whose name he or she speaks. There is thus a double paradox in the testimony of humanitarian psychiatry. On the one hand, it refers less to clinical expertise in trauma than to the common understanding of suffering. On the other, it indicates more about the moral sentiment of the witness than about the experience of the victim.

Political subjectivation as I have outlined it here is related to this representation of victims and their cause. On both the Palestinian and the Israeli sides, social agents tend to construct their presence in the public arena in terms of affects. Trauma, to which claim is increasingly laid, largely escapes from the confines of its psychiatric definition to articulate a much less clearly defined psychological condition. From this point of view, the victims are not only rhetorical figures; they also become political subjects. To say this is in no way to imply a presumption that individuals consider themselves victims. Such a generalization, which is often made, has little meaning on the empirical level, for not only do experiences vary but above all they remain largely inaccessible to ethnographic investigation: What do we know about what people facing these violent situations think and feel? However, we can say that humanitarian testimony contributes to forming victim subjectivities to which social agents must make reference, including when they seek to make a demand for justice heard—in other words, precisely when they wish to move beyond the logic of compassion. Thus political subjectivation passes through a twofold operation in which the rules of the game are imposed (humanitarian psychiatry defines a legitimate way of presenting one's cause in the language of trauma and victimhood) and through which these rules can be appropriated or even diverted (local actors adopt but adapt the vocabulary and representation they have not chosen but of which they still can make use). Humanitarianism was tending to produce a form of subjectivity devoid of historical subject. Palestinians took over this subjectivity precisely in order to demand what they were being denied: the status of political subjects.

9. Hierarchies of Humanity

Intervening in International Conflicts

> Since man no longer believes that a God is guiding the destinies of the world as a whole, or that, despite all apparent twists, the path of mankind is leading somewhere glorious, men must set themselves ecumenical goals, embracing the whole earth.
>
> FRIEDRICH NIETZSCHE, *Human, All Too Human*

When the Czech president and the British prime minister described the NATO bombing of Kosovo, during spring 1999, as a humanitarian act, many analysts considered that a threshold had been crossed in the definition of just wars.[1] The subsequent Western army interventions in Afghanistan in 2001 and Iraq in 2003 confirmed this impression, demonstrating that humanitarian language could be mobilized at the heart of military operations. This development manifested a phenomenon that had been emerging over the preceding two decades. Humanitarian action has in fact become a major modality and a dominant frame of reference for Western political intervention in scenes of misfortune throughout the world, whether they involve armed conflict or natural disasters, or their more or less direct consequences in the form of epidemics, famines, disability, or trauma.[2] Previously the prerogative of nongovernmental organizations and intergovernmental bodies, humanitarianism has also become a policy instituted at state level, with many countries implementing their own activities within this domain (for example, the Secretariat of State for Humanitarian Action in France, and the Overseas Development Administration in the United Kingdom). A form of governmentality that its supporters view as a substitute to the order of Cold War realpolitik is being deployed throughout the globe. The new language of humanitarianism produces a distinct intelligibility regarding world affairs and a particular form of collective experience. The way that armed interventions such as those in Somalia are justified and international crises like Darfur are qualified, how the part played by military peacekeepers in the massacre of Srebrenica is scrutinized and the management of refugee camps in the African Great Lakes region is examined, and ultimately our assessment of international policy itself, have been profoundly altered by the repertoire of images and actions supplied by the humanitarian movement.

One common interpretation of this new configuration tends to distinguish and contrast politics and humanitarianism, declaring that the latter is gradually replacing the former, or even announcing the advent of humanitarianism and the end of politics. "Humanitarianism is not a political issue, and it should remain apart from political maneuvering," asserts Rony Brauman, a former president of Médecins Sans Frontières.[3] Giorgio Agamben offers a still more radical version of this thesis, arguing that "the separation between humanitarianism and politics that we are experiencing today is the extreme phase of the separation of the rights of man from the rights of the citizen."[4] Yet one may doubt whether there exists, in our society or any other, a space devoid of politics or even a space outside politics. Everything suggests, on the contrary, that rather than becoming separate, humanitarianism and politics are tending to merge—in other words, humanitarianism is indeed a politics. In France particularly, three former presidents or vice presidents of Médecins Sans Frontières have been appointed ministers; several have been elected to political office, and others have become high-level civil servants—not only in the traditional aid sector but also in health and social welfare. Conversely, former ministers of social affairs or of health have become presidents of large organizations such as Action contre la faim (Action against Hunger) and the French Red Cross.[5] At the international level the process is even more marked: since the Rwandan genocide and the French army's belated Operation Turquoise, Western military action in scenes of disaster and conflict has been conducted under the banner of humanitarianism, and increasingly insistent efforts are being made to bring nongovernmental organizations on board. When they intervened in Kosovo and Iraq, the governments allied respectively within NATO and around the United States spoke of humanitarian emergency, thus confirming that the legitimacy of interventions had shifted from the legal realm (since they did not have the support of the United Nations) to the moral sphere—the defense of human rights and even, more restrictively and more specifically, of humanitarian law. We can speak of the humanitarianization of international crisis management and the parallel politicization of the nongovernmental humanitarian field. This evolution has been criticized by the humanitarian movement, which sees in it a loss of its moral purity or simply of its independence, but the larger implications for the politics of life are less clearly perceived: they nevertheless lie, as we shall now see, at the heart of the tensions that divide nongovernmental organizations.

On March 28, 2003, as on the last Friday of every month, the Administration Board of Médecins Sans Frontières met between 5:00 and 11:00 p.m., at the organization's headquarters on the first floor of a Parisian building situated near La Bastille. On that particular evening a heady atmosphere of anticipation and excitement reigned. There was the customary overview of the situation in a number of "missions" in various parts of the world, followed by a more in-depth examination, with discussion of several specific topics relating to the running of the organization and its activities. The construction of the "international movement"—the network of branches in twenty countries, six of which were actually in a position to conduct operations, which strives to ensure a coherence of identity and policy in the work of each national body beyond the specifics of local history and culture—was discussed. The Drugs for Neglected Diseases Initiative (DNDi) was also addressed: this was a unique program initiated two years earlier in order to establish, in international collaboration with private foundations and public partners, an activity of research and development for drug treatments deemed unprofitable because of the poverty of the Third World patients who needed them.

The monthly meetings of the Administration Board are open to the public. All members of the organization can participate, including the staff. Usually, attendance gradually thins out as the evening wears on. But on that March 28, many stayed, waiting for the last item on the agenda. The subject was the state of operations in Iraq. Eight days earlier, U.S. and British troops had begun their bombardment of the country, ending the long run-up to a war that was declared in a climate of growing international tension and division. Médecins Sans Frontières had a complex history with the Iraqi state, having refused to aid earlier—even when the United Nations Children's Fund (UNICEF) was publishing the most alarming statistics about the hundreds of thousands of children dying as a result of the international embargo—so as to avoid succumbing to what it considered to be the manipulation of international humanitarian sentiment by the criminal Baathist regime. Nevertheless, the organization decided, after long and difficult deliberations on its Executive Committee, to maintain a team of six people in Baghdad during the onset of the war. According to the head of programs in Paris:[6]

> Intervening in a war zone is not easy. Six expatriate volunteers are working in one of the thirty-two hospitals in the city. Basic needs have been secured (stocks of water, food, drugs, sandbags), they keep travel to a minimum, and they are very careful to identify themselves to the two sides. But everyone is aware of the risk. After evaluating the

situation in the field, a reduced team decided to stay. Analyzing the balance of risk and action, we felt our presence was appropriate.

Should the six members of Médecins Sans Frontières then remain there, given the danger they would face both from the Iraqi regime and its cornered military and from the American army and its rain of bombs, and given that their presence was likely to be of limited efficacy, considering the extensive Iraqi health care facilities available in Baghdad? Should the lives of aid workers be risked to save other lives among local populations? The discussion that arose about the presence of the team in Iraq was, by all accounts, the most intense debate the organization had experienced in recent years. However, it skirted the most painful truth—the ontological inequality underlying this transaction in human lives, between those that are imperiled and those that are saved.

I take this scene as a starting point for raising the question of humanitarian action in terms of the politics of life that underlie it.[7] What I term politics of life are politics that bring into play differentiated meanings and values of human lives. These politics are distinct from biopolitics as defined by Michel Foucault, who analyzes the technologies applied rather than meanings and values, and who is interested more in populations than in lives.[8] Humanitarian action is indeed a biopolitics in the sense that it uses techniques of management of populations in setting up refugee camps, establishing protected aid corridors, making use of modes of communication around public testimony to abuses perpetrated, and conducting epidemiological studies of infectious diseases, malnutrition, trauma, and even violations of the laws of war. But humanitarian action is also a politics of life in the sense that, first, it takes as its object the saving of lives, which presupposes not only risking others but also selecting those that have priority for being saved (for example, when drug supplies are insufficient); and second, it champions causes publicly, which implies not only neglecting other ones but also constructing them by choosing the best way of representing the populations assisted (for instance, as victims rather than resistance fighters).

Biopolitics and politics of life are therefore neither superimposed on one another nor opposed to one another. This study focuses on the latter. In the politics of life, moral issues become central. What kind of life is at stake, explicitly or implicitly, in humanitarian intervention? This is the question that interests me here. My aim is not to take an overview or pronounce judgments,[9] but to enter as it were the heart of humanitarian activity, to analyze the consequences of choices made and practices implemented—in short, to follow humanitarian logic to its end.[10] I explore a triple lifeline: that which runs between the sacrificeable lives of populations and the freely sacrificed lives of aid workers; that which separates the sacred lives of Western soldiers from the sacrificeable lives of local civilians; and finally, that which distinguishes the valued lives of expatriate volunteers from the devalued lives of local staff. All three can have tragic consequences. Thus I attempt to identify the features of an ontological inequality that contravenes the principle of common humanity defended by humanitarianism by producing implicit hierarchies. I do so by recourse to a traditional dramaturgical form with its unities of place, time, and action, returning to the scene that took place at the beginning of the Iraq War.

AN ETHICS IN ACTION

During the months leading up to the 2003 Iraq War, Médecins Sans Frontières, like many other humanitarian organizations, undertook "exploratory missions" in Iraq and neighboring countries with the aim of predicting the consequences of military intervention, in terms both of injured and sick within Iraq and refugees outside the country.[11] In particular, delicate negotiations were conducted with the Iraqi Ministry of Health and the Red Crescent to establish an official framework for the mission so as to obtain the necessary work permits and ensure independent operation. The memo issued by Médecins Sans Frontières on March 11, 2003, makes reference to two proposals that were agreed to by both sides and gave the organization this mandate: assist in a hospital in the south of Baghdad, and take responsibility for the care of a potential twenty million displaced people. But in the days following the signing of this agreement, the Iraqi authorities proved unwilling to keep their side of the contract, forbidding the volunteers from entering hospitals to evaluate the health situation.

On March 18, U.S. president George W. Bush issued a solemn appeal to Saddam Hussein, calling on him to leave Iraq within forty-eight hours. As the last flights evacuating the expatriate staff of international agencies and nongovernmental organizations were leaving Baghdad, six members of Médecins Sans Frontières—including a surgeon, an anesthetist, and a general practitioner—decided to remain despite the imminent danger. This small group included one of the organization's most public figures, the president of the international movement. But they were not the only ones to have made that choice: in addition to the International Committee of the Red Cross, Première Urgence and Caritas maintained a reduced presence. On March 20, U.S. and British troops launched their attack and the bombing of the Iraqi capital began. Intense and intermittent, it lasted several days, during which Médecins Sans Frontières' team in Baghdad had very little chance of leaving their hotel. Several bombs fell nearby, a brutal reminder of the reality and proximity of the danger. However, the hospital where they were supposed to work received only a handful of patients with minor injuries, for which they supplied some surgical equipment. The mission coordinator in Paris reported to the Administration Board: "At the moment the team feels that it is not very useful, but it is preparing for what may come."

This landscape of risk and uncertainty formed the backdrop for what the minutes of the March 28 Administration Board meeting call a "debate on the controversial decision to establish a team in Baghdad" within the French branch of the organization.[12] There was a lively discussion about the safety of the team, as there had been a few days earlier at the meeting of the Executive Committee, which had taken the decision to stay in Iraq. Conflicting opinions were expressed and deep divisions emerged as to whether it was justified to maintain a humanitarian presence in this context: the issues raised concerned both the evaluation of the danger and the anticipated efficacy of the intervention. As the president, who was himself in favor of the team staying, indicated, the stake was the same in every situation of humanitarian intervention: for those who are on site, once the conflict is under way, "there is no guaranteed emergency exit," he said, and this is one of "the occupational hazards of our profession." Remaining in a country at war, he suggested, always bore a cost, if not in actual human losses, then at least in terms of the possibility of casualties. Nevertheless, he concluded that "the level of risk we run in Baghdad does not seem any greater than in other places where we operate," pointing out that "we have many teams in danger zones." Some on the Administration Board were less sanguine about the peril to which the local team was exposed and its psychological capacity to deal with it. But the issue of security, which was highlighted in the debate, was obviously overshadowed by another, even more difficult, question: Why stay? If the risks were high, what was their justification? What use were members if they were confined to a dangerous place? It was the usefulness of the mission that generated the most heated exchanges.

Some argued that wherever in the world Médecins Sans Frontières volunteers exposed themselves to objective danger, they did so to bring "real, concrete assistance." In the case of Iraq, the potential contribution of a team of three medical doctors was obviously modest compared with the hundreds of health professionals working in the thirty-five hospitals in Baghdad, or even, within the specific context of the team's activity, compared with the sixty physicians, surgeons, and anesthetists, with seventeen operating theaters, in the sole hospital where the team planned to offer assistance. Nevertheless, efficacy was the officially accepted justification for the decision to stay. According to the president: "The reason we have representatives in Baghdad is so that they can bring aid. That is the criterion on which we based our decision. We send teams when we think they can offer concrete help, not just in the name of an ideal. That needs to be stated clearly and unambiguously." Many, however, remained unconvinced, particularly given the small number of staff relative to the casualties that were anticipated. One long-standing member of the organization offered his own interpretation on this point, relativizing the efficacy but defending a principle: "It is part of our charter to be present in war zones. But war surgery itself is inefficient, because it saves only ten percent more people than if there were no intervention. The question therefore is, to be or not to be there? And my answer is: if we were not there, I would wonder why." Weighing the various arguments, one administrator underlined: "That's the nub of it—the constant dialogue between the principles in our charter and genuine efficacy. Some put more emphasis on the principles, others on efficacy; you often find that within the teams." Finally, as the atmosphere of the discussion became increasingly tense, a young member of the staff attempted some kind of synthesis between the logic of efficacy and that of principles: "It seems to me," he said, "that what Médecins Sans Frontières represents is an ethics in action. It's impossible to separate the two, and we are always aware of the limits of our activity. What is part of our principles is that each life saved counts, and that some actions save lives. I think that in Baghdad that space will emerge very soon." His diagnosis was probably correct, but not his prognosis: events would cruelly prove him wrong.

Four days after this meeting, two of the six members who had remained in Baghdad, together with their driver, were taken by agents of the Iraqi intelligence service to an unidentified location. For more than one week there was no news of them. Médecins Sans Frontières refrained from describing them publicly as hostages or releasing their names to the press, in order to avoid any additional risk. Anxiety mounted within the organization, as Western troops approached, conditions in Baghdad grew increasingly unsafe, and finally the hospital where the team had hoped to work was looted, leaving the four volunteers who were still at liberty with no possibility of action. The coordinator of the Iraq mission in France deplored the absurdity of the situation in a memo dated April 10: "We have had to suspend our activities at the very moment when Baghdad's hospitals are overrun with casualties." After being held for nine days, the two volunteers and the driver were freed. Seventy-two hours later, U.S. and British troops occupied the center of Baghdad. Humanitarian aid poured in, especially from organizations that had accumulated staff and equipment on the other side of the border in expectation of refugees who never arrived. It seemed obvious that Médecins Sans Frontières was now able to reach its hospital and finally provide real assistance to the victims of the war, who were rapidly increasing in number.

On April 28, however, the French branch of the organization made the decision to leave Iraq—before it had even started its humanitarian work. Having come to help "populations at risk," at a time when many had decided to remain out of a country deemed much too dangerous, the team was therefore leaving without having been able to intervene, just when most others, including the Belgian and Dutch branches, were choosing to return or to stay. This retreat was not understood by those who had taken serious risks during the bombing and found themselves summoned home precisely when serious needs were emerging. The French team thus left disillusioned. Meanwhile, in the Paris headquarters, the official position was to deride other aid organizations that, it was claimed, had been too ready to exaggerate the seriousness of the situation in order to sensitize their donors. "Desperately seeking humanitarian crisis," one former president of Médecins Sans Frontières and a desk coordinator commented ironically, in an article published a few months later. "No humanitarian crisis in Iraq," declared the president of the organization in a French daily newspaper.[13] These comments seemed to make little case of the other two branches of the organization that had remained.

Even among the French members, consensus did not exist. Bernard Calas, the head of the mission and one of the hostages, noted in the report produced for the organization's General Assembly in May 2003: "The French branch's decision to leave Baghdad seemed to me very hasty, and I think was based on debatable arguments constructed in order to justify the decision. As if the end of the war would automatically be followed by a period of reconstruction. Because we were unable to define this crisis, we dismissed it, without going further into the needs of the people and the alternatives of negotiation and speaking out. Ironically, you could say we've come full circle and owing to lack of foresight, our intervention was marked from beginning to end by hasty decisions." His analysis was severe, but it is true that by the end of this operation, even though it conformed to the spirit and letter of the organization's charter, which states that members "provide assistance to populations in distress" and "understand the risks and dangers of the missions they carry out," Médecins Sans Frontières certainly did not appear to have had the efficacy invoked as the justification for maintaining a team in Baghdad, and in particular had not "saved lives" as they anticipated. But what merits attention, more than this relative "failure," which was in the end recognized as such,[14] are the emotions this mission aroused within the Executive Committee as well as the Administration Board.

THE SENSE OF SACRIFICE

If we accept the hypothesis that crisis in an institution erupts when a situation touches directly on its core principles, we then need to examine what underlies the conflict about the decision to remain in Iraq. In this confrontation between principles and efficacy, what is at stake is the very meaning of humanitarian medicine. The clash of arguments that paradoxically reinforces that final formulation of an "ethics in action" effectively opposes two figures of life: the life that is saved (that of the victims), and the life that is risked (that of the aid workers). Physically, there is no difference between them; philosophically, they are worlds apart. They bear witness to the dualism conceptualized by Giorgio Agamben and discussed earlier, between the bare life that is to be saved and the political life that is freely risked, between the *zoē* of "local populations" who can only passively await both bombs and humanitarian workers, fearing the former and mistrusting the latter, and the *bios* of those "citizens of the world," the aid workers who come, with courage and devotion, to render them assistance.[15] Recognizing the inequality between these lives at the level of their very meaning—even more than in terms of the objective threats they face—is not to question either the validity of a specific humanitarian action undertaken in the name of victims' rights, or the good faith of individual humanitarian actors who defend those rights. It is rather to attempt to understand the anthropological configuration in which the two are located—a configuration in which the sacred no longer resides in man as master of his existence, but in life itself. What it signifies is, for humanitarian actors, the freedom to sacrifice themselves for a just cause, and for local populations, the condition of being sacrificeable in the war. In contemporary societies this inequality is perhaps both the most ethically intolerable, in that it concerns the sense given to life, and the most morally tolerated, since it forms the basis for the principle of altruism.[16] And this is the truth that humanitarianism revealed in Iraq.

Humanitarian politics presents itself as a resolute bias in favor of "victims." The world order as portrayed by this politics comprises the strong and the weak. Humanitarian workers operate in the space between the two, assisting the weak while denouncing the strong. They intervene in places "where life is not worth a dollar."[17] They focus on those considered at risk of physical disappearance and incapable of maintaining their own existence. Of course, not all "survival" situations, as these actors often describe them, are equally dramatic or involve the same risks to life, but the core of humanitarian action is indeed existence under threat. "Saving strangers"[18]—in other words, people one does not know—simply on the grounds of their common humanity is the supreme mission that humanitarian organizations undertake. Such an objective presupposes that victims are identified. This might appear simple, given the way we perceive conflicts or the way they are presented to us. It nevertheless involves a double elision.

First, in a war there may be victims on both sides, and often outside of either: the usual moral dichotomies, obviously based partly on political reality, on the contrary imagine a simplification of the world in which victims and their aggressors must be identifiable and namable: Biafrans, Tamils, Chechens, Kosovars, set against Nigerians, Sri Lankans, Russians, Serbs. Reality sometimes escapes these confines when, for example, Tamils massacre Sri Lankan farmers, Chechens abduct a European aid worker, or Albanian Kosovars become the persecutors of Serbian families who stayed in Kosovo. Second, depicting a group or a people as victims imposes a status on its members that they do not necessarily recognize as their own: the individuals represented as victims may regard themselves as combatants or militants, or as politically dominated and territorially expropriated, but will often bend to the category assigned to them, understanding its logics and anticipating its advantages. However local people consider themselves, this construction of victims is viewed by humanitarian organizations as both necessary, since it identifies the target of intervention, and sufficient, in that the perspective of the populations is never required. Nongovernmental organizations are nevertheless led to reflect when divergences of interpretation emerge between them, as happened in Darfur when some called for a military intervention to stop what they qualified as a genocide, whereas others interpreted the events as part of an internal conflict in which intervention would bring about more harm than good.

This dichotomic moral conception of the world and the role that aid workers should play within it can easily be set within the genealogy of "pastoral power" as Michel Foucault characterized it, in reference to the Hebrew and the Christian shepherds.[19] In the French philosopher's view, what characterizes this power is first that it is exercised not over a territory but "over a flock," second that it presents itself as "fundamentally beneficent," and finally that it is "individualizing"—leading the shepherd to be "prepared to sacrifice himself for his flock." Similarly, the humanitarian power is exercised over a population that must be aided, essentially for the good of the collectivity, and even more specifically for the good of each individual. Here we clearly see that collective action toward the population (in a refugee camp, for example) is in no way opposed to the individual action that is the very substance of it (each life saved counts, it is argued). It is thus easy to understand that remaining in Baghdad meant feeling responsible in the abstract for a people under bombardment, but also concretely for the individuals that the aid workers could save, however few in number. This responsibility may not extend to sacrificing oneself, but at least to taking that risk. Hence the founding inequality of the humanitarian gesture resides in this asymmetry of lives, between those whose life is passively sacrificeable, because they are at the mercy of the bombs, and those whose life can be freely sacrificed, because they decided to stay. For the former, the gift can have no counter gift, since it is assumed that they can only receive: they are the beholden of the world. For the latter, the gift may even be the gift of the self—at least in theory.

Up to this point, on the scene of war, one protagonist is missing. I have presented the humanitarian agents standing beside the victims they assist. I now need to situate them in relation to the military powers involved in the conflict.

THE PRICE TO BE PAID

The representation of the protagonists offered by Jean-Hervé Bradol is probably the darkest. "Humanitarianism can make resistance to the elimination of one part of humanity into a way of life based on the satisfaction of unconditionally offering a person whose life is at risk the assistance that allows him to survive," he writes.[20] His moral geography of the world contrasts two continents—that of the "established political powers" whose function is "to decide on human sacrifice, to divide the governed between those who must live and those who may die" and that of the "humanitarian project," which has "taken the arbitrary and radical decision to try to help those that society sacrifices." The former derives from the "cannibal ideal," since "the edification of the international order always requires its quota of victims." The latter proceeds from a "subversive dimension," because "humanitarian aid is primarily addressed to those whose demand to live is confronted by the indifference or open hostility of others." This binary world therefore opposes a politics of death (that of criminal states) to a politics of life (that of humanitarian actors).[21] Thus defined entirely in moral terms, politics is a new war between an axis of good and an axis of evil. By a surprising paradox, at the very moment when some countries, first and foremost the United States, were throwing themselves into a moral crusade against their demonized enemies, some in nongovernmental organizations were adopting an equally Manichaean discourse. Yet this is less surprising than it appears, and while here the formulation is cast in radical terms, it still articulates a vision of the world that is broadly shared within the humanitarian sphere, at least among French organizations. Moreover, the language of sacrifice refers explicitly to the religious origins of pastoral power: condemning "human sacrifice" and saving "those that society sacrifices," to the extent of paying with one's person, reconnects with the tradition of both Abraham (the one who sacrifices) and Christ (the one who sacrifices himself). Beyond the rhetoric, there is in this representation of humanitarianism a sort of genealogical truth.

Without necessarily accepting the moral division of the world proposed by Médecins Sans Frontières' former president, one can understand the decision to stay in Baghdad and the risks it involved for the embedded team as a resistance to the way in which states at war treat the lives of their soldiers, their enemies, and even civilian populations. In this respect, the moral economies of the Western military leadership, influenced by the general evolution of the value attached to human life, underwent a profound change over the twentieth century: from the carnage of the First World War battlefields to the collective trauma of the Algerian war (for France), and above all Vietnam (for the United States), we have moved to maximum avoidance of military losses.[22] But the corollary of the "zero death" doctrine, as it has developed over the past twenty years in the West, and as it has been theorized by U.S. military experts, is the rhetoric of "collateral damage," which forms the necessary counterpoint. Reducing the risks on one's own side implies increasing them on the enemy's side, including—in conflicts putatively launched for the purposes of "liberating" or "protecting" populations— among civilians. This logic reached its apogee with the NATO bombing of Kosovo in 1999. Not only did the strategic choice of an aerial operation make it possible to limit losses among the Allied forces, at the expense of the human casualties that bombing often involves, but the tactical decision to have the aircraft fly at high altitude so they would be inaccessible to Serb antiaircraft defense necessarily entailed a reduced level of ballistic accuracy: aircraft targeting errors killed more than five hundred civilians among the Kosovar populations the operation was supposed to protect, but not one pilot died.[23] Certainly, for the intervening powers these human losses were undesirable, but they were unavoidable in light of the military choices made.

Although it was less efficient because it involved ground operations and especially the deployment of a substantial long-term presence, inevitably resulting in military losses, the Iraq War of 2003 gave a new twist, and above all an unprecedented breadth, to this doctrine. In addition to the fact that the massive bombardment that preceded and prepared for the invasion generated large numbers of casualties among Iraqis, including many civilians, the subsequent measures to ensure the security of U.S. and British troops resulted in widespread preventive use of firearms, again in order to reduce the risk of soldiers being killed. Only a few particularly bloody or tragic episodes were reported. However, discrepancies in mortality were huge. By October 2004, more than a year after military operations began, the army of occupation had suffered 1,000 deaths, versus the 100,000 estimated by a British epidemiological study of the Iraqi population. Two years later, in October 2006, Allied military losses numbered 2,925, while the same epidemiologists put the number of lives lost on the Iraqi side at 655,000, of which 601,000 were directly linked to violence, a third of them caused by the coalition forces.[24] These marked disparities, with deaths occurring exclusively among the military for the intervening forces and mainly among civilians in the Iraqi population, offer an a posteriori measure of the implicit politics of a differential valuing of human beings.

This politics was established before the event through the strategic choices made by senior military commanders, aimed at limiting the toll in lives of the coalition forces, even if that was at the price of a very high number of deaths among the local population. Arithmetically, the life of a Western soldier was worth two hundred times more than the life of an inhabitant of the country where the former was intervening in order to "liberate" or "protect" the latter: sacrificing the lives of several hundred local people was the condition for preserving the sacred life of one individual. This calculation would seem cynical had it not effectively been made for the purposes of estimating the compensation to be paid in the event of death: the "tariff" was set by insurance companies at $400,000 for a U.S. soldier killed at the front, while the U.S. government paid $2,500 for each Iraqi civilian killed in error.[25] Here the valuation is 160 times higher— not far from the previously estimated ratio for casualties.

There is, of course, rarely any public proof that this idea of the price to be paid is really behind the reasoning of those governing. This is what makes a statement by Secretary of State Madeleine Albright particularly remarkable. In a television interview in 2000, a journalist asked Albright if she thought the half million Iraqi children estimated by UNICEF to have perished as a result of the economic blockade was an excessively high price to pay for exerting pressure on the Baathist regime: "This is a very hard choice but we think the price is worth it," she said.[26] We could in fact consider it a sort of moral progress, to use a phrase inherited from the Enlightenment, that during the 2003 Iraq War the counting of lives lost on both sides, and thus the calculation of the ratio of deaths, was even possible. By contrast, at the time of the First Gulf War, estimates of Iraqi deaths varied from a few thousand to several hundred thousand, but no serious attempt was made to arrive at a more precise number, either by the victorious Allied troops or by the defeated Iraqi regime. When no one counts deaths, it means that lives no longer count. The famous statement of General Tommy Franks, head of the coalition forces, in 2003—"We don't do body counts"— probably says more about the reality of distant conflicts than he himself realized at the time.[27] For even if, as I have noted, we have mortality figures from epidemiological studies, which are not beyond critique, there are no reliable government statistics that could not only provide a precise number of deaths but also—at least—give the deceased individuals a name.

Médecins Sans Frontières' decision to remain in Baghdad when the bombing was about to begin issues a challenge to this politics of lives that "don't count." By exposing themselves to danger, the team raised the question of the equality of lives in a concrete, immediate way: all lives apparently became equal again—that is, equally vulnerable for the Iraqis and for the humanitarian agents assisting them. The sacrifice to which they consented (risking being killed) shifted the radical inequality between the sacred life of those on one side (Western soldiers) and the sacrificed lives of those on the other (local civilians). By this heroic act, the humanitarian politics of life offered a striking counterpoint to the military politics of life. At least, that was the intention.

THE VALUE OF LIVES

In effect, this equality did not long withstand the test of reality. The kidnapping during the first days of the coalition intervention forced the humanitarian ideal to face the harsh fact of the value of lives. The abduction of three members of the team paralyzed not only their three colleagues but also the entire organization, which initially halted all activity, and then resolved to withdraw the mission. On the Iraqi side, not one life was saved; not even one injury was treated. Above all, it became clear that Médecins Sans Frontières could not countenance risking lives: when the danger moved from hypothetical to real, the intervention was suspended to avoid further risk to the abducted, and when they were released by the kidnappers, at a time when other aid organizations were just getting to work, the French branch of Médecins Sans Frontières left Iraq, arguing that the health situation was not after all great cause for concern and additionally the conditions of operation were not satisfactory.[28] In reality, the trauma of the abduction had highlighted the contradictions inherent in a declared policy of risking lives that could not be maintained in the face of real danger.

The Iraqi episode, which fortunately ended happily, is indicative of the fragility of humanitarian organizations regarding kidnapping. The only remarkable feature of it is that those within the organization had a difficult time articulating the simple truth that the lives of aid workers sent into the field are an absolute priority. This is understandable: after expending so much energy to demonstrate that the workers should stay despite the risk, it was not easy, particularly after the event, to admit that they were leaving the country because of the danger. More generally, the vulnerability to abduction, which has become routine in several parts of the world, influences the activities of aid organizations—a phenomenon that obviously extends beyond them and is also a serious concern for Western governments. A number of other Médecins Sans Frontières members have been kidnapped in recent years, and each time the result has been paralysis not only of the mission concerned but also of the entire organization. Whether it be in Colombia, Chechnya, Dagestan, Somalia, or the Democratic Republic of Congo, after each hostage taking, aid to the local population has been suspended and the organization has concentrated entirely on a single aim—saving the abducted colleague. Fortunately, this goal has been achieved in every case.

The paramount concern to protect the organization's own staff should be no surprise, especially since the abducted members are almost always expatriates and have established friendships not only within the local teams but also in the European offices. Moreover, the protagonists in conflicts are well aware of the West's sensitivity to kidnapping, and in some regions of the world, especially central Asia, take cynical advantage of it, unconcerned about the difference between soldiers and aid workers, private security guards and foreign journalists, forcing governments and nongovernmental organizations into protracted and difficult negotiations in which the value of the lives of those who have been abducted is assessed and translated into cash terms. The case that most concerned Médecins Sans Frontières in recent years, that of Arjan Erkel, the Dutch head of mission in North Caucasus, offers a prime example. Only after twenty months in captivity, without any indication as to who had ordered the kidnapping, was he released following the payment of a 1 million euro ransom by the Dutch government, which then sought in vain to reclaim the money from the organization.[29] The publicity surrounding this transaction not only confirmed that money had been paid but also revealed the amount, and it therefore made clear the value that might be placed on the life of an aid worker—or more precisely, the life of an expatriate aid volunteer, for even among the members of these organizations, not all lives are of equal value.

The most common distinction Médecins Sans Frontières makes in its missions (like all foreign organizations, whether working in aid or development) is between "expatriates" and "nationals." Expatriates come mostly from Western countries (although recently efforts have been made to incorporate some from the Third World) and are members of the organization, while nationals come from the local community and are considered paid employees. To justify this difference in status, Médecins Sans Frontières has long asserted that while expatriates were committed to the humanitarian project, nationals simply needed a job—in other words, volunteers on one side, mercenaries on the other. But the argument was reversed when it came to negotiating pay scales. It was put to the local staff, who were on short-term contracts and sometimes even employed by the day, that the service they rendered to the local populations should be their real reward. By contrast, the financial situation was much better for expatriates whom, it was said, had to continue paying their housing expenses in Europe. There are many other disparities. Expatriates participate in the general assemblies and vote for their representatives, while nationals are kept outside of the organization's democratic process. In the field, authority rests with the expatriates, even when they are inexperienced volunteers working with experienced local professionals. Outside of work, the expatriates live together in accommodations provided by the organization, often separated off from the local community, whereas nationals return to their homes each evening.

This means of managing missions, with the categorization of staff on the basis of their origin, was until recently taken for granted in aid circles. Essentially, it was considered that the humanitarian venture involved well-intentioned men and women from Western countries devoting themselves to populations in peril but needing local assistance to perform their good works, just as colonial administrators might have need of local chiefs—and anthropologists of informants. The nationals, who were never part of the central administrative staff or represented among the senior management, not only had no voice in the organization, but even remained invisible: no one in the headquarters knew them, because air transport was paid only for expatriates, and they were rarely taken into consideration in the field, not being involved or even consulted in decisions. It was only a decade ago, thirty years after the creation of Médecins Sans Frontières, that this discrimination, which obviously contradicted the organization's founding principles, began to pose problems and elicit criticism, partly because of the practical obstacles it presented to operation. Amanda Harvey, the head of human resources for the field teams, made rectifying the situation a priority:[30] "We have reached the limits of a system based on a corporatist 'expat' functioning that no longer corresponds to the reality of MSF today. The improvements we are able to bring will remain marginal unless we question our organization. How can your work in the field in Sudan be effective if you never ask the opinion of the Sudanese people?" Several projects for reform were therefore drawn up, but never implemented despite the repeated protests of local professionals who hoped they would at last be recognized.

Yet the disparity in status between expatriates and nationals has major practical consequences. As we have seen, there are differences in salary and above all in contractual terms, since nationals are often employed for short periods, even on a daily basis: moreover, the precariousness of these contracts is heightened by the fact that they are concluded in the missions and therefore at the discretion of expatriate staff. The vulnerability of local employees is accentuated still further by the very unequal levels of social protection afforded. While medical coverage for expatriates is equivalent to that provided under the French social security system, nationals often do not have insurance, and when they are sick, generally receive neither treatment nor sickness benefit. At the general assembly of 2000 this issue was finally raised and a motion was passed calling on Médecins Sans Frontières to provide health insurance to cover treatment and care for national employees with AIDS. This motion was a response to the disturbing paradox that while the organization championed the provision of antiretroviral drugs and criticized Western states and international bodies for their failure to address this issue, many in their own staff were being neglected.[31] It took a long time for the motion to be translated into action, and three years after it was passed, the president was still expressing concern about the problems of implementation.

The issue of the protection of national staff took on an even more tragic dimension in conflict situations, as unlike expatriates they had no institutional immunity. One study revealed that almost six of every ten deaths among aid workers over the past twenty years were of national staff, but this is a very substantial underestimate, because on the one hand, as we have seen, many of them are employed on a casual basis and therefore do not appear on staff lists, and on the other, in Rwanda, where there was a particularly high death rate among aid workers, few figures differentiating national staff are available.[32] In other words, even within humanitarian organizations—as in development and cooperation organizations— distinctions are systematically instituted between foreign staff, almost always Western and white, and local employees. These distinctions relate not only to status, power, responsibilities, type of contract, salary level, and marks of esteem, but also to the protection of their lives, or their very survival, whether they were threatened by disease or war. Both the AIDS epidemic and the Rwandan genocide cruelly exposed these discriminations and their consequences.

Thus within the arena of humanitarianism itself, hierarchies of humanity were passively established, though rarely identified for what they were—a politics of life that, at moments of crisis, resulted in the constitution of two groups of individuals: those whose condition of expatriate protected the sacred character of their lives, and those who, because they belonged to the society receiving aid, were paradoxically excluded from this protection. For a long time, humanitarian workers, so preoccupied with saving "others," did not even realize that alongside them the national staff, perhaps too close to be considered as part of the otherness of victims but at the same time too distant to be deemed to belong to their humanitarian community, were not being afforded the same right to live for which the expatriates advocated in the international arena. But the protagonists in conflicts had clearly seen this blindspot. Their calculations took into account the fact that not all lives bore the same price. When they abducted aid workers, they knew that only foreigners had a substantial market value that they could negotiate fiercely, but also a political price that they would pay heavily for if they ended up killing their hostages. Their compatriots locally employed, by contrast, whose lives the abductors did not imagine could be valued in cash terms and whose death they realized would cost them nothing, were generally simply executed.

Humanitarian action by nongovernmental organizations, from the birth of the International Committee of the Red Cross to the emergence of the movement inaugurated by Médecins Sans Frontières, has historically been constructed in response to the inhumanity of war, as a way of restoring the basic idea of humanity itself. Whether its origins are Christian, as among the charitable religious orders, or secular, as with the philanthropic societies, there are two aspects to this principle, which refer to the two senses of the word itself: humanity as mankind (an idea) and as humaneness (a sentiment). This paradigm, which is today broadly accepted, has been established in contrast to others that either institute natural distinctions between human beings (through the idea of race, for example) or promote indifference to distant others (particularly in the stoking of nationalist sentiment).

In contemporary conflicts, the military forces that intervene, in the name either of their country or of higher concerns (leaving aside the question of whether this often largely rhetorical distinction is real), do not reject the idea and sentiment of humanity in principle; however, their practice calls it into question. The discourse of their governments and their senior officers generally leads them to construct the enemy as a category of humanity sufficiently distant to be killed in large numbers and without compassion. The injustice of contemporary war no longer resides, as in earlier times, in carnage shared roughly equally between the opposing sides, but rather in the unequal value accorded to lives on the battlefield: the sacred life of the Western forces of intervention, in which each death is counted and honored, versus the sacrificeable life of not only the enemy troops but also their civilian populations, whose losses are hardly tallied and whose corpses sometimes end up in mass graves. In the face of these inhuman politics of life—inhuman in the sense that they run counter to both the idea and the sentiment of humanity—humanitarian organizations call for a politics of life that reestablishes solidarity between human beings and gives equal value to lives.

But this politics unwittingly introduces a dual sort of inequality—one relating to the people on whose behalf they intervene, and the other to the individuals with whom they work. First, at the very moment when it restores the equal value of all humans through a solidarity extending as far as potential sacrifice in the field, the humanitarian gesture in fact introduces a distinction between those whose lives may be risked (humanitarian workers) and those whose lives are actually at risk (the people on whose behalf they intervene). The former are political subjects actively committed to their aid mission, while the latter only have their recognition as victims passively subjected to the event. The relationship established between them is less one of solidarity than of obligation, in which the gift of life is at stake. This contract is not upheld, however, in the full extent of its implications, because when danger becomes real (through hostage taking, in particular), the mission is suspended. The abstract, and ultimately moral, distinction between political subjects and putative victims becomes a concrete, even physical inequality between those who may decide to leave and those who have no option but to stay. Second, at the point when humanitarian action is deployed in the field in the name of helping the most vulnerable, it fails to recognize the difference established within its organizations between those who come from far to render assistance (expatriate volunteers) and those who enable them to achieve this task (national staff): the former are deemed to be working out of devotion, the latter out of necessity. A contractual, financial, and political hierarchy, which is also a hierarchy of status, is established between them. The corollary of this is the different levels of protection from disease and danger, which institutes an inequality in the symbolic and therefore economic value of lives, which participants in conflict use to their advantage.

The first of these two inequalities is at some level inherent in humanitarian intervention: it points to the fact that not all lives are accorded the same value and that in the end it is possible to save lives only as long as there is no real risk to one's own. Ultimately, it does derive from the principle of our conception of the sacredness of human life, but like charity, this conception begins at home. The second inequality, however, is an unconscious form arising in humanitarian action: it reveals the truth of a hierarchy of lives that is usually hidden, but which is brought into the open with the realization that a local employee is just an auxiliary in an enterprise emanating from the West and thus cannot be part of this generous venture. It thereby articulates the basis of the humanitarian movement: an impulse of moral sentiments from the rich toward the poor countries, from a world at peace to a world at war. The two inequalities are bound together: the inequality between expatriates and nationals represents the manifestation within humanitarian organizations of the inequality between benefactors and victims. It would obviously be wrong to ignore the extent to which both these inequalities, far from being unique to humanitarian actors, are set within contemporary moral economies: the inequality of lives, often invisible, is one of their foundations.

Conclusion

Critique of Humanitarian Reason

> We must go beyond the outside-inside alternative; we must be at the frontiers. Criticism means analyzing limits and reflecting on them.
> MICHEL FOUCAULT, "What Is Enlightenment?"

What is a critical thinking? How can it help us in comprehending the world, and possibly acting on it? These are the questions social sciences have been asking since their inception. Although Émile Durkheim promoted a positive science of society, he was nevertheless profoundly engaged in a critical reflection, often more moral than political, about the world and its transformations—not only in his public life but also in his intellectual life. Long regarded as the defender of axiological neutrality, Max Weber still considered the exercise of critical thought as perhaps even more essential to research than to action—far from the overly simple antinomy between science and politics with which he is often credited. Even though he was involved in the natural sciences before he turned to anthropology, Franz Boas placed his disciplinary knowledge at the service of a demanding social critique—even to the detriment of his own official standing.[1] The question is therefore not new. In the past as today, the vocation of social scientists often emerges from a combination of interest in the permanent process of invention of which societies are both the source and the product, and judgment about the state of affairs as they encounter them in the social world. Critical thinking sits at the crossroads between the two, between curiosity and indignation, between the desire to understand and the will to transform. Thus involvement, as addressed by Norbert Elias, is not just a constraint imposed on social sciences and need not make them envious of or nostalgic for the detachment of the natural sciences: it is what makes them unique, and even indispensable.[2] Ultimately, the social sciences can only be critical.

Provided that we accept this premise—and who would defend the idea of any science that is not grounded in critical thinking?—the question is merely displaced: What is the foundation of critique? Or, how is it to be

243

deployed? In a famous article published in the last year of his life, Michel Foucault discusses a text written by Kant in 1784 in response to the question raised by a Berlin newspaper: "What is enlightenment?"[3] Paraphrasing Kant's argument very freely, in order, as was his custom, to make the author he commented on say what he himself thought, he notes: "The hypothesis I should like to propose is that this little text is located in a sense at the crossroads of critical reflection and reflection on history. And, by looking at it in this way, it seems to me we may recognize a point of departure: the outline of what one might call the attitude of modernity." In other words, the birth of critique in the modern age emerges from this questioning of the present, which is no longer taken as a given, but as a historical moment, true engagement with which paradoxically consists in viewing it from a distance. Where the self-evidence of the social world imposes itself through current affairs and everyday life, a capacity for surprise needs to be maintained.

This is the method I have tried to adopt in this book, by identifying, over a range of social contexts, a general logic that I have proposed to call humanitarian reason, and which I believe throws some light on the multiple facets of a moral history of the present. But this exercise is not without its difficulties. It is in fact especially delicate because it is addressed to what appears not only to go without saying but also to be morally imperative. Listening to excluded and marginalized individuals, assisting the poor and disadvantaged, granting recognition to sick immigrants and asylum seekers, showing compassion for AIDS orphans and disaster victims, testifying on behalf of populations afflicted by wars—these are all attitudes and actions that we automatically believe to be good, for causes that we deem just in and of themselves. In questioning this moral self-evidence, by taking it as an object of study rather than an object of judgments and emotions, we drive a wedge into what is generally the subject of consensus. In analyzing it while attempting to maintain a distance from evaluation and emotion, we risk being accused of relativism (since we are recalling that these actions and attitudes considered as deriving from absolute imperatives are in fact historically and culturally situated) or cynicism (because we are establishing that moral sentiments are compatible with political considerations, ideological positions, and even practical interests). It is thus particularly difficult to apply a critical reflection to these questions, which tend to be placed beyond debate. Humanitarian reason is morally untouchable.

But once we attempt to go beyond this intellectual taboo, the question becomes: What is the correct distance from which to study it? Or perhaps, more precisely, what is the correct position for critique? Since Plato's allegory in Book VII of *The Republic*, one classic—and ultimately, heroic—response has consisted in the affirmation that the social function of critics is to bring men the light of truth. Thus, having succeeded in emerging from the cave where his companions in misfortune are held back, the philosopher can tell them that there is a sun outside and that they are living amid the illusion of the shadows they take for reality. He brings them knowledge of what they ignore, and critique of what they believe they know. To do so, he must venture outside the cave. Michael Walzer proposes an opposite conception:[4] "Some critics seek only the acquaintance of other critics; they find their peers only outside the cave, in the blaze of Truth. Others find peers and even comrades inside; in the shadow of contingent and uncertain truths." He points out how the position adopted influences the politics of critique: frequently lofty radicalism outside the cave, readily complacent understanding inside it.

Most social science studies straddle this line between outside and inside. One must choose one's position. For some, the task is to unveil. For the others, it is to translate.[5] Those on the outside denounce the social order. Those on the inside offer a grammar of social worlds. Among sociologists, the tension between the two is expressed between those who make criticism a tool of their radicalism and those who take it as the object of their analysis: critical sociology versus the sociology of criticism. In anthropology, the boundary is often drawn between those who challenge the structural violence of the world and those who seek to give an account of the unique ordering of each society: critical anthropology versus culturalist anthropology. Ultimately what we encounter here is the difference between two approaches to ideology:[6] that of Karl Marx, who sees ideology as what deforms, disguises, and even inverts reality for us by masking the logics of domination and class interests, and that of Clifford Geertz, who views it as the cultural system by which we make sense, particularly political sense, of social relations. In Marx's version ideology is dissimulating and exploits us; in Geertz's it is integrative and constitutes us. We could therefore approach humanitarian ideology in the first case on the basis of what it hides about the reality of the world, and in the second on the basis that it has become our means of apprehending that world. At first sight the two viewpoints contrasted in this series of binaries seem irreconcilable: one cannot be both inside and outside, reveal what agents cannot see at the same time as translating what they know better than we do. But I would venture a reformulation of this duality by suggesting the possibility of a critical thinking located "at the frontiers"[7]—on the threshold of the cave, to return to the allegory, at the point where one step to either side takes us out into the light or plunges us into the darkness.

It is this position at the frontiers that I have sought to defend in this book. I have not situated myself above actors, looking down on them from a place where criticism is easier because it is never put to the test. I have therefore assumed that the validity of the discourse on suffering, the benevolence of politics of compassion, and the reduction of persons to the status of victim should not be taken for granted. I have tried to grasp what this humanitarian reason means and what it hides, to take it neither as the best of all possible governments nor as an illusion that misleads us. It seems to me that by viewing it from various angles (from situations nearby to distant scenes, from listening centers to war zones) and by examining a range of objects (from the administration of the poor to the management of disasters, from the question of asylum to the issue of testimony) we can render the global logics of humanitarian reason more intelligible. Above all, in these sites, I have moved between the inside and the outside of the social worlds I studied, remaining attentive both to the discourses and practices of their members and to the facts and stakes of which they seemed unaware, closely marking their limits but also their spaces of freedom. My critique has thus been supported by the lucidity and reflexivity of actors—many of whom demonstrate their ambivalence or disappointment in relation to the policies they implement—without abandoning the autonomy of a sociological and anthropological approach that strives to explore areas to which they are blind. I knew from experience that it was possible to obey this dual injunction: having drawn up medical certificates for undocumented immigrants at the same time as criticizing the humanitarianization of immigration policy, and having worked in humanitarian organizations while maintaining a critical position within them, I was conscious of the possibility and even the necessity—but also the difficulty—of this negotiation between involvement and detachment, which, rather than being a sort of schizophrenia, simply proceeds from an ethical and intellectual rigor in which respect for informants does not preclude the exploration of areas where they are unable or unwilling to go.

The critique I argue for is thus a critique that includes us—individually and collectively—and not one that leaves the social scientist alone outside the cave. This, I believe, is a truly radical critique.[8] But since I have engaged in this dialogue with philosophers, I have to add that unlike them, we sociologists and anthropologists—at least those who have an ethnographic practice—produce our critique on the basis of studies in which individuals think and act, groups form and oppose one another, interests exist and come into conflict. We work not in the pure realm of concepts, but in the day-to-day reality of life, and therefore have to deal with the "irreducible empiricism" pleaded for by Olivier Schwartz.[9] This means that things are somewhat more complicated, for behind ideas and ideologies there are people with their contradictions and doubts, who belong successively or simultaneously to different worlds, who support varying positions and take their place within different logics; there are also situations in which the interpretations are delicate and the issues uncertain, in which relations of power shift and are even sometimes reversed. Facing these actors and these facts, which resist all attempts at reduction, critique must precisely give an account of this irreducibility. The fragility but also, without doubt, the greatness of the social sciences lie in the fact that they must always come to terms with realities that are complex and even indeterminate simply because they result from human intentions and actions. Given these conditions, how can a critique of humanitarian reason be constituted?

If we accept, following Charles Taylor, that the "social imaginary" of an era "is not a set of ideas; rather it is what enables, through making sense of, the practices of a society," we may say that humanitarian reason represents a powerful social imaginary of our time.[10] Yet it seems to escape in part the Canadian philosopher's analysis: he argues that "central to Western modernity is a new conception of the moral order of society," at the heart of which he places certain social forms including "the market economy, the public sphere, and the self-governing people, among others." In my view, humanitarian reason deserves greater emphasis than that "among others": it occupies a key position in the contemporary moral order. I hope to have shown it in operation in this book, analyzing how it has been mobilized in the practices of our societies, from the treatment of poverty, asylum, and endangered children to the justification of public actions, political causes, and even wars. This humanitarian reason is embedded within our long modernity, but also in our immediate present. In this respect the distinctive feature of contemporary societies is without doubt the way that moral sentiments have become generalized as a frame of reference in political life. This is the phenomenon I term "humanitarian government." Let us return once more to its distinguishing features.

We need to return to the two senses of the word "humanity," which in French remain undifferentiated, using the same term for both, but which are semantically distinguished in English and German.[11] As *Menschlichkeit* or "mankind," humanity is the entirety of men and women, and what distinguishes them from other living beings. As *Humanität* or "humaneness," humanity is the sympathy one feels for one's fellows, particularly for those who are suffering. The first sense describes the idea of a human species; the second denotes a moral sentiment with respect to human beings. The two are linked by a simultaneously inclusive and exclusive principle, which is a fundamental feature of the Enlightenment. It is inclusive in that it incorporates all human beings within a single category that is not only biological but also political. It is exclusive in that it separates human beings from the animal kingdom and allocates them a specific status. As idea and sentiment, humanity presupposes an equality of rights and of concern among human beings: this was a major shift from earlier paradigms, as Reinhart Koselleck has shown.[12] More precisely, humanity, if we take it in its double meaning, implies that all lives are equally sacred and that all sufferings deserve to be relieved.

Humanitarian government derives from this premise: it is a politics of life and a politics of suffering. The two are not exactly aligned with one another. This book commences with the latter, as it is displayed in the listening centers, and closes with the former, as it plays out in zones of conflict. In fact, the whole volume is organized around this duality, which is also a complementarity. Equivalence of lives, equivalence of suffering: clearly this is the central issue in France's humanitarian justification for granting residence to immigrants suffering from serious illness, in the humanitarian exception declared in Venezuela wherein the poor and the wealthy were presumed equal in the face of natural disaster, in humanitarian psychiatry during the Second Intifada with the attempt to place the victims on both sides on the same level, and in the humanitarian organizations' decision to stay in Iraq, exposing their members to the bombing just as the inhabitants of Baghdad were exposed.

Historically, but also genealogically, humanitarian reason thus defined is embedded in a Western sociodicy. Historically because its key episodes—from the abolitionist movement in Britain two centuries ago to the U.S. interventionism of the past two decades, from the founding of the Red Cross to the birth of Médecins Sans Frontières—belong to the history of Europe and North America. And genealogically because the ethos from which it proceeds has its source in the Christian world—in terms of both the sacralization of life and the valorization of suffering—although, of course, there are other traditions of compassion and charity, from Islam to Confucianism to Buddhism. The two dimensions, historical and genealogical, are clearly conjoined in contemporary humanitarian expansionism. We need to grasp the anthropological implications of this expansionism.

The "end of religion" has long been considered in the Nietzschean terms of the death of God, and the Weberian sense of the disenchantment of the world. Recent analyses, conversely, have highlighted the "return of religion," in the form of Muslim, Jewish, and Christian fundamentalisms but also via the proliferation of churches and sects, in America and Europe as well as in Africa and Asia. Without underestimating this movement of religious renaissances, we need to consider another development, less visible but perhaps more profound, which is manifested in the secularization of the religious, "the religious after religion," as Marcel Gauchet puts it.[13] This analysis suggests that the contemporary presence of religion is most effectively manifested where it is least identifiable, where it becomes so self-evident that we do not even recognize it for what it is any more. In this view, the ultimate victory of religion lies not in the renewal of religious expression throughout the world, but in its lasting presence at the heart of our democratic secular values.

The idea of human life as the highest good appears to us an inviolable principle that we believe to have been decisively won by our modernity—despite the fact that the United States, the country that makes greatest use of the humanitarian argument to justify its wars, is among the few that have yet to abolish the death penalty. But this principle derives from an older one, as Hannah Arendt points out:[14] "The reason why life asserted itself as the ultimate point of reference in the modern age and has remained the highest good of modern society is that the modern reversal operated within the fabric of a Christian society whose fundamental belief in the sacredness of life has survived, and has even remained completely unshaken by, secularization and the general decline of the Christian faith." I have proposed the term "biolegitimacy" for this recognition of life as the highest of all values—life that must be understood in the sense of being alive. This life lies at the core of humanitarian government, in the relative privilege accorded to the undocumented seriously ill over all other immigrants and even asylum seekers, or the universal consensus regarding the intervention of organizations working in emergency aid rather than social justice programs, not to mention protests or riots. Conversely, it is also what makes policies that prioritize the collective interests of public health over benefits for individual patients, and on a quite different level, the gesture of combatants who sacrifice themselves in suicide attacks against their enemies, simultaneously unintelligible and intolerable to most people.

In Western societies the paradigm of romantic engagement with the world has thus shifted from the figure of the volunteer risking his or her life alongside liberation movements to the figure of the humanitarian saving lives in spaces set apart from the fighting. Although the same concept of "life" is invoked, it refers to different truths: in the first case the political life of the one who fights, and in the second the physical life of the one who is aided. My point here is not to suggest that one is more valuable than the other, but first to indicate that a major shift has taken place, one we are not altogether aware of, and second to note that among all the possible meanings we could ascribe to the human condition, the one we have placed at the summit of our system of values is that which relates to the most restricted but also the most unarguable definition of life: what Walter Benjamin[15] calls "life itself," or maybe more explicitly, the simple fact of being alive. That the question is no longer contested does not mean that we cannot still discuss the issues involved.

Alongside this development, contemporary moral economies have been constituted around a new relation to suffering, which makes it a central element of our public life. We must emphasize this paradox: while the spectacle of suffering has disappeared completely from the public places where the physical punishment inflicted on criminals was previously exhibited, the representation of suffering through images and narratives has become increasingly commonplace in the public sphere, not only in the media, whose propensity for exposing intimate details of pain is well known, but also in the political arena, where it furnishes an effective justification for action. This fascination with suffering also derives from a Christian genealogy. Although it is found in many traditions of thought, Stoicism being just one example, the valorization of suffering as the basic human experience is closely linked to the passion of Christ redeeming the original sin, a passion that was repeated over several centuries through the torments of martyrs and the mortification of the saints. The singular feature of Christianity in this respect is that it turns suffering into redemption. However, modernity marks a turning point in this genealogy of redemptive suffering, both in literature and in politics. As Hannah Arendt suggests,[16] "History tells us that it is by no means a matter of course for the spectacle of misery to move men to pity; even during the long centuries when the Christian religion of mercy determined moral standards of Western civilization, compassion operated outside the political realm and frequently outside the established hierarchy of the Church." With the entry of suffering into politics, we might say that salvation emanates not through the passion one endures, but through the compassion one feels. And this moral sentiment in turn becomes a source of action, because we seek to correct the situation that gives rise to the misfortune of others.

Humanitarian government is the heir to this active protest against the suffering of the world. But it alters it in two essential ways: first by renouncing violence, only agreeing to intervene in spaces that have previously been pacified (the protected corridors aid organizations demand from parties to war), and second by substituting its own action for the potential action of the suffering masses (the latter no longer express their condition directly). Nevertheless, beyond these changes over time, one must emphasize the persistence of the place of suffering in the moral space of Western societies, and still more, its valorization as an experience of individual or collective salvation. This valorization is ambiguous, as even Saint Augustine remarked,[17] because the spectacle of the other's suffering evokes both horror and pleasure: one feels sadness when one sees the misfortune of others, but cannot detach oneself from this vision because, he writes, we love to feel pity. This emotional duality of empathy remains a characteristic trait of humanitarian reason. We need only examine the iconographic exposure of emaciated bodies and imploring gaze in advertising campaigns for aid to the Third World to grasp the persistence of this double valence of suffering, which simultaneously repels and attracts. Similarly, the narrative of the hardship of the unemployed applying for financial assistance, of the asylum seekers soliciting refugee status, of the children suffering from AIDS in South Africa, and of adolescents in the Second Intifada forms part of this logic of the exhibition of suffering in which, it is believed, the mobilization of moral sentiments offers access to the transcendent truth of the victims.

The constitution of life as sacred and the valorization of suffering thus make contemporary humanitarian government a form of political theology. As Carl Schmitt's famous dictum states: "All significant concepts of the modern theory of state are secularized theological concepts."[18] While the generalization inherent in this proposition may be debatable, and the analogy between the state of exception and the Christian miracle not entirely convincing, it might be seen as having a more specific relevance around the diptych of life as highest good and suffering as redemptive ordeal. Humanitarian government, because it establishes these two foundations of Christian thought in the political space, clearly represents the religious aspect of the contemporary democratic order. The dual politics it lays claim to and promotes—of life and of suffering—prolongs and renews the Christian legacy. Acknowledging this legacy makes it possible to draw out the full meaning of the expansion of humanitarian reason.

Ultimately, this is one of the answers to the question that Claude Lefort poses about the "permanence of the theological-political" in the contemporary world:[19]

Instead of searching in democracy for a new episode in the transfer of the religious into the political, should we not consider that the theological and the political have become detached from one another; that a new experience of the institution of the social has emerged; that the revival of religion occurs at its points of weakness; that its efficacy is no longer symbolic, but imaginary; and finally that it does no more than testify to democracy's difficulty, no doubt unavoidable, no doubt ontological, in making itself legible for itself—and equally to the difficulty that political and philosophical thought have in addressing the tragedy of the modern condition without misrepresenting it?

This is my argument in this book: humanitarian reason corresponds to this ultimate theological-political recess at the "points of weakness," where "the tragedy of the modern condition" can no longer be eluded.

From this perspective, I therefore propose that we consider humanitarian government as the response made by our societies to what is intolerable about the state of the contemporary world.[20] In the face of violence, disasters, and epidemics, and also poverty, insecurity, and misfortune, what is intolerable is not only the presence of the tragic but the inequality in which it is embedded. As we have seen, the lives of the Palestinian youth, the Iraqi civilian, the ill African, or the unskilled immigrant worker in France have much lower value than, respectively, the lives of the Israeli child, the American soldier, the European patient, or the French professional. The suffering of the unemployed man, the refugee, and the disaster victim is not simply the product of misfortune, it is also the manifestation of injustice. Humanitarian reason, by instituting the equivalence of lives and the equivalence of suffering, allows us to continue believing—contrary to the daily evidence of the realities that we encounter—in this concept of humanity which presupposes that all human beings are of equal value because they belong to one moral community. Thus humanitarian government has a salutary power for us because by saving lives, it saves something of our idea of ourselves, and because by relieving suffering, it also relieves the burden of this unequal world order. Of course, we may consider that it is being put to cynical use, when U.S. planes drop food parcels on Afghan populations at the same time as bombs, in an effort to gain some support in the population, or when a French nongovernmental organization, taking advantage of the confusion of the war in Darfur, tries to abduct Chadian children from their parents so that they may be adopted abroad. But these misuses of humanitarian reason should not divert us from its deeper significance, which may be no less troubling. It is crucial to understand the logics of this social imaginary and its ethical and political implications.

For humanitarian government does more than just preserve our conception of the human: through the moral sense it credits us with, it endows us with our own share of humanity. We become more fully human via the manner in which we treat our fellows. I am not thinking here of the individual affect of the generous donor or the devoted volunteer, but of a collective sentiment through which our societies can imagine themselves in solidarity with the weight of the world, whether it be close or distant. If, as Zygmunt Bauman writes,[21] the production of "wasted lives" is "simultaneously a most harrowing problem and a most closely guarded secret of our times," the defense of humanitarian reason represents the ethical counterpoint, because it challenges this logic by asserting the principle of the equal value of all lives.

However, on the global scale it is obvious that humanitarian government displays a dual model. In poor countries it deals with large and often undifferentiated populations, for whom mass initiatives are set in place. In rich countries, it is faced with individuals, whose narratives it examines and whose bodies it scrutinizes. Refugees represent the paradigmatic expression of the former, and asylum seekers the emblematic figure of the latter. For refugees there are the huge camps where thousands are gathered, protected, and assisted. For asylum seekers there is the subtle legal argument through which decisions are parsimoniously made about which of them may be granted protection under the law. But in order for this double register of humanitarianism to work, both the territorial and the moral boundaries between the two worlds must be sealed as tightly as possible—for example, preventing refugees from the South from claiming the prerogatives granted to asylum seekers in the North. The cases of the Sangatte "camp" and the shipwreck of the *East Sea* are exemplary of this endeavor, showing the importance for Western societies of opening their democratic space as little as possible, while preserving the possibility, as a last resort, of granting consideration to those who succeed in entering our world, but on the basis of humanitarianism rather than as of a right.

And this ultimate choice reveals a profound truth: in the shift from the "right of the receiver" to the "obligation of the giver," as Georg Simmel suggests in his analysis of responses to poverty (which can be generalized to all forms of aid),[22] it institutes a radically unequal order that is the mark of the humanitarian relationship—a structural fact, in other words, regardless of the motivations of actors. This inequality is unavoidable, precisely because it is socially instituted, not the result of individual choices or conducts. The point is not only demonstrable in theory: it is also empirically validated. My aim in presenting the studies I have discussed is to try to establish it much beyond the places where humanitarianism customarily finds its legitimate space—that is, within nongovernmental organizations involved in emergency aid and international bodies devoted to the protection of refugees.

Of course, it could be remarked that the introduction of humanitarian reason into the management of asylum and immigration in France, assistance for AIDS orphans in South Africa, or aid to the victims of disaster in Venezuela makes possible a proximity between the humanitarian agents—whether they be volunteers of nongovernmental organizations, officials of the state, or employees of an international agency—and the people being aided, who may even sometimes acquire a degree of embodied presence. Thus the asylum seekers whose story is validated by a scar that testifies to the persecution endured, the illegal immigrants whose serious illness establishes legitimate grounds for obtaining documents, the South African orphans who benefit from the concern of international institutions, the Venezuelan woman saved from natural disaster by the military, all become, by the grace of humanitarian reason, simply a little more human for us. And this is no small thing, given the dehumanization of which they are frequently the object.

However, the very gesture that appears to grant them recognition reduces them to what they are not—and often refuse to be—by reifying their condition of victimhood while ignoring their history and muting their words. Humanitarian reason pays more attention to the biological life of the destitute and unfortunate, the life in the name of which they are given aid, than to their biographical life, the life through which they could, independently, give a meaning to their own existence.[23] The administrator of the French social fund for the unemployed who marveled at applicants' ability to describe their hardship and justify their request, and the journalist sent to the Palestinian territories who expressed surprise that the bold stone throwers wet their bed at night, both believed they had made an important discovery about the subjectivity of the poor (in the first case) and of combatants (in the second). It is likely, though, that at the very moment of their epiphany, they were failing to recognize those of whom they were speaking for who they were, and what they meant by doing what they did.

There is a truth here that is less anodyne than it appears. Ultimately, what is lacking in humanitarian government is perhaps that, beyond life as sacred and suffering as value, it fails to recognize the Other as a "face," to use Emmanuel Levinas's term,[24] this face "present in its refusal to be contained," this face that resists any attempt to possess it even in the name of good. From this point of view, recognizing a face also means recognizing

a right beyond any obligation, and hence a subject beyond any subjection—
even to humanitarian reason.

By way of epilogue, allow me to recall a tragic event that will plunge us a
last time into the contradictions and paradoxes, strengths and weaknesses,
of humanitarian reason. On August 2, 1999, when the Sabena flight from
Conakry arrived in Brussels, two bodies were found in the plane's undercarriage.[25] These deaths—from hypothermia or suffocation, experts opined—
would probably have gone unnoticed, as had several others that occurred in
similar circumstances within a few months, if they had not been children,
aged fourteen and fifteen, and particularly if the following letter had not
been found in the hand of one of them:

Your Excellencies, members, and officials of Europe.

It is a distinctive honor and deep trust to write this letter to talk
to you about the aim of our trip and our suffering—we the children
and the youth of Africa.
First of all, we bring you our greetings—the sweetest, the most
adorable and respectful greetings of life. To this end, please be our
support and help. You are for us, in Africa, those whom we should
solicit to obtain aid. We beseech you, for the love of your continent,
for the sentiment you have for your people and above all for the
love of your children that you love so dearly like life. Moreover,
think of the love and kindness of the creator, God, the Almighty,
who has given you the good experiences, wealth, and power to
construct and organize your continent so well that it has become
the most beautiful and admirable of them all.
Members and officials of Europe, we are appealing to your
graciousness and solidarity to come to our rescue. Please, help us.
We are suffering enormously in Africa. We have problems and
suffer from lack of children's rights.
The problems we have are: war, disease, malnutrition, etc. As for
children's rights, in Africa, and especially in Guinea, we have
plenty of schools but a great lack of education and teaching. Only in
the private schools can one get good education and good teaching,
but it requires quite a lot of money, and our parents are poor, they
must feed us. Then, we do not have sports facilities such as soccer,
basketball, tennis, etc.
Therefore, we Africans, especially we, the African children and
youth, are asking you to set up a great, effective organization for
Africa so that it might make progress. And if you find that we
expose and sacrifice our lives, it is because we suffer too much in
Africa. We need your help to combat poverty and put an end to war

in Africa. Our greatest wish, though, is to study, and we ask that you help us to study to become like you in Africa.

Finally, we beseech you to forgive us for daring to write such a letter to you important people whom we truly respect. Do not forget that it is to you that we must complain about the weakness of our strength in Africa.

> Written by two Guinean children, Yaguine Koita
> and Fodé Tounkara

The emotion aroused by this tragedy, particularly in Belgium, where a few months earlier a young woman from Niger was suffocated by the police charged with returning her to her country, was not only a response to the fatal outcome of this intercontinental journey made by two children trying to escape the poverty and violence in their homeland. It related to the singular quality of the letter, which, one could say, touched the heart of Western societies. Contrarily to what it seems, it is not a "humiliating appeal to a superior" asking "pathetically for paternalistic neocolonial benevolence."[26] Beyond the cultural and literary code of supplication, which it would be wrong to reduce to a "neocolonial" relationship (especially given that such supplication is still a reality, even in France among French people as developed earlier), it is remarkable that this letter uses throughout the language of humanitarian reason, the language of suffering and aid ("help us, we are suffering enormously"), the language of life and sacrifice ("you find that we expose and sacrifice our lives"), within humanitarian reason's own field of engagement ("to combat poverty and put an end to war"). The reason these boys' words affect us so powerfully is therefore because they turn back toward us the image we want to present to the world, and because their death puts our powerlessness to the test. Thus if they demonstrate mimicry, it does not consist in imitating what we are, but what they think we would like them to be. We must therefore hear, behind their words, their voices, as Veena Das suggests:[27] "voice may give life to frozen words"—and her formula could not be applied more literally or more tragically here.

Remarkably, however, in a final reversal, the emotion we feel—here again, I stress, not individually but collectively—seems to testify to our humanity. Despite their terrible fate, we can perceive these Guinean children as still our fellows, our brothers. But our compassion for their demise can only reassure us about ourselves on the condition that we forget that several weeks earlier, a Senegalese teenager who had miraculously survived an almost identical odyssey from Dakar to Lyons was sent back to his country, where a second attempt to stow away, hidden again in the undercarriage of a plane, resulted in his death; and that a few months later, a Cuban opposition activist who had similarly risked his life to flee his country had his request for asylum rejected without examination in the transit zone in Roissy airport, and was brutally expelled to be returned to the authorities in Havana—just two among many similar episodes in the political history of contemporary hospitality.[28] Yaguine Koita and Fodé Tounkara probably gave Western ideals, the distant echoes of which reached them even in their poverty-stricken neighborhood in Conakry, more credit than they should have. For had they survived their fatal journey, the reason of state would once again have prevailed against them—over the humanitarian reason to which they appealed.

Chronology

France	World
1944 Battle of Normandy and liberation of Paris	1944 International Committee of the Red Cross Nobel Peace Prize
1945 End of the Second World War	1945 Liberation of Auschwitz concentration camp
Setif and Guelma massacres by French troops	U.S. atomic bombs on Hiroshima and Nagasaki
1946 Fourth Republic	
	1948 UN Declaration of Human Rights
	1949 Foundation of NATO
	1950 Establishment of UNHCR
	1951 Geneva Convention on Asylum
1954 Algerian war of independence begins	
1958 Fifth Republic, Charles de Gaulle president	
	1960 Independence of Senegal
1962 Algerian war of independence ends	
1965 Charles de Gaulle reelected president	1965 Vietnam War begins
	1967 Six Day War in the Middle East
	(continued)

259

France	*World*
1968 Protests and strikes in May	1968 Biafran war in Nigeria Massacre of My Lai by U.S. soldiers in Vietnam Invasion of Czechoslovakia by the Soviet Union
1969 Georges Pompidou president	
1971 Foundation of Médecins Sans Frontières	1971 Indian intervention in Bangladesh
1972 Foundation of GISTI	
1974 Giscard d'Estaing president	
	1975 Cambodian genocide by the Khmer Rouge Fall of Saigon and departure of U.S. troops
1979 Humanitarian Operation Ile-de-Lumière Foundation of COMEDE	1979 Boat people in China Sea
1980 Foundation of Médecins du Monde	1980 Beginning of Iran-Iraq war
1981 François Mitterrand president Urban riots in Les Minguettes near Lyon	1981 UNHCR Nobel Peace Prize
	1982 Invasion of Lebanon by Israel
	1984 Famine in Ethiopia Band Aid founded by Bob Geldof
1986 Jacques Chirac prime minister Secretary for Human Rights created	
1988 François Mitterrand reelected president Secretary for Humanitarian Action created Michel Rocard creates the minimum guaranteed income (RMI)	1988 UN Peacekeeping Forces Nobel Peace Prize
	1989 Massacre in Tiananmen Square Fall of Berlin Wall

France	*World*
	1991 Operation Provide Comfort in Iraq
	Croatian and Bosnian wars of independence
	1992 Operation Restore Hope in Somalia
	Creation of the European Union
1993 Edouard Balladur prime minister	
Pasqua Immigration Law	
	1994 Tutsi genocide in Rwanda
	First democratic elections in South Africa
1995 Jacques Chirac president	1995 Massacre of Bosnians in Srebrenica
Foundation of the Centre Primo Levi	
	Foundation of Oxfam International
1996 Undocumented immigrants occupy a church in Paris	
1997 Lionel Jospin prime minister	
Social movement of the unemployed	
1998 Chevènement Immigration Law	1998 Extradition denied for Augusto Pinochet
	TAC founded in South Africa
1999 MSF Nobel Peace Prize	1999 Peacekeeping operation in East Timor
	NATO bombing of Kosovo
	Vargas tragedy in Venezuela
2000 Universal medical coverage (CMU) created	2000 Second Intifada in Palestine
2001 *East Sea* runs aground on French Riviera	2001 Attacks in New York and Washington, DC
	Military intervention in Afghanistan
	Health exception in TRIPS Agreement in Doha

(continued)

France	World
2002 Jacques Chirac reelected president	2002 International Court of Justice created
	2003 Military intervention in Iraq
	2004 Humanitarian crisis in Darfur Tsunami in Southeast Asia
2005 Urban riots and state of emergency	2005 Responsibility to protect voted by UN
2007 Nicolas Sarkozy president Ministry of Immigration created	
	2008 Earthquake in Sichuan Israeli attack against the Gaza Strip
2010 Deportation of Roma	2010 Earthquake in Haiti Floods in Pakistan

Note: This succinct chronology is an attempt to order some of the landmarks in the recent history of humanitarian reason. Although my case studies have the 1990s and the first decade of this century for a time frame, I think it useful to circumscribe a long second half of the twentieth century to provide a broader historical perspective. The end of the Second World War is an arbitrary but significant starting point: it offers the sort of ambiguities that constitute the heart of this volume. The facts and events listed here are of varying importance and meaning, but they are all relevant to the content of the book.

Notes

INTRODUCTION

1. Most particularly since Adam Smith, whose *Theory of the Moral Sentiments* (1759: 1–2) begins as follows: "How selfish soever man may be supposed, there are evidently some principles in his nature, which interest him in the fortune of others, and render their happiness necessary to him, though he derives nothing from it, except the pleasure of seeing it. Of this kind is pity or compassion, the emotion which we feel for the misery of others, when we either see it, or are made to conceive it in a very lively manner." In his history of moral philosophy, John Rawls (2000) links Smith to Hutcheson, Shaftesbury, Butler, and Hume as belonging to a mainly Scottish "moral sense school."

2. The parable is recounted by Luke (10: 30–37). It is Jesus's response to an "expert in law" who asks, "Who is my neighbor?" In his study of "distant suffering," Luc Boltanski (1999 [1993]: 11) sees this scene as a paradigm that in his view is distinct from pity and compassion, and that he describes as "communitarian." Various translations of the gospels nevertheless state indifferently that the Samaritan "took pity on" the injured man or "was moved to compassion." Thus neither the identity of the Samaritan nor his involvement in an act of assistance justifies this distinction.

3. As proposed by Michel Foucault (1989: 154) in the summary of his lectures at the Collège de France of 1979–1980, titled "The Government of the Living": according to Foucault, this consists of the "techniques and procedures designed to direct the behavior of men," and he significantly speaks of "government of children, government of souls or consciences, government of a household, of the state or of oneself."

4. Inherited from the Enlightenment, and more specifically from the philanthropic societies of the late eighteenth century analyzed by Catherine Duprat (1993: xiv), who follows the definition offered by François-Vincent Toussaint in 1748: "By humanity I mean the interest that men take in the fate of their fellows in general, merely because they are men like them. This sentiment

engraved in their hearts is responsible for the other social virtues and supposes them likewise imprinted." This text incorporates both the English terms to which the word "humanity" refers: "mankind" (the species) and "humaneness" (concern).

5. See Nicolas Sarkozy, "Discours pour la France qui souffre" [Speech for the France that suffers], December 18, 2006, http://www.u-m-p.org/site/index .php/s_informer/discours/nous_allons_faire_revivre_l_espoir, and, in the case of George W. Bush, "President Promotes Compassionate Conservatism," April 30, 2002, http://www.whitehouse.gov/news/releases/2002/04/20020430-5.html (both consulted in February 2010).

6. See the amended version of the decree of November 2, 1945, on the conditions of entry and residence for foreigners in France, issued on November 25, 2004, particularly article 12b, paragraph 11, http://www.legislationline .org/legislation.php?tid=137&lid=2124&less=fals, and Tony Blair's speech in Chicago on April 22, 1999, where he defined what later came to be known as the "Blair doctrine" justifying armed intervention abroad, http://www.opende mocracy.net/globalization-institutions_government/article_1857.jsp (both consulted in January 2009).

7. The most radical form of this affirmation of inequality of moral sentiments is found in Nietzsche, who does not distinguish between compassion and pity, and in whose view, as Gilles Deleuze (2003 [1962]: 141) notes, "pity is the love of life, but of the weak, sick, reactive life: it is militant, and announces the final victory of the poor, the suffering, the powerless and the small."

8. Myriam Revault d'Allonnes (2008: 17) finds a key to interpretation in Tocqueville's formula of "the equalization of conditions" and evokes a "democratic compassion."

9. The two phenomena—hostility on one side, resentment on the other— could be described in reference to Shakespeare's *The Tempest*, or even more explicitly, to the version of the play rewritten by Aimé Césaire (1980 [1969]), as respectively the Prospero and the Caliban syndromes: "I pity you," says Prospero to Caliban; "And I hate you," Caliban replies (act 3, scene 5).

10. At least within the political space under consideration here or, as Martha Nussbaum (2001: 401) writes, in the relationship between "compassion and public life." I am not dealing here with compassion in the private sphere, as felt by a mother for the pain of her child, for example.

11. In the wake of the events of September 11, 2001, and their aftermath, and drawing on a discussion of the thinking of Emmanuel Levinas, Judith Butler (2004: xvii) proposes an ethics of precarious life "based upon an understanding of how easily human life is annulled." It is possible to expand this reflection beyond murderous physical violence by considering the vulnerability of lives and the way they are governed.

12. According to Alain Rey (2006 [1992]: 2898), "precarious is borrowed from the legal Latin *precaria*, 'obtained through prayer.' This signification, which implies an intervention from above and hence the absence of inevitability, results in the sense of 'unstable, passing.'" Consequently, "this legal term

describes something that is granted, something exercised only by concession, by a permission that can be rescinded by the person who granted it." In other words, from the etymology, *precarious* does not correspond to the static description of a condition, it involves a dynamic relation of social inequality.

13. Although we have studies of various aspects and moments in the history of humanitarianism, very few provide a synthetic vision in the *longue durée*. Michael Barnett's *Empire of Humanity* (2011) is an exception, going back to the antislavery and missionary movements in the nineteenth century.

14. This thesis is defended and illustrated by Charles Taylor in his *Sources of the Self* (1989: ix), which he describes as "an attempt to articulate and write a history of the modern identity."

15. A recent examination of the history of slavery and antislavery on a global scale, with a specific focus on Britain, France, and the United States, can be found in Seymour Drescher's *Abolition* (2009).

16. The deeper history of humanitarian intervention has been investigated in Gary Bass's *Freedom's Battle* (2008), which situates the roots of this political and military practice in the early nineteenth century.

17. The distinction between the two temporalities and my choice to focus on the recent transformation of humanitarianism proceed from a similar preoccupation as that of Samuel Moyn's *The Last Utopia* (2010), which insists on the rupture of the 1970s in the history of human rights and the singularity of the contemporary problematization of the issues in the public sphere.

18. It is impossible to present an exhaustive bibliography of the considerable literature on these questions. We can cite, in France, works by Pierre Bourdieu (1999), Luc Boltanski (1999), and Jean-François Laé (1996) for sociology, by Vincent de Gauléjac (1996) and Christophe Dejours (1998) for psychology; and in the United States, studies by Arthur Kleinman (1988), Nancy Scheper-Hughes (1992), Paul Farmer (1992), and Philippe Bourgois (1995) for anthropology, and David Morris (1991), Cathy Caruth (1995), and Ruth Leys (2000) for literary studies. A partial analysis of this corpus appeared in an earlier review (Fassin 2004c).

19. I refer respectively to the 950-page volume *La Misère du monde* (Bourdieu 1999 [1993]) and the edited trilogy *Social Suffering* (Kleinman et al. 1997), *Violence and Subjectivity* (Das et al. 2000), and *Remaking a World* (Das et al. 2001). Significantly, in a concession to this current concern, the English edition of Pierre Bourdieu's *The Weight of the World* bears the subtitle *Social Suffering in Contemporary Society*, thus using a lexicon absent from the French title but, as we will see, not from its subtext.

20. This language has entered the higher echelons of the French state, particularly (under the influence of sociologists representing very diverse schools of thought) the Commissariat Général du Plan (General Planning Commission), responsible for strategic planning (Fassin 1996). Although it is unlikely that the porosity between intellectual and political worlds is the same in both countries, a similar logic is noted in the United States, where the ethos of compassion has taken a foothold in political arenas (Berlant 2004).

21. There is a considerable body of literature on the construction of social problems (Schneider 1985). However, in my use of the concept of problematization I am aligning myself essentially with the view of Foucault (1994: 669–670) who, at the end of his life, came to see his entire philosophical work as relating to a succession of "problematizations" of the social world (around madness, the clinic, prisons, sexuality, etc.): "Problematization does not mean representation of a preexisting object, nor the creation by discourse of an object that does not exist. It is the totality of discursive or nondiscursive practices that introduces something into the play of true and false and constitutes it as an object for thought."

22. A concept proposed by the historian Edward Palmer Thompson (1971) and taken up by the political scientist James Scott (1976) in his interpretation of popular uprisings, moral economies have been interpreted in various ways. Adopting but significantly reformulating their acceptation to insist on the moral rather than economic dimension, I have proposed to view moral economies as "the production, dissemination, circulation and use of emotions and values, norms and obligations in the social space: they characterize a particular historical moment and in some cases a specific group" (Fassin 2009b: 1257).

23. The symbolic gesture made by Nicolas Sarkozy on May 17, 2007, offers a telling example of this development and its ambiguity: very shortly after his election as president of France, he organized a solemn ceremony at which the letter written by the young Resistance fighter Guy Môquet to his mother just before he was executed by the Gestapo in 1941 with twenty-six of his unfortunate companions was read aloud. Sarkozy announced that henceforth the reading of the letter would become compulsory in classrooms at the beginning of every school year. The first lines are well known: "My darling little mother, my adored little brother, my beloved little father, I am going to die!" It was through the pathos of this farewell that the French president chose to articulate the consensual voice of "national identity," devoting the new Ministry of Immigration to the celebration of this concept. When this controversial measure was implemented, the Réseau éducation sans frontières (Education without Borders Network, a French nongovernmental organization supporting illegal immigrant children and their parents) denounced the policy of expelling foreigners without residence rights implemented by this same ministry, stating: "If we are to be worthy of the 27 [Resistance fighters including Môquet] who died at Chateaubriant, we have to oppose the hounding of undocumented immigrants." See http://www.republique-des-lettres.fr/1644-nicolas-sarkozy.php, http://www.lepost.fr/article/2007/10/22/1040150_lecture-de-la-lettre-de-guy-moquet-resf-vs-dati.html, and Éric Fassin's article "Guy Môquet et le théâtre politique des émotions" [Guy Môquet and the political theater of emotions], Mouvements, October 21, 2007, http://www.mouvements.info/spip.php?article186 (all three consulted in February 2010).

24. The opposition between two publications by French moral philosophers that appeared in the same year clearly reveals this tension. Emmanuel

Renault's *Souffrances sociales* [Social suffering] (2008) offers an example of the first attitude: he documents the suffering produced by society and defends those who strive to relieve it. Extending the work of Christophe Dejours, he sees the "neoliberal" organization of labor as the source of this new "social pathology." In his view the historicity of the category and the politics that it mobilizes is without object. Myriam Revault d'Allonnes's *L'homme compassionel* [Compassionate man] (2008) illustrates the second stance. The author questions the routine adoption of the language of suffering, and following Hannah Arendt, sees the "politics of pity" as denaturing the sentiment of humanity, and "compassionate democracy" as a form of contemporary devotion in the public space. In her perspective, emotions form part of a political theater.

25. See Bourdieu (1999 [1993]: 4 and 614); in this book, the sociologist moves from an analysis of the social reproduction of inequality to a study of the "poverty of position," for the victims of which "the experience is no doubt all the more painful when the world in which they participate just enough to feel their relatively low standing is higher in social space overall," and he replaces the objectivation of objectivation, which was formerly the keystone of his method, with the subjectivation of subjectivities, following a "conversion of the way we look," described as a genuinely "benevolent disposition" to the "sufferings" of his informants.

26. See Boltanski (1999 [1993]: xiv and 179–182); after developing a distanced approach throughout the book, the sociologist significantly ends by unexpectedly bursting into the political arena in defense of humanitarianism and particularly of its hero Bernard Kouchner, who ironically became a few years later Nicolas Sarkozy's minister and was therefore associated with the French president's infamous policy against immigrants and the Roma. "Criticism is easy, but art is difficult," writes Boltanski. "It is therefore fitting to ask the critics what they want and what they propose. Those to whom we have referred do not tell us clearly." And for good measure, he does not hesitate to compare these critics of humanitarianism with "the young members of *Action française*" (a far-right movement of the 1930s in France) who, in another era, also denounced the excessive use of pity in the public space.

27. See the pioneering work of Larry Minear and Thomas Weiss (1992), Nicholas Wheeler (2000) on "humanitarian intervention in international society," and Mark Duffield (2001) on the "new humanitarianism in global governance," and the considerable literature published since.

28. Among those holding the formalist view, significant writings include Stanley Hoffmann's (1996) work on the "ethics of humanitarian intervention" and Hugo Slim's (2002) on "humanitarian philosophy": both propose ways of making so-called humanitarian intervention, particularly on the part of states, better—that is to say, essentially more legitimate. Representative examples of the critical position include the analyses of Anne Orford (1999) on "muscular humanitarianism" and Vanessa Pupavac (2001) on "therapeutic governance": the former sees the very principle of intervention without the sanction of

international law as problematic, while the latter is interested in the mobilization of psychiatric categories such as posttraumatic stress in the description of violence and in the effects of the pathologization of victims of war.

29. With the help of Save the Children, political scientist Alex de Waal (2005 [1989]) has studied the famine in Darfur and the difficulties of intervening to combat it. Reviewing her experience as head of mission for Médecins Sans Frontières, Fiona Terry (2002) proposes in parallel an analysis of the paradoxes of humanitarian action, particularly regarding the Tutsi genocide in Rwanda.

30. The anthology edited by Nancy Scheper-Hughes and Philippe Bourgois (2004) offers numerous revealing examples of the changes at work in North American anthropology.

31. See Mariella Pandolfi's "Laboratory of Intervention" (2008). In a more recent text (2010), she discusses the permanent state of emergency that is prevailing in contemporary conflicts.

32. See Peter Redfield's "Doctors, Borders and Life in Crisis" (2005). In a later essay (2010), he underlines the specificity of humanitarian intervention in contexts of abandonment rather than war or disaster.

33. As did Richard Rechtman and I (2009 [2007]) in our study of trauma when we explored the political uses of this category in the South of France after an industrial disaster, in the Palestinian Territories during the Second Intifada, and among asylum seekers soliciting a refugee status in Europe.

34. In a similar vein, Signe Howell (1997) brought together a series of case studies of local moralities in the United Kingdom, Zimbabwe, Argentina, Mexico, Mongolia, North Yemen, and Papua New Guinea.

35. Returning to the formula of the collection I edited with Alban Bensa (2008) to show the epistemological but also ethical problems of the politics of fieldwork today.

36. Introducing his seminar at the École des Hautes Études en Sciences Sociales, Pierre Bourdieu, in his dialogue with Loïc Wacquant (1992: 220–221), stated: "The *summum* of the art, in the social sciences, is, in my eyes, to be capable of engaging very high 'theoretical' stakes by means of very precise and often apparently very mundane, if not derisory, empirical objects." Using the certificate of schooling as a basis for "studying the effects of the monopoly of the state over the means of legitimate symbolic violence," he added: "What counts, in reality, is the rigor of the *construction* of the object. The power of a mode of thinking never manifests itself more clearly than in its capacity to constitute socially insignificant objects into scientific objects."

CHAPTER 1

1. See the volume edited by Joëlle Affichard and Jean-Baptiste de Foucauld (1992) for the Commissariat Général du Plan (General Planning Commission). The expression "fracture sociale," adopted by Jacques Chirac, has been attributed to demographer Emmanuel Todd or to philosopher Marcel Gauchet, an-

other illustration of the role played by the social sciences and humanities on the forging of a political lexicon to replace the Marxist vocabulary of class.

2. Jacques Chirac's opponent in the second round of the 1995 presidential election, the Socialist Lionel Jospin, sought in vain to seize the theme of a "divided France," adding his own personal touch as he declared unconvincingly that he preferred the idea of a "rift" to that of "fracture." See "Une 'fracture sociale,' deux théories économiques" [One "social fracture," two economic theories], Les Echos, May 2, 2007, http://www.lesechos.fr/info/france/300166117 .htm (consulted in February 2010).

3. This research, conducted at five of these facilities in Paris and its outskirts, has been published in Fassin (2004b). It was based on interviews and observation at the various sites, two of which were studied by Zahia Kessar (the center for adolescents in Saint-Denis) and Blandine Boulenger (the center for unemployed in Paris).

4. Médecins du Monde had launched a "France mission" in 1986, soon followed by Médecins Sans Frontières; their purpose was to help those who had no access to welfare support. In a symmetrical but ultimately complementary shift, people who had previously campaigned for local causes were becoming involved in action around more distant issues (Collovald 2001). Xavier Emmanuelli himself, cofounder of Médecins Sans Frontières and subsequently of the "Samu Social" (emergency services for the homeless), published a book titled La fracture sociale [Social fracture] a few years later.

5. An assessment of only those structures set up under the terms of the 1997 circular listed sixty-seven of them, with a total budget of 167 million francs (US$30 million). See the report prepared by Élisabeth Jacob et al., Évaluation des points écoute jeunes et/ou parents [Evaluation of support centers for youth and/or parents], OFDT, Étude no. 23, 2000.

6. A detailed account of this center appears in "Un dispositif d'observation psychologique" [A facility for psychological observation], from Fassin (2004: 83–102), where excerpts and statistics from the report of this center can be found.

7. However, the report by the Haut Comité de la Santé Publique (High Committee for Public Health) titled La souffrance psychique des adolescents et des jeunes adultes [Psychic suffering among adolescents and young adults], published in February 2000, advises caution in making the link between suffering and violence: "The notion of the psychic suffering of young people is vague," warn the authors. "There is too much of a tendency to confuse it with some of its effects, cobbled together in the equally vague category of 'youth violence.'" See http://www.sante.gouv.fr/htm/actu/36_000200.htm (consulted in February 2010).

8. See Pierre Rosanvallon (1995) and Robert Castel (1995), who share a similar focus. The "social question" is an expression used in the nineteenth century to account for the pauperization of the proletariat and its emergence as a political problem. The current "new social question" also combines the two dimensions: the economic reality and its expression in the public sphere.

9. Hélène Thomas (1997) underlines the role played by the books *Les exclus* [The excluded] by René Lenoir (1974) and *Vaincre la pauvreté dans les pays riches* [Defeating poverty in rich countries] by Lionel Stoléru (1977) to formulate the persistence of poverty in an affluent society.

10. Philippe Robert (2002) notes that the theme is of less recent date than is generally supposed, since it first appeared in the late 1970s.

11. The controversy revolved around the rights to the image, because the woman asked that her photo not be published. Her protest was encouraged by the Algerian authorities, who were accused in turn of wanting to evade the question of their responsibility in the massacre, since the army in a nearby barracks had failed to intervene. The photographer, Hocine Zaourar, was awarded the World Press Photo Prize that year for this "Madonna of Benthala," as she is often described. See http://www.humanite.fr/1998-02-14_Cultures_-La-Madone-de-Benthala-photo-de-l-annee-1997 (consulted in February 2010).

12. See *Télérama*, no. 2553, December 16, 1998, 8–9, and *Le Monde*, April 9, 1998, 9. Many other articles also appeared during this period, including "Thou Shalt Labor in Pain," *Libération*, April 20, 1998, and "Stress and Depression Empty Offices," *Libération*, October 10, 2000. Magazines issued special features: among others, *Santé mentale* [Mental health] reported on "psychic suffering" in December 1998, *Santé et travail* [Health and work] on "the suffering of women at work" in April 2000, and *La Pensée* [Thought] on "suffering at work" in March 2002.

13. See "Surmenage et limites du médecin" [Overwork and doctors' limits], workshop for general practitioners conducted on January 20, 1999. The theme was taken up in an editorial in *Le Monde* on January 2, 2002, titled "Suffering Medicine," which was in fact related to the general practitioners' strike calling for an increase in the fee for a basic medical consultation to twenty euros, and for a home visit to thirty euros: suffering was an argument for better fees. Here again, however, the doctors' problems were seen in relation to their patients' misfortunes: "The campaign has a lot of support, translating a general distress. Doctors are complaining not just about their income, but about their working conditions," having "become the first port of call in a society where individuals are suffering most of all from isolation."

14. See "Les téléspectateurs jugent le journal télévisé" [The public judge the news on television], *Le Monde*, November 27, 2001. The study was based on techniques (graded questionnaire, focus groups, representative sampling) supposedly guaranteeing that it was scientific.

15. In her essay *On Revolution* (1962), Hannah Arendt distinguishes between the abstract pity felt for the masses and the concrete compassion for the beggar. This distinction is taken up by Luc Boltanski in *Distant Suffering* (1999 [1993]). Today, media have the power to individualize the masses and make distant scenes seem close, thus transforming pity into compassion.

16. This review, in *L'Homme* (1999, 149: 214–215), of *Social Suffering*, edited by Arthur Kleinman, Veena Das, and Margaret Lock, can be compared with another commentary on the same book by Vincanne Adams, in *Ameri-*

can Anthropologist (1998, 100: 1064), asking a different question: "Why is this imperative to elicit, expose and position ourselves in relation to suffering so important? One might ask whether this imperative is not also culturally specific in origin. What is the cultural and philosophical basis for the imperative of this volume? Curiously, if suffering is recognized as an inevitable outcome of state and modern social formations, then why is *only* suffering so representable in our discipline these days?"

17. See, among many others and with an increasing audience, Christophe Dejours (1998), Dominique Lhullier (2007), and Isabelle Méténier (2010).

18. In his study, Alain Ehrenberg (1998: 180) focuses on the man who "becomes depressed because he must imagine that everything is possible for him." He took up his argument a few years later in the journal *Esprit* (2004): rejecting phenomenological approaches to psychic suffering, he sees the invocation of it as "the public expression of the tensions felt by a type of individual who is still required to be disciplined and obedient, but now above all autonomous, with a capacity to act and decide for himself."

19. See, for instance, and with somewhat distinct orientations, Chaumont (1997), Erner (2006), and Eliacheff and Soulez-Larivière (2006).

20. Recognizable here is the Foucauldian analysis that Hacking acknowledges as his approach (1995: 3–4): "As a research strategy I have always been much taken by what Michel Foucault named archaeology. I think that there are sometimes fairly sharp mutations in systems of thought and that these redistributions of ideas establish what later seems inevitable, unquestionable, necessary."

21. In his book on "mad travelers," Hacking (1999) suggests that this model of the "ecological niche" can be applied to a whole series of diseases and patients who might be said to exist only for a time.

22. Through repeated use during the 1980s, the two terms became accepted usage. They should however be considered in a critical perspective, and a considerable body of scientific writing has already been devoted to this. For a presentation of these two notions and their empirical validation, see the books by Serge Paugam (1991) and Christian Bachmann and Nicole Le Guennec (1997).

23. As the study Hervé Hudebine and I conducted in the Parisian region illustrates, the compassionate discourse around heroin users had infiltrated the police's viewpoint and way of working to such an extent that they spoke of them with a sort of commiseration, and systematically avoided stopping them so that they could get to their needle exchange sites in peace. See *Politiques de la drogue et gouvernement des villes: Les scènes locales de la réduction des risques* [Drug policy and urban local government: Local scenes of risk reduction], report, Bobigny, CRESP, 2002. For an analysis of policy at national and local levels during this period, see Bergeron (1999) and Lovell (1998), respectively.

24. During the same period, the common view of people with AIDS shifted radically. Disapproval of the practices of homosexuals and, as we have seen, of drug users, which had so strongly marked the first years of the epidemic in a

logic of "victim blaming," gave way to a concern for "public goods," as Nicolas Dodier (2003) notes, referring to individual and public health, of course, but also the combat against stigmatization, and the valorization of self-fulfillment.

25. As Isabelle Astier (1998) shows in her study of job-finding committees, this policy was based on a process of delving into people's private details.

26. See notably the contributions by Jacques Donzelot and Joël Roman (1991) and by Alain Touraine (1992) to collective volumes by the Éditions Esprit. The reports by the Commissariat Général du Plan are *Exclus et exclusions: Connaître les populations et comprendre les processus* [Excluded and exclusions: Identifying populations and understanding processes] for Philippe Nasse's report and *Cohésion sociale et prévention de l'exclusion* [Social cohesion and preventing exclusion] for Bertrand Fragonard's report. At this time relations between this planning body and the intellectuals associated with the journal *Esprit* were close and organic (personal links, working groups, copublished reports). For a sociohistorical analysis of the concept of exclusion, see Fassin (1996).

27. As Alain Bihr and Roland Pfefferkorn (1999) recall, in 1998 unemployment reached 4.5% among professional classes compared with 21.9% among unskilled workers in France; the proportion of short-term contracts and temporary employment was 2.9% for professionals and 19.2% for unskilled workers.

28. The physical presentation of the volume was in itself remarkable. On the dust jacket of the French edition (1993), the book's title was overlaid by the two words "france speaks" in giant red "typewritten" letters. However, when the book was fully opened, the word "france" became "souffrance" (suffering). Éric Maigret (2002: 172) recounts how he was approached by the organizers of the study: "As a student, I was invited to contribute to the research; I remember I found the invitation reductive not in terms of the subject, but because of the substantialist way it was defined: we had to find someone we knew who was 'really suffering' through his or her life." The "instruction" was that "only suffering would be audible."

29. The first elements of this collective research had already been presented in the issue of *Actes de la Recherche en Sciences Sociales* titled simply "Suffering," which appeared in December 1991. It is rather moving to see Pierre Bourdieu discover, not without a certain degree of naivety, the "lives of others." He himself recognized this and stressed how this research had formed a turning point in his scientific project: "I had to get to the age I am and develop a little more social nerve in order to commit this transgression."

30. The report is significantly titled *Une souffrance qu'on ne peut plus cacher* [A suffering that can no longer be hidden]. In the terms of reference, Delarue stated that his institution is "kept regularly informed of the problems that hinder the implementation of policies for combating exclusion," and that "these difficulties relate particularly to a state of ill-being or more specifically to the mental health of particular groups." Thus the notions of social exclusion and mental health were linked from the outset. The report, written by Hélène Strohl, came out as a typed document in 1995.

31. In one of his courses, John Langshaw Austin (1962: 23) jokingly gives the following example of infelicity in a performative utterance: "Suppose, for example, I see a vessel on the stocks, walk up and smash the bottle hung at the stern, proclaim 'I name this ship the *Mr. Stalin*' and for good measure kick away the chocks: but the trouble is, I was not the person chosen to name it."

32. Proceedings of the conferences were published: J. Furtos et al. (eds.), *Déqualification sociale et psychopathologie: Devoirs et limites de la psychiatrie publique* [Social marginalization and psychopathology: The obligations and limits of public psychiatry], Lyons, ORSPERE, 1994; and J. Furtos et al. (eds.), *Souffrance psychique, contexte social et exclusion* [Psychic suffering, social context and exclusion], Lyons, ORSPERE, 1997.

33. The forty-seven members of the interdepartmental working group included seven psychiatrists considered expert in groups deemed to be challenged. One of them, Jean Maisondieu, a former army doctor and hospital psychiatrist in Poissy, was a pioneer of the clinical practice of exclusion.

34. In his early works, Castel (1981: 155) speaks of a "psychological culture," that is, a "cultural stance that tends to see insertion in the psychological as the achievement of the vocation of the social subject."

35. Of particular note here is the influential report by Eric Piel and Jean-Luc Roelandt, *De la psychiatrie à la santé mentale* [From psychiatry to mental health], for the minister for health, Paris, 2001.

36. The core of the network around which the working group was structured was made up of researchers and professionals who had met within the framework of a community health project in the Franc-Moisin district of Saint-Denis, led by Lazarus and sociologist Michel Joubert. The house-to-house survey conducted among the residents of the project had revealed the frequency of depressive-type mood disorders, found among 59% of those interviewed. The authors of the investigation (Joubert, Bertolotto, and Bouhnik 1993: 112) therefore posited "a socioepidemiology of ill-being," which was to "form the basis of a clinical practice of the everyday," but in their research report they were not yet using the term "suffering."

37. The book's very title, *Souffrance en France*, echoed *La misère du monde*, to the point that Dejours (1998), in a rhyming play on words, adopted, perhaps unconsciously, the phrase ("souffrance"/"france") that appeared, as mentioned earlier, on the dust jacket of Bourdieu's book.

38. A special issue of *Esprit* titled "A quoi sert le travail social?" [What use is social work?], published the same year, examined this development whereby analysis of social work had shifted from condemnation on the grounds of the control it was deemed to exert over the dominated, in the 1970s, to criticism of its failures to meet the expectations of users, in the 1990s. Where previously they were accused of doing too much, social workers were now reproached for not doing enough.

39. The wealth of writing by psychiatrists and psychologists on the topic of suffering is certainly not limited to the Lyons school of "psychosocial practice," even if this trend unquestionably played the predominant role in constructing

a legitimate space for suffering in public policy. A number of networks and organizations, variously more psychoanalytic or more ethnocultural in orientation, were also exploring this social dimension of suffering.

40. The quotes are from Jean Furtos's lecture to the 1997 conference, *Souffrance psychique, contexte social et exclusion*, and the ORSPERE report *Points de vue et rôles des acteurs de la clinique psychosociale* [Points of view and roles of actors in psychosocial practice], Ministère de l'Emploi et de la Solidarité / Fédération nationale des associations d'accueil et de réinsertion sociale, 1999.

41. In 1999 the national network Souffrance psychique et précarité (Psychic Suffering and Precariousness) was set up on the initiative of the Lyons team: it was chaired by Xavier Emmanuelli, a founder of Médecins Sans Frontières, with Antoine Lazarus as one of its administrators. In 2000 the journal *Rhizome: Bulletin national santé mentale et précarité* [National bulletin on mental health and precariousness] was launched, with the support of the Ministry for Employment and Solidarity. Edited by Jean Furtos, it became one of the main organs of promotion for the cause of psychic suffering and of debate on the future of mental health practice. In 2002 ORSPERE became a national observatory.

42. In the *Tractatus* (1922 [1921]), and even more specifically in the *Philosophical Investigations* (2004 [1953]).

43. The research report by Pierre Vidal-Naquet, Irène Amiel, Sophie Trévant, and Sylviane Touzé, *Lieux d'écoute et prévention des toxicomanies* [Listening facilities and prevention of drug abuse], Conseil général de la Seine-Saint-Denis, 1997, offers plenty of evidence of the very wide variety of facilities: between the center for the unemployed providing services to job seekers, which took advantage of the circular to recruit a "shrink who hangs around," as the psychologist called himself, and the drug users' support and treatment facility that engaged in "street work" with youth leaders, state funding was the only common feature that allowed for comparison and, potentially, the retrospective constitution of a "community" of specialists in listening.

44. This unit has been described in "Une rencontre improbable entre des psychanalystes et des chômeurs" [An unlikely meeting between psychoanalysts and unemployed] from Fassin (2004b: 143–149), from which excerpts of interviews are taken.

45. According to Taylor (1989), the "sources of the Self" should be sought further back than the moral philosophy of the Enlightenment, going as far as Locke, Descartes, and even Augustine.

46. From this point of view the emblematic scene of this shift is the atrocious execution of the failed regicide Damiens, who attempted to kill King Louis XV of France. His death by drawing and quartering is recounted, not without a certain relish, by Michel Foucault at the beginning of *Discipline and Punish* (1977 [1975]). This was the last public execution in France.

47. See Taylor (1989).

48. In the first volume of *The History of Sexuality* (1979 [1976]). In contrast with commonsense discourse about the repression of sexual issues, he underscores their omnipresence.

49. In his book *Governing the Soul* (1989: 198). His analysis was preceded by Richard Sennett's in *The Fall of Public Man* (1977).

CHAPTER 2

1. The symbolism of Christmas is particularly strong in the history of aid to the poor. In a study conducted in Marienthal in the aftermath of the 1929 crisis, Paul Lazarsfeld and his team (1981 [1932]) evoke the parcels provided by the municipal authorities to help unemployed miners spend the holiday less miserably. The success of the 1997 movement, which was the subject of a study by Didier Demazière and Maria-Teresa Pignoni (1999), was partly a result of the public outcry at the abolition of the social funds that financed the Christmas bonus for the unemployed.

2. In 1998 the French currency was the franc, but the euro was introduced in January 1999. To facilitate interpretation of the financial aid received by the beneficiaries of the fund, figures are presented in euros. In that period the exchange rate was 1 euro = US$1.10. Therefore the amounts given in euros can be approximated to the equivalent in dollars: http://www.x-rates.com/d/EUR/USD/hist1998.html (consulted in May 2010).

3. According to the Institut National de Statistique et d'Études Économiques (National Institute for Statistics and Economic Research, INSEE), the seasonally adjusted rate of unemployment peaked between 1993 and 1997 at about 12% of the working population. To put this in perspective, until the early 1970s it had never risen above 3%. See http://www.ladocumentationfrancaise.fr/dossiers/emploi/chiffres-cles.shtml (consulted in February 2010). The social movement thus came into being at the peak of the crisis. But the rate of underemployment was much higher, and taking into account those in training who were seeking work, those working reduced hours or forced into short-term contracts, and unemployed people who had given up looking for work or had retired early, the figure rises to 6,700,000—double the official figure, and one-fourth of the active population. These were the groups involved in the mobilization of "the unemployed and the precarious." See the 1996 study discussed in Freyssinet (2004).

4. This phrase was coined by Guido Calabresi and Philip Bobbitt (1978), two legal specialists whose book *Tragic Choices* spawned a fertile field of research on what John Elster (1992) names local justice.

5. On organ transplants, see especially the study by John Elster and Nicolas Herpin (1992). Sébastien Dalgalarrondo and Philippe Urfalino (2000) study the problem posed for people with AIDS by the arrival of the second generation of antiretroviral drugs.

6. As analyzed notably by Michel Messu (1991), who shows how social support services function.

7. In this study this monthly residual income per person (the "rest for living") averaged 43 euros for the unemployed receiving ASSEDIC benefit, 65 euros for those on minimum income, and 130 euros for the "low-paid workers." See Didier Fassin and Anne-Claire Defossez, *Une charité d'État: La mise en place du Fonds d'urgence sociale en Seine-Saint-Denis* [State charity: The establishment of the Social Emergency Fund in Seine-Saint-Denis], Bobigny, CRESP, Study Report no. 1, 2000.

8. These are the terms of the 1998 report produced by Marie-Thérèse Join-Lambert, the inspector general of social affairs, at the request of the prime minister: *Rapport de mission sur les problèmes soulevés par les mouvements de chômeurs en France fin 1997–début 1998* [Report of inquiry into problems raised by the unemployed workers' movement in France late 1997–early 1998].

9. Natalie Zemon Davis (1987) has studied petitions to the king under the ancien régime in France. I analyzed the rhetoric and arguments used by applicants to the Social Emergency Fund in "La supplique" [The Petition] (2000).

10. Interviews were conducted in collaboration with Anne-Claire Defossez with the main actors involved, either directly or indirectly, in the operation of the fund: members of the allocation committee, local government officers responsible for examining applications, social workers in local communities, and representatives of unemployed workers' associations. A sample of 300 applications was drawn at random from among the 20,000 received by the prefecture services: 100 people receiving unemployment benefits, 100 receiving the minimum income, and 100 individuals engaged in salaried work. Each file contained brief sociodemographic data, an income and expenditure account, and a text in which the applicant gave grounds for her or his request, as well as the committee's decision, the amount of any aid granted, and a copy of the letter sent to the applicant; it often also included handwritten notes explaining the committee's decision.

11. In his famous study (Garfinkel 1984: 114) of the work of trial jurors.

12. As demonstrated—and, moreover, defended—by historian Pierre Rosanvallon (1995: 197, 210, and 217), who takes the view that the state must "above all take care of individuals, each in their own specific situation," rather than implementing measures universally applicable to all groups.

13. Sociologist Serge Paugam (1993: 85 and 87) notes the recurrence of this logic since the French Revolution and argues that it reasserts "the collective's obligation to guarantee sufficient resources for subsistence" for the poor: the aid system should remedy the insufficiencies of the insurance system.

14. Despite the presentation of these principles as radically different from those of social assistance, the two guidelines—individualization of aid and the principle of emergency—fit perfectly into the government approach, in the tradition of "modern assistance" that Georg Simmel (1998: 47 and 66) recognizes as being "unique as a public institution."

15. Thus Erving Goffman (1963: 11) shows that in "the routines of social intercourse," the "anticipations" people have of others insensibly become "righteously presented demands."

16. Following the definitions provided by André Lalande (1993: 75 and 182). For the noun "the arbitrary": "In the concrete sense: the individual whim of an authority; a capricious decision about a matter on which one should proceed through reasoning or by application of a rule." For the adjective "arbitrary": "Depending entirely on an individual decision, not an established order or a reason applied to all." The critical commentary notes: "The arbitrary differs from the contingent in that the latter does not contain the idea of whim." "Contingent" is defined thus: "General sense: anything conceived as being able to be or not be is contingent." Further on: "Relative sense: a fact is contingent in relation to a given general law or a given type, when it consists not in the application of that law or that type, but in some circumstance particular to a given individual object to which they apply. Any concurrence of phenomena that is not constant or even general is contingent."

17. The book was written in the period following social unrest, during which welfare provision was substantially extended in the United States. It was reissued, in an updated version, two decades later when the ideological climate and the economic situation were very different and there was widespread criticism of social welfare (Piven and Cloward 1993 [1971]).

CHAPTER 3

1. See the circular at http://www.legifrance.gouv.fr/WAspad/UnTexteDeJorf ?numjo=INTD9700104C, and the law 98-349 at http://www.legislationline .org/documents/action/popup/id/7617 (both consulted in February 2010).

2. For this study, interviews were conducted in a public hospital, north of Paris, that was founded in 1935 as Hôpital Franco-Musulman (French Muslim Hospital) for the Arab Muslim patients of Paris and its region, as part of the colonial Service de surveillance et de protection des indigènes nord-africains (Service for the surveillance and protection of North African natives). In 1978 it became the Hospital Avicenne, open to all patients, but still with a high proportion of immigrants from Maghreb and sub-Saharan Africa. I carried out my research in relation with the medical and social clinic I had created for patients without medical coverage, mostly undocumented immigrants. Rather than participant observation, one could speak therefore of observant participation.

3. And also to the title of the novel by Hervé Guibert, *The Compassion Protocol*, published in France in 1991, shortly after the author's death from AIDS. "Compassion protocol" is a term used by doctors to describe a treatment of last resort that has not gone through the usual stages of clinical testing.

4. Lecture given in 1980 at the Twenty-Second Conference of the Société de psychologie médicale de langue française (Association of French-Speaking Medical Psychologists), published in 1981 in the journal *Psychologie médicale*, and republished in *The Suffering of the Immigrant* (Sayad 2004 [1999]: 180). Tellingly, the initial title of the article, "Health and Social Equilibrium among

Immigrants," was revised in the 1999 French publication to "Illness, Suffering and the Body"—a formulation more in keeping with the contemporary pathos on these issues.

5. The term "sinistrosis" first appeared in 1908, in the language of forensic medicine in a clinical report by Édouard Brissaud, who described with this term the posttraumatic psychic consequences resulting from an accident at work. This diagnosis made it possible for the ideology of suspicion toward workers who complained of vague symptoms in these situations to become part of psychiatric nosography for more than half a century. In the 1950s and 1960s it was widely used to describe—and discredit—a pathology then focused on workers from North Africa who were suspected of seeking secondary benefits in this way, to the detriment of the French social state (on this issue, see Fassin and Rechtman 2009 [2007]: 37–38 and 64–66).

6. The emergence of the question of the *sans-papiers* (undocumented) out of the social movement that started with the occupation of the Church of Saint Hippolyte in Paris in June 1996 is examined in a collective volume I co-edited (Fassin, Morice, and Quiminal 1997). The expression "the useless in the world" is Geremek's (1980).

7. The Groupe d'information et de soutien aux immigrés (Immigrant Information and Support Group, GISTI) published analysis on the circular in July 1997 and on the law in July 1998: *Sans-papiers: Régularisation? Analyse de la circulaire du 24 juin 1997* [Undocumented foreigners: Legalization? Analysis of the circular of June 24 1997] and *Entrée, séjour et éloignement des étrangers après la loi Chevènement* [Entry, stay and removal of foreigners following introduction of the Chevènement Act].

8. In its December 1995 *Rapport suivi d'un avis sur la situation des personnes atteintes par le VIH de nationalité étrangère et en irrégularité de séjour* [Report and opinion on the situation of HIV-positive foreign nationals without residence rights], the Conseil National du Sida (National AIDS Council) condemned the policies toward undocumented immigrants living with HIV/AIDS.

9. The statistics relating to applications submitted in the Seine-Saint-Denis *département* come from the Directorate of Health and Social Welfare (DDASS). The national data on the application of the new law were provided by the offices of the Ministry of the Interior at the Observatoire du Droit à la Santé des Étrangers (Observatory for Foreigners' Right to Health Care, ODSE), a collective of seventeen organizations including Médecins du Monde, Service oecuménique d'entraide (Ecumenical Service for Solidarity, CIMADE), Comité médical pour les exilés (Medical Committee for Exiles, COMEDE), GISTI, Aides (an AIDS support organization), Act Up Paris (an AIDS advocacy organization), and the Centre Primo Levi (Primo Levi Association, an organization assisting victims of torture), http://odse.eu.org/IMG/pdf/Analyse_de_l_ODSE.pdf (consulted in February 2010).

10. By "social condition," I mean an objective situation that, unlike the "human condition" as understood by Hannah Arendt (1958), is historically consti-

tuted but also sociologically differentiated: rather than a human being, this is a social—and political—subject (Fassin 2001).

11. The seven-page memo, dated February 11, 1997, was titled "La procédure des autorisations d'extension de prolongation de séjour pour des raisons sanitaires: Le role du médecin inspecteur de santé publique, ou les mains sales?" [The procedure for authorizing extensions of permission to remain on health grounds: The role of the public medical officer, or dirty hands?].

12. For her dissertation at the École Nationale de Santé Publique (National School of Public Health), titled Le maintien des étrangers pour raison médicale sur le territoire français [Allowing foreigners to stay in France on health grounds], submitted in April 1999, Dominique Delettré analyzed the statistics and interviewed DDASS medical inspectors in the Île-de-France region—that is, Paris and the eight surrounding départements, which represent by far the most populous region of the country.

13. This table is freely inspired by that proposed by Howard Becker in his well-known book Outsiders (1963), wherein he discusses the four configurations of deviance, depending on whether or not the act was committed and if it was recognized.

14. During the 1990s ethnopsychiatry enjoyed unprecedented popularity in France, going well beyond psychological circles, in the realm of medicine, social action, judicial practice, and public policy, and even infiltrating intellectual and media circles (Fassin 1999 and 2011a).

15. This represents a seventeenfold increase: by comparison, the total number of applications, as opposed to the permits granted, for medical assessment rose progressively from 1,500 in 1999 to 5,678 in 2001; 33,133 in 2003; and 40,940 in 2005. These figures, issued by the Ministry of the Interior, were published by ODSE: http://odse.eu.org/IMG/pdf/Analyse_de_l_ODSE.pdf, and COMEDE: http://www.comede.org/UserFiles/File/Rapport_Comede_2006.pdf (both consulted in February 2010). However, the increase should also be viewed in relative terms: on December 31, 2005, official statistics showed 23,605 people legally resident in France on medical grounds, representing 0.72% of the total migrant population.

16. See Case of N. v. the United Kingdom (Application 26565/05, Judgment Strasbourg, May 27, 2008), Lawtel, http://www.isd.salford.ac.uk, and the commentary by Canadian lawyer Caroline Lantero, "La Cour européenne des droits de l'homme et les étrangers malades: Le ton se durcit," July 2008, at http://www.cerium.ca/La-Cour-europeenne-des-droits-de-l,7451 (both consulted in February 2009).

CHAPTER 4

1. These statistics come from the United Nations High Commission for Refugees: http://www.unhcr.fr/cgi-bin/texis/vtx/statistics/opendoc.pdf?tbl=STATISTICS&id=42b283744, and from OFPRA: http://www.ofpra.gouv.fr/documents/OFPRA_Rapport_2004.pdf (both consulted in February 2010).

2. Suspicion of refugees is of course neither a uniquely French phenomenon nor entirely new. The collective book *Mistrusting Refugees*, edited by Valentine Daniel and John Knudsen (1995), offers a range of examples and interpretations.

3. According to COMEDE's 2005 report (http://www.comede.org/IMG/pdf/rapp_comede05.pdf), Sri Lankans represented the largest group of foreigners seeking the center's help in cases of torture, and second largest (behind Sudanese) in cases of violence. The figures and the following quotation are taken from OFPRA's 2005 report: http://www.ofpra.gouv.fr/documents/OFPRA_Rapport_2005.pdf (both consulted in February 2010).

4. In the following text I use CNDA except when I refer precisely to an event related to its previous version as CRR.

5. To use the formula that Michel Foucault (1994: 20) proposed, notably at a round table where he discussed his work with historians on May 20, 1978.

6. The study is grounded on interviews conducted with members of several nongovernmental organizations and judges from the CNDA. It was complemented by the analysis of a corpus of 250 randomly selected medical certificates that I realized in collaboration with Estelle d'Halluin. It is also informed by my own involvement with the question of asylum and certification when I later became president of COMEDE.

7. The scene is described in "Terror as Usual: Walter Benjamin's Theory of History as State of Siege," in the collection of essays *The Nervous System* (1992: 33).

8. The catalogue of the exhibition, *Maux d'Exil* [Exile sickness], photographs by Olivier Pasquiers and testimonies gathered by Jean-Louis Levy (Paris: Bar Floréal, 2000), brings together the two series of documents, images, and accounts, obviously without linking them for reasons of confidentiality.

9. As noted by Pierre Clastres (1977 [1974]: 157) in relation to the Mandan and Guayaki Indians, whose painful tattoos represent "the inscribed text of primitive law," and Maurice Godelier (1986 [1982]: 78) in relation to the prescriptions of the Baruya of New Guinea, which constitute "the commands of the domination of men over women and the submission of the young to their elders."

10. Véronique Nahoum-Grappe (1996: 283) sees collective rape as serving the political program of "elimination of a community"; Jackie Assayag (2004: 283) argues that hyperbolic evil is brought into play through "biopolitical practices on human material."

11. This is the famous thesis of *Discipline and Punish* (1977 [1975]: 16). Our modernity is characterized by a displacement of the punishment from the body to the soul and by a shift in the inquiry of truth from the act committed to its explanation and signification.

12. For a history of the policies of asylum and an analysis of the role of the nongovernmental organizations, see Estelle d'Halluin's dissertation (2008).

13. This was how Arnaud Veïsse (2003: 32) put it, adding that "the medical certificate should never be the deciding factor in awarding refugee status."

14. Which "gives asylum to foreigners banished from their homeland in the cause of freedom," as Sophie Wahnich (1997: 27) reminds us, emphasizing nevertheless the atmosphere of suspicion in which this principle of hospitality was applied during the revolutionary period.

15. As Hannah Arendt writes in her study of imperialism (1951: 269): "Those whom persecution has called undesirable become the *indésirables* of Europe."

16. See Michael Marrus's book on the history of refugees in the first half of the twentieth century. In his epilogue (1985: 371), he announces "the apparent end of a European refugee problem," because "refugees are relatively few in number." History is never written in advance, and both the sharp rise in requests for asylum since the beginning of the 1990s and, even more, the political stakes that have crystallized around the refugee issue show that the "problem" remains far from over.

17. As Gérard Noiriel (1991) showed in his study of the national debates that preceded and followed the signing of the Geneva Convention, particularly in France.

18. For an analysis of this issue, see Patrick Weil (1991) on the policies and Vincent Viet (1998) on the institutions.

19. In 2006 OFPRA's rate of positive decisions was 7.8%. This figure represented a reduction over the previous year's level of 8.2%. This is all the more remarkable given that the number of requests had fallen by 26% during this period, from 51,391 to 37,986. The decrease in the rate of acceptance is often ascribed to an increase in applications, suggesting that a larger proportion of applications are judged unfounded. The inverse development of a fall in applications, due mainly to much stricter control at the points of exit from country of origin and entry into France before any application can be submitted, thus did not result in a corresponding increase in the rate of acceptance. To the refugees accepted by OFPRA should be added the 4,425 adults who were granted refugee status in 2006 by the CRR; this figure represents a 54% decrease over 2005. In total, 7,354 asylum seekers were granted asylum in 2006: http://www .ofpra.gouv.fr/documents/rapport_Ofpra_2006.pdf (consulted in February 2010).

20. We have already noted this in relation to residence permits, to which illegal migrants who were denied a permit attached an almost magical power of social integration (Fassin and Morice 2001). No sooner had they been granted one than they realized its limitations in terms of getting work, housing, and simply a place in French society: the undocumented thus discovered that while they were nothing without "documents," they were little more even when they did possess them.

21. Her article "Paroles de victims et vérité certifiée par l'expert" [The words of victims and the expert-certified truth], *Mémoires*, no. 25, October 2004, is a revised version of a paper that appeared in the same journal in June 2003 (no. 22) under the title "Le mythe de la preuve" [The myth of proof]:

http://www.primolevi.asso.fr/web/fr/file_pdf/articles_Memoires/Memoires
_25.pdf (consulted in February 2010).

22. Élisabeth Didier's article "Torture et mythe de la preuve" [Torture and the myth of proof] (1992) is often cited by actors involved in asylum.

23. British anthropologist Anthony Good (2007), who acted as an expert witness for the British asylum service, offers a detailed analysis of aspects of the interpretation of the 1951 Geneva Convention, particularly in relation to "well-founded fear" and the conditions of implementation of this criterion, on the basis of the United Nations High Commission for Refugees' *Handbook on Procedures and Criteria for Determining Refugee Status,* which discusses the subjective dimensions of such fear.

24. Richard Rechtman and I (2009 [2007]) have examined the specific history of trauma and its usage in the construction of psychological proof of torture and violence.

25. According to Max Weber (2008: 198): "All ethically oriented action can follow *two* totally different principles that are irreconcilably opposed to each other: an ethic of 'conviction' or an ethic of 'responsibility'. This is not to say that the ethic of conviction is identical with the lack of responsibility, or that the ethic of responsibility is identical with lack of conviction."

26. What we could describe, following Nikolas Rose (1989), as the "ethical-political" domain in which, he argues, the techniques required for the exercise of responsible government and the negotiation between duties to oneself and to others are brought into play.

27. In his study of bureaucratic practices of asylum in Sweden, Mark Graham (2003) gives an example of the emotional involvement of agents of government.

28. See Nathalie Berger's analysis (2000) of the convergence of European policies on asylum and immigration. What struck me when I attended the Paris Conference was the moral rhetoric European ministers in charge of immigration issues (mostly ministers of the interior) were employing to maintain the illusion that asylum was treated differently from immigration, in spite of the increasing evidence to the contrary. I wondered how much cynicism entered these discourses.

29. In his study on U.S. immigration service agents, particularly on the Mexican border, Josiah Heyman (1998) offers another example of these ethical issues.

30. This question arises for all those who write about violence, as Veena Das (1997) observes in relation to Indian women who suffered extreme brutality during the partition of India.

31. The long descriptions with which Jonathan Spencer (2000) reports scenes of violence in the Sri Lankan civil war, through the story of a young Sri Lankan man, offer a marked contrast to this style.

32. This phenomenon goes beyond the situation analyzed here, as Liisa Malkki (1996) observes, arguing that the administrative-legal status of refugee in some sense eliminates the individual's condition.

33. As Michael Pollak (1990) writes in relation to the interviews he conducted with three women who escaped Nazi concentration and extermination camps.

34. In the chapter "The Decline of the Nation-State and the End of the Rights of Man" (Arendt 1951: 277).

35. To use the phrase coined by Allen Feldman (1994: 407), who seeks to analyze how this massification is also constructed through the images disseminated by the media.

36. As Talal Asad (1997: 289) emphasizes, distinguishing clearly between the idea (which he does not agree with) that "civilization" has led to a decline in torture, and the idea (which he defends) that torture is declared "uncivilized," leading to the practice of it becoming secret.

37. This tragic story was publicized by Simone Fluhr, who supported the young man through the asylum request process and brought together all the elements of his application after his death: "En mémoire de Mr. Elanchelvan Rajendram," *Recueil Alexandries, Collections Reflets*, May 2007, http://terra .rezo.net/article572.html (consulted in February 2010).

CHAPTER 5

1. See "Un non-lieu pour des gens de non-droit" [A non-place for people with non-rights], report of a study carried out by the Comité catholique contre la faim et pour le développement (Catholic Committee against Hunger and for Development, CCFD), the Service oecuménique d'entraide (Ecumenical Service for Solidarity, CIMADE), the Groupe d'information et de soutien aux immigrés (Immigrant Information and Support Group, GISTI), the Syndicat des avocats de France (French Lawyers' Union, SAF), and the Syndicat de la magistrature (Magistrates' Union, SM) on October 12 and 13, 2000: "We describe it as a 'camp' rather than a 'center' because of the living conditions prevailing there and the uncertain legal status of this 'thing' which has no precedent other than the camps for Spanish Republicans in the late 1930s." See http://www.gisti.org/spip.php?article655 (consulted in February 2010).

2. Sarkozy continued to refer back to this decision in the period that followed. Returning to Calais three years later, he declared: "Sangatte will hold a very important place in my life in government office." When he stood for election to the French presidency, he made the camp the symbol of his courageous stand on immigration control, stating at a press conference on December 11, 2006: "In 2002, the sinister Sangatte hangar was recognized throughout Europe as a symbol of the Jospin government's laxity and irresponsibility on immigration. There were two or three thousand migrants crammed in there, in conditions unworthy of our country, hoping to get to the United Kingdom." See http://discours.vie-publique.fr/notices/063004436.html (consulted in May 2011).

3. See, for example, "Fermer le camp ne résoudrait pas la question des réfugiés" [Closing the camp would not solve the refugee problem], *Le Monde*,

May 30, 2002, and "Le camp de la Croix-Rouge doit fermer fin décembre" [Red Cross camp to close at the end of December], *Libération*, December 3, 2002.

4. I reconstructed it on the basis of interviews with local people and an analysis of the local press. See also "Des milliers de fantômes en camp" [A camp full of thousands of ghosts], summary of study visit by CCFD, CIMADE, GISTI, SAF, and SM on October 12 and 13, 2000, http://www.gisti.org/spip.php?article654 (consulted in February 2010).

5. In his *Indo-European Language and Society*, Émile Benveniste (1973: 75–78) explains his method: "The vocabulary of Indo-European institutions holds important problems, the terms of which have in some cases not yet been posed. They can be discerned through the revealing words of an institution whose traces can often only be glimpsed fleetingly in a given language."

6. In his seminar at the École des Hautes Études en Sciences Sociales of January 10, 1996, titled "The Foreigner Question" (Derrida 2000 [1997]: 53–54).

7. It is worth remembering that the rate of refugee status accepted by the Office Français de Protection des Réfugiés et des Apatrides (French Office for the Protection of Refugees and Stateless Persons, OFPRA) fell from 95% in 1976 to 7.8% in 2006. For an analysis of the discourse of legal differentiation in the 1990s, see the collection *Les lois de l'inhospitalité* [The laws of inhospitality], which I coedited with Alain Morice and Catherine Quiminal (1997). For a discussion of the politics of legitimate discrimination in the first decade of the twenty-first century, see the collection edited by Claire Rodier and Emmanuel Terray (2008).

8. The empirical approach of this chapter involved an analysis of the press, a series of interviews, and an observation in the center of Sangatte, but it was also an endeavor to include the treatment of the issues at stake via cinematographic and performing arts.

9. For a study of ZAPI 3 (Zone d'attente pour personnes en instance), the waiting zone for persons pending decision on their application for entry at Roissy where foreign arrivals holding documents not considered valid are held while their case is investigated in more depth and a decision is made, usually to send them back to their country, see Makaremi (2009).

10. Henri Courau, a Red Cross member at the time, who was studying for a doctorate in anthropology, expressed his disappointment in the July 2002 issue of *Forced Migration Review*: http://www.fmreview.org/FMRpdfs/FMR14/fmr14.9.pdf (consulted in February 2010).

11. See *Dignity or Exploitation: The Choice Is in Your Hands*, International Organization for Migration, 8 pages, http://www.gisti.org/dossiers/sangatte/documents/index.html#dignity (consulted in February 2009).

12. For detailed statistics about the center, see the study based on the data from the Red Cross conducted by Romain Liagre and Frédéric Dumont (2005).

13. Following this incident, even Eurotunnel, the company running the Channel Tunnel, called for the Sangatte center to be closed. See Rebecca Pave-

ley, "500 Immigrants Storm Chunnel," *MailOnline*, http://www.dailymail. co.uk/news/article-91930/500-immigrants-storm-Chunnel.html (consulted in February 2010).

14. In her book on Haiti, Erica Caple James (2010) gives a gripping account of the insecure conditions in Port-au-Prince and the indefinable boundary between civil and political violence.

15. OFPRA's annual report of activities for 2001 notes: "Applications from Haitians, which have increased by 45%, constitute the third largest proportion of asylum seekers. Of 2,713 cases logged, 324 came from the Cayenne Prefecture in French Guyana [a territory where many Haitians fleeing their country try to find refuge]. In view of the remoteness of this office and the consistently high number of applications (which were given priority), OFPRA organized a two-week mission to examine cases in June 2001, backed up by video interviews and a second series of video interviews in September. These interviews showed that the requests for asylum were largely unfounded under the terms of the Geneva Convention, since they related essentially to the general lack of security but also to economic difficulties." It is likely that Marie's account was interpreted in terms of general lack of security and economic hardship. Moreover, rape is a crime known to be virtually impossible to prove very long after the event—although the subsequent development of this case tragically offers a corrective to that assumption. See http://www.ofpra.gouv.fr/documents/OFPRA_Rapport_2001.pdf (consulted in February 2010).

16. As demonstrated by the memo drawn up by Françoise Galabru, technical adviser at the Department for Population and Migration, on the impact of Article 12a11 of the ordinance of November 2, 1945, amended by the law of 1998 relating to the entry and residence of foreigners in France, a year after it was introduced. See unpublished and untitled document, Department for Population and Migration, June 26, 2000, 10 pages.

17. See the report by the French Senate Enquiry Committee, which includes minutes of the hearings organized during 1998: http://www.senat.fr/ rap/l97-47021/l97-47021_mono.html (consulted in February 2010).

18. In *Homo Sacer* (1998 [1995]: 4), Agamben interprets Aristotle's uses of *bios* and *zoē* to make this distinction foundational of his theory of biopolitics. Reformulating Michel Foucault's concept, he writes that "the entry of *zoē* into the sphere of the *polis*—the politicization of bare life as such—constitutes the decisive event of modernity and signals a radical transformation of the political-philosophical categories of classical thought."

19. This story is recounted in an article I wrote on the "social condition" of immigrants with AIDS (2001): it represents an ideal-type of the figure of the "legitimate body."

20. The concept of "biological citizenship," introduced by Adriana Petryna (2002) in relation to the victims of the Chernobyl explosion who were given social rights provided they could demonstrate the pathological consequences

of the accident, is useful in thinking about the situation of the sick given residence rights on the sole basis of their diseased body, as long as we do not lose sight of the fact that ultimately—and ironically—what is acquired is a social citizenship.

21. Quotations from Bertrand Delanoë and Philippe Seguin, at that time respectively Socialist and Conservative candidates for the mayoralty of Paris. Opposite—and hence more expected—opinions were of course voiced; for example, by the former right-wing minister of the interior Charles Pasqua, who pejoratively qualified the Cambodians as "economic refugees" and said that to welcome them would "open the floodgates." Conversely, Marie-Georges Buffet, general secretary of the Communist Party, expressed sympathy for "these people driven by poverty and lack of status." All quotations from articles in *Le Monde* on February 18, 19, 20, 21, and 23, 2001.

22. The poll was conducted by Conseil sondage analyses (CSA) on February 21 and 22, 2001: http://www.csa.eu/multimedia/data/sondages/data2001/opi20010221a.htm (consulted in May 2011).

23. The dramatic developments of this contemporary Exodus have been recounted by Solenn de Royer (2002).

24. See Pierre Georges, "Épuration clandestine?" [Purging the illegals?], *Le Monde*, February 22, 2001. See also the opinion column by Nathalie Ferré, then chair of GISTI, "Europe et l'exil" [Europe and exile], *L'Humanité*, February 23, 2001.

25. See "Droit d'asile" [Right to asylum], editorial, *Le Monde*, February 22, 2001: "In terms of government responsibility, the concern expressed by the Prime Minister and other Socialist ministers was no doubt legitimate. But it could not hide their inability to find the words of humanity and generosity one would have expected in such a situation. The discourse on the refusal to accept all the misery of the world is one thing. The instinctive reaction when this misery is suddenly presented in the flesh, with the terrible image of the shipwrecked ship and its human cargo, is another." Thus instincts are mingled with emotion.

26. Quoting John Hope Simpson, Arendt (1951: 280–281) also emphasizes that despite all efforts to draw legal distinctions between the two categories, "all refugees are for practical purposes stateless."

27. One Iranian actor in the company explained: "We committed ourselves to testify for the refugees. They are always in my mind as we are improvising." Another, Russian, said: "Here I've seen the living history of the world today emerge through the body, the gaze, the soul. The actors reconstituted the refugees' accounts with love. Sometimes I can't act any more, I'm so moved by the testimony. The boundary between real world and theater disappears for me." See "Le Théâtre du Soleil porte la voix des réfugiés" [The Théâtre du Soleil carries the voice of refugees], *Le Monde*, April 1, 2003.

28. In Australia, however, the distinction was emphasized and the treatment of the survivors of the *East Sea* contrasted with the rejection of the pas-

sengers on the *Tampa*. Former prime minister Malcolm Fraser declared in 2001, at a conference at the University of Perth: "Recently, when 1,000 Kurdish refugees were beached on the southern French coast, we saw a French Minister moving to the place to see that the refugees were properly treated. . . . It was a humane and sympathetic approach. The refugees were treated with dignity and esteem. On Australia's record of recent times, our reaction would have been very different." See http://www.safecom.org.au/detention. htm (consulted in February 2010).

29. Significantly, Smaïn Laacher, author of the only monograph on Sangatte (2002), referred to it as a "center" in his book, which resulted from a study funded by the Red Cross in 2001, and as a "camp" in the title of his lecture for the Ligue des Droits de l'Homme at the École des Hautes Études en Sciences Sociales in 2003. His vocabulary was more prudent in front of his funders than with human rights activists.

30. This route of investigation has been the subject of an illuminating exploration by Marc Bernardot and Isabelle Deguines: "The whole collective memory of the village of Sangatte seems to be called into question. The village archives have been neglected and are incomplete. Do the inhabitants of Sangatte have something to forget? One might well wonder, for although it has not been mentioned in interviews with residents or in the very many articles devoted to the center, Sangatte has already been home to a camp, but a Nazi camp, in 1942. . . . One cannot help thinking that the installation of the Red Cross center on the same sea front, opposite the farm that served as the Nazi camp, must have contributed to reviving ghosts and old wounds." See "Cohabiter à Sangatte" [Cohabiting in Sangatte], *Plein Droit*, 2003, 58, http://www.gisti.org/doc/plein-droit/58/cohabiter.html (consulted in February 2010). There is a parallel that can be drawn with the disappearance of all traces of the infamous Second World War French transit camp portrayed in Arnaud des Pallières's 1997 film *Drancy Avenir*, in which a history student seeks out this invisible and forgotten site of memory.

31. The pioneering studies by Liisa Malkki (1995) and Jennifer Hyndman (2000), on refugee camps in Tanzania and Kenya, respectively, come to mind.

32. This structural analysis is not, for Peschanski (2002: 97), contradictory with historical and political differentiations between Republican, Nazi, Vichy, and Liberation camps.

33. It is developed in *Homo Sacer* (1998 [1995]: 166 and 174), where he reviews the genealogy of camps from those set up by the Spanish in Cuba in 1896 and the British in South Africa in 1901.

34. In an attempt to clarify his position and discard some misunderstandings, Giorgio Agamben (2009) published a short piece to answer the question, "What is a paradigm?" stating that the parallels he had drawn did not mean to be historiographical accounts. However, most of his followers have been more literal in their interpretation of the continuity between the various forms of camps.

35. See Agier (2004: 121). Although in this article Agier assimilates the different forms of internment, his primary aim is to show the continued presence of a political life in these camps where refugees appear reduced to bare life.

36. At the end of *Homo Sacer* (1998: 188) Agamben asserts: "There is no return from the camps to classical politics." And at the beginning of *State of Exception* (2005: 4), he writes in relation to the Guantánamo detainees: "The only thing to which it could possibly be compared is the legal situation of the Jews in the Nazi *Lager*, who, along with their citizenship, had lost every legal identity."

37. In his book on camps, Marc Bernardot (2008: 119) takes a similar approach, distinguishing camps where the aim is repression from those whose function is principally to protect.

38. In *Hatred of Democracy* (2006: 51 and 27), Rancière asserts: "The democratic scandal simply consists in revealing this: there will never be, under the name of politics, a single principle of the community." He also criticizes the " 'democratic' equivalence of everything" that permits "all phenomena to be placed on one and the same plane in being related to one and the same cause."

39. See in particular "La préfecture dément que des policiers aient arrosé d'essence un blockhaus servant d'abri aux migrants près de Sangatte" [The prefect's office denies that police sprayed gasoline over a pillbox in which migrants were sheltering near Sangatte], *Le Monde*, November 26, 2002, and the testimonies of members of Collectif After Sangatte, particularly in the field journal, where the entry for April 28, 2006, begins: "Last night we weren't gassed." See http://after.sangatte.free.fr/article.php3?id_article=7 (consulted in February 2010).

40. For this superposition and confusion of internal boundaries and external borders, see the book I edited on the "new frontiers of French society" (Fassin 2010a), as well as the two volumes published without author under the title *Cette France-là* (2009 and 2010).

41. As Zygmunt Bauman (1998: 18) notes: "Rather than homogenizing the human condition, the technological annulment of temporal/spatial distances tends to polarize."

42. See the article by Olivier Clochard, Antoine Decourcelle, and Chloé Intrand on waiting zones (2003), and the statistics relating to foreigners at the border published by ANAFÉ in November 2008: http://www.anafe.org/down load/generalites/stats-za-nov2008.pdf (consulted in February 2010).

43. See the article by Olivier Clochard, Yvan Gastaut, and Ralph Schor on camps for foreigners (2004) and Claire Rodier's paper "Les camps d'étrangers, nouvel outil de la politique migratoire en Europe" [Camps for foreigners: A new tool of immigration policy in Europe], September 2003, http://www.mig reurop.org/article205.html (consulted in February 2010).

44. At the 2003 Berlin Film Festival, *In This World* was awarded the Golden Bear, the Peace Prize, and the Jury Prize. In spite of these awards, however, it

was largely ignored by the public in Europe. By contrast, *Welcome* was relatively successful in France.

CHAPTER 6

1. Data drawn principally from the following reports: UNAIDS, *Aids Epidemic Update*, December 2000; Department of Health, *National HIV and Syphilis Sero-prevalence Survey in South Africa*, 2001; Medical Research Council, *The Impact of HIV/ Aids on Adult Mortality in South Africa*, September 2001.

2. For a history of the AIDS epidemic and the controversies surrounding it, see my book *When Bodies Remember* (2007b [2006]). Where necessary, I use the terms "African" and "white" as they are used in South Africa, the other two "racial" groups being "colored" (mixed race, mostly in the Cape Town area) and "Indian" (Asian, mainly in the region of Durban). Paradoxically, at the very moment when the racial barriers inherited from apartheid were being broken down, these categories continued to be recorded, if only for the purposes of combating their effects in terms of segregation and discrimination. But just a few years after the end of apartheid, beyond the needs of evaluation, the racial categories remained deeply present in the social life of South Africa, as the controversy around AIDS revealed.

3. The SABC3 TV channel's program *100 Greatest South Africans* organized a national televised poll in September 2004. Nkosi Johnson appeared at number 5 on the list, after Nelson Mandela, heart surgeon Christiaan Barnard, the last president under apartheid Frederik de Klerk, and Mahatma Gandhi, but before Thabo Mbeki—in a sign of the times, Hendrik Verwoerd, the architect of apartheid, featured one place above Chris Hani, the hero of the struggle against the white supremacist regime. See http://en.wikipedia.org/wiki/SABC3%27s_Great_South_Africans (consulted in February 2010). A book by Jim Wooten about Nkosi Johnson took as its title the last sentence of his speech: "We are all the same."

4. For the full text of the speech, see "An Arrow Straight from the Heart," *Star*, July 11, 2000.

5. A renown that quickly transcended South Africa, since Johnson entered the pantheon of the educational project "My Hero," based in California, which aims to "celebrate the best of humanity." He is listed there as an "Angel Hero," a status corresponding to "foreigners who lift up our souls or give us hope through their acts of kindness." The citation refers to Johnson's speech at the International AIDS Conference: "A tiny figure in a shiny dark suit and sneakers, nervously holding a wireless microphone, Nkosi Johnson, all of 11 years old, held an audience of 10,000 delegates in rapt, occasionally tearful silence as he told the story of his birth and his life." See "Angel Hero: Nkosi Johnson," http://www.myhero.com/myhero/hero.asp?hero=nkosi (consulted in February 2010).

6. As Nancy Scheper-Hughes and Carolyn Sargent (1998: 1) write: "The cultural politics of childhood speaks to the political, ideological and social uses of childhood."

7. For this research, fieldwork was conducted on an intermittent basis from 2000 to 2007. It was based on interviews and participant observation in the African townships of Alexandra and Soweto, in the province of Gauteng, and the former African homelands of Gazankulu and Lebowa, in the province of Limpopo, with the collaboration of Frédéric Le Marcis and Todd Lethata. It also included a study in the emergency department of the Chris Hani Baragwanath Hospital of Soweto, with Duane Blauuw, Loveday Penn-Kekana, and Helen Schneider, from the Centre for Health Policy of the Witwatersrand University in Johannesburg. Details can be found in Fassin (2007b [2006]), including the references on the empirical elements evoked here.

8. Quotations and headlines are taken respectively from the *Saturday Star,* January 30, 1999; the *Weekly Mail and Guardian,* October 16, 1998, and May 14, 1999; the *Cape Times,* February 22, 1999; the *Sowetan,* April 5, 2002; the *Sunday Independent,* June 25, 2000; the *Saturday Star,* July 8, 2000; and the *Star,* July 12, 2000. Accusations of genocide and holocaust are from "Probe Manto and Mbeki for Genocide," *Sapa,* February 23, 2003; interview with Malegapuru William Makgoba, *Weekly Mail and Guardian,* October 6, 2000; "AIDS Denial and Holocaust Denial," Justice Edwin Cameron, Edward Smith Annual Lecture, Harvard Law School, April 8, 2003; Zachie Achmat's speech to the AIDS in Context conference, April 2001.

9. In the famous expression coined by German biologist Paul Ehrlich, awarded the Nobel Prize for Medicine in 1908, to describe his discovery of a treatment for syphilis based on arsenic. The phrase has become common usage for all treatments that combine the qualities of simplicity, efficacy, harmlessness, and low cost. Allan Brandt (1985) recounts this story. For an analysis of the development of nevirapine, see Alton Phillips's study (2010) and my "political biography of a magic bullet" (in press).

10. As it was termed by Richard Horton, editor-in-chief of *The Lancet* (1996), in his account of the theories of leading dissident Peter Duesberg, a professor at Berkeley.

11. The child's doll-like face was blazoned across the front page of the *Weekly Mail and Guardian* on October 19, 2001, under the headline: "Taking Silence to Court: Thirty rand could have prevented baby Tinashe contracting HIV." This was an explicit reference to the theme of the Durban conference: "Breaking the silence" referred to both the battle against stigmatization and the fight for treatment.

12. The story of Magda A., a woman who suffered sexual abuse since childhood and now has AIDS, which Frédéric Le Marcis, Todd Lethata, and I reconstructed (2008), shows how closely the conditions of production and reproduction of such violence are linked to a social, economic, and political context rather than to the expression of a South African nature or culture.

13. Programs for reducing maternal and infant mortality that Anne-Claire Defossez and I studied in Latin America (1992) offer a further illustration: on the one hand, only infant mortality was taken into account for a long time, despite the fact that the inequalities in maternal mortality were much greater; on the other, when the latter was made the target of specific measures, the argument used to justify the initiative was often at least partly the benefit to the children of being brought up by their mothers.

14. The study conducted in South African maternity hospitals by Rachel Jewkes, Naeemah Abrahams, and Zodumo Mvo (1998) is revealing in this respect.

15. The articles quoted appeared in the *Star*, September 9, 2002; *Pretoria News*, April 19, 2005; the *Saturday Star*, September 3, 2005; *Sapa*, September 4, 2000; and the *Independent*, November 25, 2005.

16. In comparison, in the United States 1.9% of women state that they have suffered sexual abuse before the age of twelve. The figures cited here are drawn from a review of the statistics on sexual violence by Rachel Jewkes and Naeemah Abrahams (2002). See also the article by Jewkes et al., "Rape of Girls in South Africa," and the commentary "Infant Rape in South Africa," *The Lancet*, 2002, 359: 274–275 and 319–320.

17. As the headline of an article in the *Pretoria News* on June 17, 2005, put it; the article cited particularly high figures: "At least 50 children per day are raped in South Africa." In fact, "children" refers here to those younger than eighteen, with most of the rapes being committed on girls older than fifteen—in a country where the first sexual experience usually occurs at a fairly young age, this represents a sadly unremarkable sexual violence.

18. The testimony was published in the *Weekly Mail and Guardian* on April 7, 2000: "How Lucky I Am to Be Heard" and "A Society of Rapists." Despite the customary criticism of the legal system for its laxity, her young black rapist was condemned to thirty-two years in prison by an Afrikaner judge.

19. The literature on the imaginary of African sexuality includes the pioneering work of Sander Gilman (1985) and the more recent work of Elsa Dorlin (2006). On South Africa, Alexander Butchart's book (1998) is illuminating. I have studied the reformulation of this imaginary in the time of AIDS with Jean-Pierre Dozon (1989), and the theme has been also explored by Gilles Bibeau (1991).

20. See particularly "Why Children Are Raping Other Children," *Pretoria News*, October 23, 2006, and "Now Even Children Are Committing Rape," *Cape Times*, April 2, 2007.

21. See "Mbeki: No Special Treatment for AIDS Orphans," *Daily News*, April 4, 2007. The South African president was referring to a case that had just been mentioned to him of a household with five children, two of them receiving food as AIDS orphans but the other three getting no benefit from the program.

22. See *A Framework for Protection: Care and Support of Orphans and Vulnerable Children Living in a World with HIV and AIDS*, UNICEF, February 2004. The same figure is given at the end of the decade. See http://www

.worldaidsorphans.org/section/the_orphans_crisis (consulted in April 2010). Alan Whiteside and Clem Sunter (2000) suggest that this figure should be tripled to take into account in particular the fact that when parents become sick they are no longer able to raise their children, who then become orphaned a second time with the death of their grandparents, who often bring them up after their parents die.

23. See the USAID report *Orphans and Vulnerable Children: Meeting Report*, November 2003. The President's Emergency Program for AIDS Relief (PEPFAR), launched by George W. Bush, advocated focusing on the A and B of the "ABC" motto (Abstinence, Be Faithful, Condomize), to the detriment of the C. See http://web.amfar.org/treatment/TI/FR0704.pdf (consulted in November 2008).

24. See Rachel Bray, *Predicting the Social Consequences of Orphanhood in South Africa*, Centre for Social Science Research, Cape Town, Working Paper no. 29, 2003. The studies I refer to here, from Bray's study, are the Project for Statistics on Living Standards and Development (1993) and the Cape Area Panel Study (2002). The nationwide Nelson Mandela HSRC Study of HIV/AIDS gives virtually the same figures as the latter: 3.0% of children without mothers, 8.4% without fathers, 1.6% with neither parent. See Olive Shisana and Leikness Simbayi, *Nelson Mandela HSRC Study of HIV/AIDS*, Pretoria, HSRC, 2002.

25. In the study she conducted among young men who had suffered repression under white power, Pamela Reynolds (2000) describes the damaging effects of apartheid on families.

26. See the report by Martin Schönteich in 1999, "Age and AIDS: South Africa's Crime Time Bomb?," http://www.iss.co.za/PUBS/ASR/8No4/SchOnteich.html; and the report by Schönteich and Robyn Pharaoh in 2003, "AIDS, Security and Governance in Southern Africa," http://www.iss.co.za/Pubs/Papers/65/Paper65.pdf (both consulted in February 2010).

27. See the report by Helen Meintjes, Debbie Budlender, Sonja Giese, and Leigh Johnson, *Children in Need of Care or in Need of Cash?*, Centre for Actuarial Research, Cape Town, December 2003.

28. See "Residents Demand That AIDS Orphans Leave the Area," *Daily News*, August 23, 2001.

29. See in particular Ariès's *Centuries of Childhood* (1962 [1960]), where he develops his famous thesis according to which, if children have always existed, childhood is a recent invention.

CHAPTER 7

1. In *Negative Dialectics* (2005: 361), Adorno argues that the 1775 Lisbon earthquake (whose death toll is estimated between 10,000 and 100,000) constituted the first shattering of European metaphysics, the second being a still more devastating disaster that was not natural but social: the extermination of the Jews.

2. Experts in natural disasters (see Hoffman and Oliver-Smith 2002) have shown that they are rarely entirely natural, either because they result directly from human action (particularly through climate change) or because their extent and seriousness stems from the lack of foresight and the incompetence of rulers (particularly when the victims have suffered the consequences of building in high-risk zones).

3. In contrast, we could of course point to Hurricane Katrina's exposure of social and racial inequalities, and the effect of this revelation on the production of political conflict.

4. For a detailed analysis of the *Tragedia* and its historical context, see Paula Vásquez's inquiry in *Poder y catástrofe* (2010).

5. For an analysis of these various situations, see in particular the work of Michael Pugh (1998), Neil MacFarlane (1999), and Susan Woodward (2001).

6. This research was part of a collaborative program with the Universidad Central de Caracas. Fieldwork was conducted at a distance from the disaster with Paula Vásquez, who had previously realized the interviews quoted here.

7. I use the term as an echo of the title of the posthumous publication of Benjamin's works introduced by Hannah Arendt (1968).

8. This theory is defended by Shoshana Felman (1999: 202), who sees Benjamin as "a thinker, a philosopher, a narrator of the wars and revolutions of the twentieth century."

9. The expression is borrowed from Hegel by Francis Fukuyama (1992), who radically alters its meaning.

10. Opening the way to what John Armitage (2002: 27) sees as the foundation of a state of emergency and what George Steinmetz (2003) describes as the establishment of a global sovereignty.

11. As Bryan Turner notes (2002: 103): "While Jürgen Habermas expressed the hope that the Anglo-Saxon world would escape contagion from the Schmittian revival, his optimism was probably premature." The popular success of Schmitt's work on exception was accompanied by the production of scientific commentaries and renewed influence in some political circles.

12. Inspired by Benjamin and Schmitt, in *State of Exception* (2005 [2003]: 2 and 38) Agamben writes: "From a technical standpoint the specific contribution of the state of exception is less the confusion of powers, which has been all too strongly insisted upon, than it is the separation of the 'force of law' from the law."

13. In this respect, it is noteworthy that during the urban riots in France in 2005, the government under Prime Minister Dominique de Villepin, in which current president Nicolas Sarkozy served as minister of the interior, chose to declare a state of emergency, even though the riots provoked essentially damage to property, moreover limited to particular areas and at the time subsiding. The application of this law, which was used three times in the Algerian war of independence between 1955 and 1963 (Thénault 2007) aimed to dramatize the event, but by the same token it contributed to routinizing exception.

14. And also moving away from the traditional representation in terms of center and periphery, through what Walter Mignolo (2000) calls "local histories." Hugo Chávez's Venezuela, which the international media often deride as an exotic and anachronistic curiosity, particularly calls for this shift in perspective.

15. It is in his 1922 essay *Political Theology* (1985: 5–7) that Schmitt develops his theory of exception.

16. The "Father of the nation" functioned as an inspirational figure for the definition of a new social order that was to reject "the corrupt oligarchy" that had reigned for decades and restore the authority of the "sovereign people" that had been dispossessed of its prerogatives by the previous regime (Porras Ponceleón 2000). Bolívar thus became the repository of a "moral power."

17. Fernando Coronil (1997) uses the term "devil's excrement" to describe the feeling of moral degradation in the final days of the regime; he is quoting Juan Pablo Pérez Alfonso, a 1970s political analyst who described oil, at once natural bounty and source of corruption.

18. The "mystical fiction" is analyzed by Ernst Kantorowicz (1957) in his well-known study of theological-political history. It was in this register that Hugo Chávez placed himself when he arrogated full power to himself: on the one hand, he was the democratically elected representative of the people, and on the other, he was the incarnation of the nation in the Bolivarian tradition.

19. The formulation was coined by Larry Minear and Thomas Weiss (1992), in relation to the world situation following the First Gulf War in 1990, but is more generally applicable.

20. See the report "El desastre que nos destrozó la vida" [The disaster that destroyed our lives], on the website of the Humboldt organization, http://www .rescate.com/desastre.html (consulted in March 2005).

21. See "Todo por Jesús: Bitácora de las olas del Ávila" [Everything for Jesus: Navigating the waves of the Ávila], Comunidad de Hermanitas de los Pobres of the San José de Maiquetía Hospital, La Guaira, http://www.gumilla.org.ve/ SIC (consulted in March 2005).

22. The eruption of the volcano Nevado del Ruiz in Colombia, on November 13, 1985, was one of the major disasters in the recent history of Latin America. It killed twenty thousand of the twenty-nine thousand residents of the city of Armero. A particularly emotional event was the vain attempt to rescue a thirteen-year-old girl, followed worldwide via television, which showed her slow death after sixty hours struggling in the mud.

23. Similarly, Alice Fothergill (2003) reports how women hit by the floods at Grand Forks, North Dakota, in 1997, who were mostly from the middle class, felt that they were suffering a further ordeal when they became dependent on others for aid, and even claimed that they had got an idea of the experience of poor families living on welfare: there could be no clearer example of how exposure to charity is unequally distributed in the social world, as in the case of the two women evacuated to Barquisimeto.

24. In the view of Candace Vogler and Patchen Markell (2003: 2), the social contract effects a secular version of "redemption from violence," to the extent that the state to which power and authority are delegated brings "peace and security into a disorderly world," but at the same time that contract cannot avoid the fact that "violence persists, though often reorganized, renamed, or repressed."

25. In her study of the Canadian peacekeeping mission in Somalia, Sherene Razack (2004) describes the racist and criminal abuses perpetrated by the very people who had come as benefactors to this war-torn region of Africa. The "white knights" thus became "dark powers" for those they claimed to be helping.

26. This leads Angela Zago (1998) to call Chávez and his companions in arms "rebel angels."

27. See "El derecho a la vida no está suspendido" [The right to life is not suspended], http://derechos.org.ve/actualidad/comunicados (consulted in March 2005).

28. See "Entre el dolor y la solidaridad" [Between pain and solidarity], *Revista SJC* [Jesuit journal of the Gumilla Center], January–February 2000, http://gumilla.org.ve (consulted in March 2005).

29. The Venezuelan case is interesting in this respect, because the 1961 Constitution, which was still in force at the time of the 1999 disaster, includes five articles (240 to 244) that under the title "On emergency" refer only to the state of emergency, and even that in relatively cursory fashion. The 1999 Constitution, on the other hand, which was voted in on the day of the disaster, specifies a series of measures in Chapter II, "On states of exception," for the situations "state of alert," "state of economic emergency," and "state of internal and external upheaval," specifying the circumstances and consequences of each one. At the time of the events in Vargas, while the official reference had to be to the 1961 document, the government's intellectual reference was to the 1999 text, as the choice of the term "state of alert" indicates; this term did not exist in the earlier constitution, but was included among the "states of exception" in the later one.

CHAPTER 8

1. A heroic, if somewhat unreliable, version is recounted by Olivier Weber (1995). Bernard Kouchner and others, working for the Red Cross, witnessed what they viewed as genocide without being able to bear witness of this tragedy. Rony Brauman's reappraisal of the situation (2000 [1995]) suggests more prudence in the qualification of the crimes committed by the Nigerian army against secessionist Biafra, and Anne Vallaeys's revisionist history (2004) relativizes this issue of public testimony in the creation of the organization.

2. Médecins Sans Frontières (MSF) has published a remarkable series of documents titled "Prises de parole publiques de MSF" [Public testimonies],

which brings together the testimony of members and reactions to this testimony, focusing on the exemplary cases of the population transfers during the Ethiopian famine from 1984 onward, Salvadorean refugee camps in Honduras in 1988, and the Tutsi genocide in Rwanda in 1994 and its aftermath, to which four volumes are devoted. In her introduction, Laurence Binet, who put this collection together, speaks of "testimony, the form of action that gives MSF a distinct identity among other humanitarian organizations." In fact, while public testimony forms part of Médecins Sans Frontières' founding creed, many other organizations are equally committed to this principle, sometimes in an even broader sense, which includes human rights, as in the case of Médecins du Monde.

3. A detailed analysis of these issues can be found in my article on humanitarian organizations' construction of the "cause of the victims" (2004a).

4. In "Remedies for Melancholy," written by Christian Lachal and Marie-Rose Moro, the joint directors of mental health programs for Médecins Sans Frontières in the July 2002 issue of the organization's magazine, *Messages*.

5. In the *Philosophical Investigations* (2004 [1953]: 133), replying in the form of a negative question: "Isn't it the behaviour of people, in particular their utterances?"

6. In the introduction to the third volume (2001) of their trilogy on suffering, violence, and trauma.

7. The research is based on interviews, realized with Estelle d'Halluin, of members of Médecins Sans Frontières and Médecins du Monde who have been involved in the programs conducted by their organization in Palestine and Israel. It also benefited from informal discussions within Médecins Sans Frontières during my four years on the Administration Board.

8. My use of the term "subjectivation" refers to Foucault (1994: 307). However, I consider that social sciences are ill equipped to analyze the sort of introspection he has in mind when he speaks of a "search for the truth of the self." Rather, I am interested in the public production of subjects, by themselves and by others. For instance, I am not asking whether victims are psychologically affected by their condition of victimhood, but what difference it makes when we see them as such or when they have to present themselves as such to be recognized.

9. In his text on "the ideological state apparatuses," Althusser (1971 [1970]: 173) writes that "all ideology hails or interpellates individuals as concrete subjects"—in other words, produces a form of political subjectivation.

10. In her study of "the psychic life of power" (1997: 2), Butler emphasizes this "ambivalence at the site where the subject emerges" as a subjected subject and a subject subjectivizing himself or herself.

11. According to Émile Benveniste (1973 [1969]: 526), who also shows that this semantic distinction exists in all Indo-European languages.

12. What historian Annette Wieviorka (2006 [1998]) calls the "era of the witness"—that is, as she defines it, an era in which written, recorded, and

filmed testimonies of the Holocaust have proliferated—thus corresponds to the emergence of the second figure, the "survivor," who can, and must, bear witness precisely because he has lived through an ordeal in which so many others perished.

13. In *If This Is a Man* (1960 [1958]: 103), Levi analyzes this absolute limit. The only true witness is the "Mussulman," an extreme figure of dehumanization who can no longer testify. The survivor cannot speak in his name. In this sense, as Giorgio Agamben (2002 [1998]: 34) observes, "the value of testimony lies essentially in what it lacks."

14. And therefore "acting and speaking, providing care and bearing witness, would be their watchwords," as the former president of Médecins Sans Frontières Rony Brauman put it (2000 [1995]: 60).

15. Within this history of trauma, Allan Young (1995) has traced the complex and ambiguous routes by which American psychiatry forged alliances with pressure groups, particularly war veterans, to gain recognition for posttraumatic stress disorder as a diagnostic entity that paved the way to compensation.

16. Richard Rechtman and I (2009 [2007]) recounted the journey of humanitarian psychiatry; in particular, we demonstrated the role of Armenian psychotherapists after the earthquake in Leninakan.

17. The *Diagnostic and Statistical Manual of Mental Disorders* (DSM) is a classification established by the American Psychiatric Association. Since the first publication in 1952, there have been five revisions. The DSM-III, in 1980, introduced a new entity—the posttraumatic stress disorder, a normal reaction to an abnormal event.

18. As Émile Benveniste writes (1973 [1969]: 422): "The term *auctor* is applied to the person who in all walks of life 'promotes', takes an initiative, who is the first to start some activity, who founds, who guarantees, and finally who is the 'author'." Authority in the sense of the "validity of a testimony" derives from this.

19. As Agamben (1999 [1998]: 26) notes, adding that the word *martirium*, coined to designate the death of persecuted Christians, derives from this term.

20. According to statistics published on the websites of the Palestinian Red Crescent, http://www.palestinercs.org, and the Israeli human rights organization B'Tselem, http://www.btselem.org (both consulted in February 2007).

21. As Laetitia Bucaille (2004 [2002]: 139) suggests, this development reveals an Islamization of society—or rather, an inscription of religious language into the political discourse—which is sanctioned by the new canon of martyrs: "Hamas . . . has succeeded in spreading its ideology by setting up the martyr-figure as the definitive model for Palestinian struggle." Formerly a victim, the martyr can thus become a hero.

22. See Alexandra Schwartzbrod's article "Les maux de la peur à Hebron: Avec une psychologue de MSF dans la ville palestinienne sous couvre-feu"

[The diseases of fear in Hebron: Traveling with an MSF psychologist in the Palestinian town under curfew], *Libération*, March 9, 2001.

23. As recalled by Julie Peteet (1994), the violence suffered by young Palestinian men at the hands of the Israeli occupying forces when they are beaten up or arrested now forms part of the rite of passage that establishes the construction of virility and more generally the conditions of war.

24. As John Collins (2004: 36) puts it, establishing a sort of topography of this discursive field in which political, religious, literary, and now psychiatric interpretations come together.

25. The Gaza Community Mental Health Program's annual report, from which these figures are taken, can be read at http://www.gcmhp.net (consulted in December 2007).

26. The *Palestinian Chronicles* were published as a supplement of Médecins Sans Frontières' magazine *Messages* in July 2002, under the title *Trapped by War*. The excerpts presented here correspond to testimonies (pages 25–42).

27. As Agamben (2002 [1998]: 27–29) explains, the Church Fathers constructed this doctrine in response to heretics who contested the need for self-sacrifice; it later give rise to the construction of the term "holocaust."

28. The chronicles begin with an unequivocal text by Jean-Hervé Bradol, president of Médecins Sans Frontières, on the meaning of humanitarian aid: "Aid to people affected by conflict cannot be limited to food, shelter, and repairing their bodies. Only those directly affected can determine the limits of what is acceptable when it comes to an attack on human dignity. On this point, the Palestinians' response is clear: they do not accept the situation they are in and many say they are ready to die for their cause."

29. In an article on witnessing, François Hartog (2005: 200) points out the importance of this concept: "The *histor*, who intervenes in a dispute, is summoned by both parties; he listens to both, whereas the *martus* is only concerned with one side, or rather, for him there is only one."

30. This document, *Les civils israéliens et palestiniens victimes d'un conflit sans fin*, in French, published in 2003, is composed of two reports: *Opération "Mur de protection" Naplouse* [Operation "Protective Wall" Nablus], written in 2002, and *Les civils israéliens victimes des attaques des groupes armés palestiniens* [Israeli civilian victims of attacks by armed Palestinian groups], added a year later.

31. In this respect Avram Bornstein (2001) has shown how the public representation of Palestinian prisoners in Israeli prisons changed in the mid-1990s, as they shifted from being fighters in the liberation struggle to victims who required professional support for rehabilitation.

32. As the published Gaza diary of a pediatric psychiatrist working with Médecins Sans Frontières expresses in its own way: "These are the lessons I have learned from the people here: above all never think of them as victims, even if they are victims of historical misunderstandings that overtake them." See "Journal de bord de Maryvonne" [Maryvonne's log book], photocopied document, 14 pages, June 2004.

CHAPTER 9

1. According to the president of Médecins du Monde, "Never, before the North Atlantic Treaty Organization's aerial intervention in the Federal Republic of Yugoslavia, had the level of confusion between war and humanitarianism been so evident. The fact that a man as respectable as Václav Havel could assert that 'the air attacks, the bombs are not promoting a material interest; they are exclusively humanitarian in character' (*Le Monde*, April 29, 1999) reveals the extent of this confusion." See Jackie Mamou, "Au nom de l'humanitaire" [In the name of humanitarianism], *Le Monde Diplomatique*, June 1999. Other heads of state, notably Tony Blair, made use of the same argument. In this regard the evolution from the conception of the war in Bosnia (Pugh 1998) to the vision of the intervention in Kosovo (Woodward 2001) should be noted.

2. For an analysis of this expansion of humanitarianism on military terrains, see the collective book I coedited on contemporary states of emergency (Fassin and Pandolfi 2010).

3. Pointing to the reemergence of nongovernmental humanitarianism during the 1970s and 1980s, at a time when communism's star was waning, Brauman (2000 [1995]: 61) even sees in this new configuration a sort of historical fluid mechanics: "It's as if, during these periods when the ideological tide is going out, humanitarian action comes to occupy the space left vacant by politics."

4. Seeing humanitarianism, insofar as it distances itself from the figure of the nation-state, as a form of renunciation of politics, Agamben (1998 [1995]: 133) adds that the image of the refugee has become "the most significant sign of bare life in our era," and the refugee the "biopolitical paradigm."

5. The most high-profile example is that of Bernard Kouchner, cofounder of Médecins Sans Frontières and then of Médecins du Monde, who became secretary of state for humanitarian action, minister of health, and eventually minister of foreign affairs in the governments respectively of Michel Rocard, Edith Cresson, and Pierre Bérégovoy, under the presidency of François Mitterrand, and in that of Lionel Jospin, under the presidency of Jacques Chirac, and finally in the government of François Fillon, under the presidency of Nicolas Sarkozy, following a two-year interlude as head of the United Nations Interim Administration Mission in Kosovo. But Claude Malhuret and Xavier Emmanuelli also became secretaries of state, in the governments of Jacques Chirac and Alain Juppé, respectively (the tropism toward the rightwing of humanitarian workers turning to politics is worth noting). Conversely, Georgina Dufoix and subsequently Jean-François Mattéi, ministers in the governments of Pierre Mauroy and Jean-Pierre Raffarin, respectively, became presidents of the French Red Cross. These are just a few examples of the circulation between the humanitarian and political worlds typically encountered in the French context (Fassin 2007a).

6. See "Guerre en Irak: MSF soigne les civils sous les bombes à Bagdad" [War in Iraq: MSF treats civilians under the bombs in Baghdad], interview with Dr. Pierre Salignon by Dr. Michel Janssens, *Impact Médecine*, April 4, 2003.

7. This study is grounded on interviews, document analysis, and observant participation, by which I mean the type of knowledge acquired via my collaboration with several nongovernmental organizations, including Médecins Sans Frontières, of which I was administrator, then vice president between 1999 and 2003.

8. According to Foucault (1979 [1976]), biopower, or power over life, is made up of two processes of normalization: "anatamo-politics," or the discipline of the body, and "biopolitics," the regulation of populations. I have analyzed how, remarkably given the etymology of the word, biopolitics is not fundamentally a politics of life (Fassin 2006 and 2009a).

9. In this respect I subscribe to Peter Redfield's (2005: 330) formula that the work of the anthropologist is not "to unveil and denounce untruths and violations" of humanitarian organizations, but I believe it is to get as close as possible to their work and issues, including contradictions and aporia (Fassin 2011b).

10. I plan to do this using a methodology combining participant observation, reviewing my experience on Médecins Sans Frontières' Administration Board, via interviews of members within the organization, supplemented by document analysis. This study obviously delimits a particular section of the humanitarian arena, set in a specifically French history (Dauvin and Siméant 2002); the debates were no doubt posed in sometimes quite different terms in other national contexts.

11. See, for example, *Reflections on the US Military's Provision of Assistance During and Immediately After Conflict with Iraq*, Médecins Sans Frontières, February 18, 2003, 7 pages.

12. See *Procès verbal de la reunion du Conseil d'administration du vendredi 28 mars 2003* [Minutes of the meeting of the Administration Board, March 28, 2003]. These monthly sessions are always recorded and later transcribed and summarized. Whereas the Executive Committee is composed of salaried directors and runs the daily life of the organization as well as making most of the important decisions for operations, the Administration Board consists of volunteers who, meeting only once a month and not involved day after day in the issues the organization is facing, discuss and define general political lines. The singularity of Médecins Sans Frontières—unique in the French world of nongovernmental organizations—is that the same person chairs both groups: the president, who is elected and salaried.

13. The comments by Rony Brauman and Pierre Salignon (2003), and the interview with Jean-Hervé Bradol in *Le Figaro* of March 24, 2003, contrast with the much more dramatic analysis offered by the United Nations and Médecins du Monde at the same point. See, for example, "L'Irak en plein chaos" [Iraq in total chaos] in the September 2003 issue of Médecins du Monde's donor journal, which refers to an "alarming situation." The French press had taken a similar line, *Le Monde* referring to a "humanitarian crisis" (April 19, 2003) and *L'Humanité* to a "humanitarian disaster" (May 6, 2003).

14. Pierre Salignon, the head of Médecins Sans Frontières' program in Iraq, stated in an interview with *Le Monde* on May 9, 2003: "Those who attempted to carry out independent humanitarian action encountered enormous difficulties, and in the end we failed."

15. This theoretical model (Agamben 1998 [1995]) has been discussed earlier. I have tried elsewhere (2010b) to show the interest and indicate the limits of this paradigm.

16. The double paradox of intolerables derives from the fact that on the one hand they appear to be eternal values, when in fact they are historical constructions, and on the other they are given as moral absolutes, when in fact tolerance of the intolerable is a routine phenomenon (Fassin 2005).

17. As Laurence Hugues put it in Médecins Sans Frontières' internal journal: "Liberia, là où la vie ne vaut pas une guinée," *Messages*, 2003, 124: 3–4.

18. To use Nicholas Wheeler's (2000) felicitous phrase.

19. "Pastoral power" appears in several texts and lectures toward the end of Foucault's life, particularly in the 1977–1978 lectures at the Collège de France titled *Security, Territory, Population* (2007 [2004]: 114–190).

20. He adds: "On this condition, victories over this politics of the worst, by definition always temporary and partial, are possible" (Bradol 2003: 32).

21. This binarism is seriously challenged when the military kills in the name of humanitarianism, as in Somalia (Razack 2004).

22. In reality we should probably also invoke another comparative perspective by introducing the colonial wars (Le Cour Grandmaison 2005). While in the two world wars the cost in human lives was extremely high, this was true on both sides. It was in the colonial wars that the devalorization of human lives was established as a politics of massacre as Hannah Arendt (1951: 185) recalls, citing the examples of the Boxer Rebellion in China, the massacres of Arabs in the Middle East, and the extermination of the Herero in Southwest Africa, among others. The essential difference from the contemporary period is that the slaughter is no longer justified in terms of the enemy's inferiority or inhumanity, but rather as the price that has to be paid in order to obtain the desired outcome.

23. Michael Ignatieff (2000) offered an analysis of this military doctrine, calling it a "new American way of war." In fact this model is used in all military interventions conducted by Western powers, which can no longer "allow themselves" deaths among their ranks, for fear of losing the support of "public opinion."

24. The official count of coalition losses is given at http://icasualties.org/ oif. The British epidemiological studies were published in one of the most highly regarded international medical journals: Les Roberts et al., "Mortality Before and After the 2003 Invasion of Iraq: Cluster Sample Survey," *The Lancet*, 2004, 364 (9448): 1857–1864; Gilbert Burnham et al., "Mortality Before and After the 2003 Invasion of Iraq: A Cross-sectional Cluster Sample Survey," *Lancet*, 2006, 368 (9545): 1421–1428. A detailed report, *The Human Cost of*

the War in Iraq: A Mortality Study, 2002–2005, by the same authors, appears at http://web.mit.edu/CIS/pdf/Human_Cost_of_War.pdf (all sites consulted in February 2010).

25. The analysis was made by historian Andrew Bacevich, in a forum at Boston University. See Bacevich, "What's an Iraqi Life Worth," *Washington Post*, July 9, 2006, http://www.washingtonpost.com/wp-dyn/content/article/2006/07/07/AR2006070701155_pf.html (consulted in February 2010).

26. Her undersecretary of state, James Rubin, insisted that one should avoid being too idealistic and that we live in a "real world." See John Pilger, "Squeezed to Death," *Guardian*, March 4, 2000, http://www.guardian.co.uk/theguardian/2000/mar/04/weekend7.weekend9 (consulted in February 2010).

27. Some media and nongovernmental organizations have tried to produce body counts. See "Counting the Civilian Cost in Iraq," *BBC News*, June 6, 2005, http://news.bbc.co.uk/2/hi/middle_east/3672298.stm (consulted in February 2010).

28. In his 2003 report as president of Médecins Sans Frontières, Jean-Hervé Bradol downplayed the seriousness of the crisis following the fall of Baghdad in comparison with tragedies in other parts of the world: "The situation was not catastrophic. I have just been talking about Angola, Congo, North Korea, Chechnya, and the difference between serious problems, which are present in Iraq, and catastrophic situations, is clear. Overall, Iraq represented a minor emergency intervention for us."

29. To hide the fact that a ransom had been paid, the Russian security services organized a spectacular fake release, but by asking for the money to be reimbursed the Dutch government publicly revealed the conditions of the release. The latter lost its case against Médecins Sans Frontières, as well as the appeal it subsequently lodged against that ruling. For an analysis of the legal and political implications of this case, see Philippe Ryfman's article "L'action humanitaire en procès" [Humanitarian action on trial], in *Messages*, July–August 2005.

30. In the August 2003 special issue of Médecins Sans Frontières' internal journal *DazibAG*, Harvey highlighted the paradox of relying exclusively on a shifting expatriate staff and neglecting a loyal national contingent: "The turnover for an expatriate member of staff is approximately 2.5 per year. We lack relevance because we rely on people we don't keep in the field for long enough. One of the major advantages of national staff is that they have a degree of distance from operations and ensure continuity of activity. When expatriates leave, national staff remain."

31. "Six Months after Barcelona, Promises Not Kept" was the title of a special report published in 2002 as a supplement to the internal journal *Messages*, referring to the International AIDS Conference that had taken place a few months earlier. It was made up of accounts and testimonies that highlighted by contrast Médecins Sans Frontières' activities throughout the world. Six months later, the president's report admitted that treatment was not usually provided to the local staff suffering from AIDS.

32. Between 1985 and 1998, 375 deaths of United Nations and nongovernmental organization personnel were recorded, one-third of them during the Rwandan genocide: 67% of the deaths were intentional, generally by shooting, and 58% were of local staff, including 13% drivers and 12% security staff. See the article by Mani Sheik et al., "Deaths among Humanitarian Workers," *British Medical Journal*, 2000, 321: 166–168. However, according to Jean-Hervé Bradol, who at the time was head of Médecins Sans Frontières' mission in Rwanda and there witnessed the murder of some of his Tutsi colleagues: "If you asked the humanitarian organizations for the list of their staff who died in the genocide, 90% of them would be unable to provide it. That gives an idea of what was done or not done to help people when they really needed help." See the special report "Le génocide des Tutsis du Rwanda: Une abjection pour l'humanité, un échec pour les humanitaires" [The Tutsi genocide in Rwanda: A source of shame for humanity, a failure for humanitarians] in the journal *Humanitaire: Enjeux, pratiques, débats*, 2004, 10: 12–28.

CONCLUSION

1. On Durkheim's moral sociology, see his 1924 text on the moral fact (1974), and on Weber's distinction between academic and political vocations, see his 1919 lectures (2008). Franz Boas, the founder of anthropology in the United States and father of the theory of culturalism, mobilized his discipline to fight against racial theories: his public stand against some of his colleagues who had secretly collaborated with the U.S. Army during the First World War resulted in him becoming the only member ever to have been expelled from the American Anthropological Association—which he had founded.

2. The distinction between natural and social sciences, affirms Elias (1987 [1956]), lies in the fact that, in contrast with the former, the latter are produced by humans studying humans, thus challenging the classical epistemological distinction between object and subject. But rather than being a mere obstacle to objectivity, this unique position of the sociologist or anthropologist can be viewed as a heuristic tension between an unavoidable involvement and a necessary detachment.

3. And Foucault (2003: 48) adds: "In what is given to us as universal, necessary, obligatory, what place is occupied by whatever is singular, contingent, and the product of arbitrary constraints?"

4. In *The Company of Critics* (1988: xix), Walzer argues "against the claim that moral principles are necessarily external to the world of everyday experience, waiting *out there* to be discovered by detached and dispassionate philosophers. In fact, it seems to me, the everyday world is a moral world, and we would do better to study its internal rules, maxims, conventions, and ideals, rather than to detach ourselves from it in search of a universal and transcendent standpoint." Thus he stands for a criticism of "insiders."

5. Useful here is the distinction proposed by Thomas Bénatouïl (1999) between the two great theoretical paradigms of the sociology of unveiling, Marxian

in inspiration, as developed by Pierre Bourdieu, and the sociology of translation, inherited from pragmatism, as defended by Bruno Latour and Michel Callon. Interestingly, Luc Boltanski moved from the former to the latter.

6. I draw here on Paul Ricoeur's (1986) systematic exploration of the concept of ideology, particularly in Marx and Engels's *The German Ideology* and Clifford Geertz's text "Ideology as Culture."

7. As Foucault suggests in the quotation cited as an epigraph to this conclusion, following up his proposal by making "the philosophical ethos" a "limit-attitude" (2003: 53).

8. According to Vincent Descombes (2008: 61), two radical attitudes are in competition: "ideological criticism," which questions everything except the possibility itself of artificially reconstructing a new ideology in place of the old one, and "intellectual criticism of our ideology," which includes questioning ourselves, and with which Descombes allies himself, much closer in this than he claims to Foucault's proposition that criticism is first directed toward ourselves.

9. In his commentary on the work of Nels Anderson (1993: 266), he states the necessity of conceiving of sociological investigation in terms of impurity: "For a practice like ethnography, invoking the empiricist dimension means first of all recognizing that, in the conditions in which it is practiced, its materials and operations necessarily incorporate a degree of 'impurity'; that is, they cannot meet the constraints of validity and scientific objectivation."

10. About the modern "moral order," Taylor (2004: 5 and 10) suggests that it is in a process of "double expansion: in extension (more people live with it; it has become dominant) and in intensity (the demands it makes are heavier and more ramified)."

11. As we are reminded by André Lalande (1993 [1926], 1:423–424), from whom I draw the different senses in the three languages fairly freely here.

12. In his study of "asymmetric counterconcepts"—Hellene vs. Barbarian, Christian vs. Heathen—Koselleck (1985: 184) shows that the recognition of the idea of humanity introduces a fundamentally new element because it implies that there is no outside to this category, "a general name comprehending all humans—*Menschheit*."

13. At the end of *The Disenchantment of the World* (1999 [1985]: 199–209) Gauchet emphasizes that there is "an ineliminable subjective stratum underlying the religious phenomenon," giving three examples of how it is manifested: an experience of thought around the mystery of the infinite, an aesthetic experience of the unspeakable, or an experience of the problem of the self. Surprisingly, he fails to recognize the singular trace of Christianity in the contemporary political and moral order. Jonathan Benthall (2008), by contrast, in his recent *Returning to Religion*, devotes a lengthy chapter to humanitarianism. But it is true that the phenomenon became much more salient over the two decades that separate these two books.

14. At the end of *The Human Condition* (1958: 313–320), Arendt seeks to understand how life has become our highest good and sees the key to this

shift in the Christian promise of immortality, adding, moreover, that individual life then replaced the life of the polis.

15. This phrase, taken from the "Critique of Violence" (1978 [1921]: 299), is well known: "Finally, this idea of man's sacredness gives grounds for reflection that what here is pronounced sacred was according to ancient mythical thought the marked bearer of guilt: life itself."

16. In her essay *On Revolution* (1962: 65 and 107), Arendt notes that suffering, however silent, has become loquacious, and even, through the revolutionary gesture, a powerful motivator for collective action: "The masses of the suffering people had taken to the street unbidden and uninvited by those who then became their organizers and their spokesmen. But the suffering they exposed transformed the *malheureux* into *enragés* only when 'the compassionate zeal' of the revolutionaries began to glorify this suffering." Arendt holds Rousseau, more even than Robespierre, responsible for this irruption of suffering into politics—a view challenged by Myriam Revault d'Allonnes (2008: 69–70).

17. Referring in his *Confessions* (III-2: 35) to the emotions he felt in response to suffering portrayed in theater, he asks: "Why is it that a person should wish to experience suffering by watching grievous and tragic events which he himself would not wish to endure? What is this but amazing folly?"

18. In chapter 3 of his *Political Theology* (1985[1922]), Schmitt adds that this is the case "not only because of their historical development—in which they were transferred from theology to the theory of the state, but also because of their systematic structure, the recognition of which is necessary for a sociological consideration of these concepts."

19. Lefort (1986: 293) offers a new formulation of this phenomenon, asking: "Rather than seeking to redefine the relations between the political and the religious, in order to grasp the degree to which one is subordinated to the other, and hence to ask whether the sensitivity of religious thought persists or not in modern society, would we not do better to posit a theological-political formation as historically and logically a primary given?" I would add that the figures underlying this formation include, in addition to the nation and the people, which have forged or legitimized many of the regimes of our modern era, the figure of humanity, which humanitarian government draws on.

20. For a definition and a discussion of this concept of intolerableness, see Fassin (2005).

21. According to Bauman (2004: 4 and 12), the notion of "wasted lives" relates or refers back to the idea of a "full planet" on which human beings are constituted as "excessive populations."

22. For Simmel (1998 [1908]: 45–46): "Once the well-being of society requires that assistance be given to the poor, motivation shifts away from this objective toward the giver, without consequently turning toward the receiver. The poor man as a person, and his own perception of his position in his consciousness, have as little importance as they have for the giver who gives alms for the salvation of his soul."

23. A distinction that Hannah Arendt (1958: 97) establishes when she writes: "Limited by a beginning and an end, that is, by the two supreme events of appearance and disappearance within the world, life follows a strictly linear movement whose very motion nevertheless is driven by the motor of biological life which man shares with other living things. The chief characteristic of this specifically human life is that it is itself always full of events which ultimately can be told as a story, establish a biography."

24. Moreover, conversely, as Levinas (1969 [1961]: 194 and 197) notes, this " 'resistance' of the other does not do violence to me, does not act negatively; it has a positive structure: ethical."

25. The story was reported on August 4, 1999, in the Belgian daily Le Soir, under the headline: "Two Schoolboys' Final Lesson." It formed the source for a play titled Atterrissage [Landing], written by Kangui Alem, which was performed in Europe and Africa. This English version of the letter is a translation from the original, since inaccurate texts have circulated.

26. Inscribing this story within the literature on mimicry, James Ferguson (2002) shows that there is more to it: the letter is a call for Western responsibilities to its former colonies and for a global moral community.

27. In her work on violence, Veena Das (2007: 8–9) is consistently attentive to the distinction between "voice" and "speech," considering it the anthropologist's compelling and impossible duty to make the voices of those of whom she speaks heard.

28. See "Passage clandestin d'un avion, un jeune Sénégalais miraculé est mort lors de sa fugue" [Stowaway on a plane: Miraculous young Senegalese survivor dies as he flees], Le Monde, September 7, 1999, and "La France expulse un jeune demandeur d'asile cubain" [France expels young Cuban asylum seeker], Le Monde, September 3, 2000.

Glossary

Centre d'accueil pour demandeurs d'asile (CADA): Reception Center for Asylum Seekers. Publicly funded French centers where accommodation, social assistance, and legal aid are provided to asylum seekers, mostly those with a family.

Centre Primo Levi: Primo Levi Association. Nongovernmental organization created in 1995 and specialized in the medical and psychological care of victims of torture and persecution.

Comité médical pour les exilés (COMEDE): Medical Committee for Exiles. French nongovernmental organization founded in 1979 that provides health, social, and legal services to immigrants and asylum seekers.

Commissariat Général du Plan: General Planning Commission. French institution that existed between 1946 and 2006 and prepared the five-year economic plans.

Cour Nationale du Droit d'Asile (CNDA): National Court for the Right to Asylum. Previously Commission des Recours des Réfugiés (Committee of Appeal for Refugees, CRR). French jurisdiction that examines on appeal the application of asylum seekers rejected by OFPRA.

Couverture maladie universelle (CMU): Universal Medical Coverage. Social welfare program established by the French Socialist government in 2000, providing a medical coverage for the entire population including free health care for the poor.

Département: Administrative territory, corresponding to the intermediate level between the municipality and the region. It is ruled by representatives of the state (the prefect and his or her administration) and an elected body (the Conseil Général). There are 101 *départements* in France.

Direction de la Population et des Migrations (DPM): Directorate of Population and Migration. French administration under the authority of the minister of social affairs, in charge of sociodemographic aspects of immigration.

Direction Départementale des Affaires Sanitaires et Sociales (DDASS): Directorate of Health and Social Welfare. French public administration in charge of health and welfare issues in any one of the one hundred *départements.*

European Court of Human Rights: Supranational court established in 1998 by the European Convention on Human Rights, providing legal recourse for individuals who consider their rights to have been violated by one of the European countries.

Fonds d'urgence sociale (FUS): Social Emergency Fund. Ephemeral public funds granted to the French unemployed and underemployed in response to the protest of 1997.

Groupe d'information et de soutien aux immigrés (GISTI): Immigrant Information and Support Group. French nongovernmental organization founded in 1972 and devoted to the legal defense of immigrants and foreigners.

Médecins du Monde (MdM): Doctors of the World. French humanitarian nongovernmental organization founded in 1980 after secession from MSF.

Médecins Sans Frontières (MSF): Doctors without Borders. The first French humanitarian nongovernmental organization, founded in 1971.

Observatoire du Droit à la Santé des Étrangers (ODSE): Observatory for Foreigners' Right to Health Care. A collective of seventeen nongovernmental organizations dedicated to health advocacy for immigrants.

Office Français de Protection des Réfugiés et des Apatrides (OFPRA): French Office for the Protection of Refugees and Stateless Persons. French administration that examines the applications of asylum seekers in the first instance.

Oxfam International: Group of fourteen organizations acting against poverty, founded in 1995 to succeed the Oxford Committee on Famine Relief created in 1942.

Posttraumatic stress disorder (PTSD): Psychiatric entity introduced in the nosography in 1980 to qualify the consequences of traumatic events.

Revenu minimum d'insertion (RMI): Minimum Guaranteed Income. Adopted in 1988 under the French Socialist government, it granted the right to a universal minimum income.

Service oecuménique d'entraide (CIMADE): Ecumenical Service for Solidarity. Previously Comité inter-mouvements pour les evacués. French charity founded by the Protestant Church in 1939 that assists immigrants in prison and detention centers.

Trade-Related Aspects of Intellectual Property Rights Agreement (TRIPS): International agreement established by the World Trade Organization and providing standards for the regulation of intellectual property.

Treatment Action Campaign (TAC): South African advocacy organization founded in 1998, promoting access to antiretroviral drugs.

United Nations High Commission for Refugees (UNHCR): United Nations agency established in 1950 with the mandate of coordinating actions to protect refugees.

Note: Small capitals are used when the acronym is pronounced as a noun (COMEDE, OFPRA), and regular capitals when letters are pronounced separately (MSF, UNHCR).

Bibliography

Adorno, Theodor W. 2005. *Negative Dialectics*. New York: Continuum [1st German edition, 1966].

Affichard, Joëlle, and de Foucauld, Jean-Baptiste (eds.). 1992. *Justice sociale et inégalités*. Paris: Éditions Esprit.

Agamben, Giorgio. 1998. *Homo Sacer: Sovereign Power and Bare Life*. Stanford, CA: Stanford University Press [1st Italian edition, 1995].

———. 1999. *Remnants of Auschwitz: The Witness and the Archive*. New York: Zone Books [1st Italian edition, 1998].

———. 2005. *State of Exception*. Chicago: University of Chicago Press [1st Italian edition, 2003].

———. 2009. *The Signature of All Things: On Method*. New York: Zone Books.

Agier, Michel. 2004. "Le camp des vulnérables: Les réfugiés face à leur citoyenneté niée." *Les Temps modernes* 59 (627): 120–137.

Althusser, Louis. 1971. "Ideology and Ideological State Apparatuses." In *Lenin and Philosophy and Other Essays*. New York: Monthly Review Press [1st French edition, 1970].

Arendt, Hannah. 1951. *The Origins of Totalitarianism*. New York: Harcourt.

———. 1958. *The Human Condition*. Chicago: University of Chicago Press.

———. 1962. *On Revolution*. New York: Penguin.

———. 1968. "Introduction. Walter Benjamin: 1892–1940." In *Illuminations*, Walter Benjamin, 1–55. New York: Harcourt, Brace and World.

Ariès, Philippe. 1962. *Centuries of Childhood: A Social History of Family Life*. New York: Vintage Books [1st French edition, 1960].

Armitage, John. 2002. "State of Emergency: An Introduction." *Theory, Culture and Society* 19 (4): 27–38.

Asad, Talal. 1997. "On Torture, or Cruel, Inhuman, and Degrading Treatment." In *Social Suffering*, ed. Arthur Kleinman, Veena Das, and Margaret Lock, 285–308. Berkeley: University of California Press.

Assayag, Jackie. 2004. "Leçons de ténèbres: Violence, terreur, genocides." *Les Temps modernes* 59 (626): 275–304.

Astier, Isabelle. 1998. "RMI: Du travail social à une politique des individus." *Esprit* (March–April): 142–157.

Austin, John Langshaw. 1962. *How to Do Things with Words.* London: Clarendon.

Bachmann, Christian, and Le Guennec, Nicole. 1997. *Violences urbaines: Ascension et chute des classes moyennes à travers cinquante ans de politique de la ville.* Paris: Albin Michel.

Barnett, Michael. 2011. *Empire of Humanity: A History of Humanitarianism.* Ithaca, NY: Cornell University Press.

Bass, Gary. 2008. *Freedom's Battle: The Origins of Humanitarian Intervention.* New York: Knopf.

Bauman, Zygmunt. 1998. *Globalization: The Human Consequences.* Cambridge: Polity.

———. 2004. *Wasted Lives: Modernity and Its Outcasts.* Cambridge: Polity.

Becker, Howard. 1963. *Outsiders: Studies in the Sociology of Deviance.* New York: Free Press.

Bénatouïl, Thomas. 1999. "Critique et pragmatique en sociologie: Quelques principes de lecture." *Annales: Histoire, Sciences sociales* 54 (2): 281–317.

Benjamin, Walter. 1968. "Theses on the Philosophy of History." In *Illuminations,* 255–266. New York: Harcourt [1st American edition, 1942].

———. 1978. "Critique of Violence." In *Reflections,* 277–300. New York: Harcourt [1st German edition, 1921].

Benthall, Jonathan. 2008. *Returning to Religion: Why a Secular Age Is Haunted by Faith.* London: Tauris.

Benveniste, Émile. 1973. *Indo-European Language and Society.* London: Faber [1st French edition, 1969].

Berger, Nathalie. 2000. *La politique européenne d'asile et d'immigration: Enjeux et perspectives.* Bruxelles: Bruylant.

Bergeron, Henri. 1999. *L'État et la toxicomanie: Histoire d'une singularité française.* Paris: Presses universitaires de France.

Berlant, Lauren (ed.). 2004. *Compassion: The Culture and Politics of an Emotion.* New York: Routledge.

Bernardot, Marc. 2008. *Camps d'étrangers.* Bellecombe-en-Bauges: Éditions du Croquant.

Bibeau, Gilles. 1991. "L'Afrique, terre imaginaire du sida: La subversion du discours scientifique par le jeu des fantasmes." *Anthropologie et Sociétés* 15 (2–3): 125–147.

Bihr, Alain, and Pfefferkorn, Roland. 1999. *Déchiffrer les inégalités.* Paris: Syros [1st French edition, 1995].

Boltanski, Luc. 1999. *Distant Suffering: Morality, Media and Politics.* Cambridge: Cambridge University Press [1st French edition, 1993].

Bornstein, Avram. 2001. "Ethnography and the Politics of Prisoners in Palestine-Israel." *Journal of Contemporary Ethnography* 30 (5): 546–574.

Bourdieu, Pierre (ed.). 1999. *The Weight of the World: Social Suffering in Contemporary Society.* Cambridge: Polity [1st French edition, 1993].

Bourdieu, Pierre, and Wacquant, Loïc. 1992. *An Invitation to Reflexive Sociology.* Chicago: University of Chicago Press.

Bourgois, Philippe. 1995. *In Search of Respect: Selling Crack in El Barrio.* Berkeley: University of California Press.

Bradol, Jean-Hervé. 2003. "Introduction: L'ordre international cannibale et l'action humanitaire." On *À l'ombre des guerres justes: L'ordre international cannibale et l'action humanitaire,* ed. Fabrice Weissman, 13–32. Paris: Flammarion.

Brandt, Allan M. 1985. *No Magic Bullet: A Social History of Venereal Disease in the United States since 1880.* Oxford: Oxford University Press.

Brauman, Rony. 2000. *L'action humanitaire.* Paris: Flammarion [1st French edition, 1995].

Brauman, Rony, and Salignon, Pierre, 2003. "Irak: La posture du missionnaire." In *À l'ombre des guerres justes: L'ordre international cannibale et l'action humanitaire,* ed. Fabrice Weissman, 275–291. Paris: Flammarion.

Bucaille, Laetitia. 2004. *Growing Up Palestinian: Israeli Occupation and the Intifada Generation.* Princeton, NJ: Princeton University Press [1st French edition, 2002].

Butchart, Alexander. 1998. *The Anatomy of Power: European Constructions of the African Body.* London: Zed Books.

Butler, Judith. 1997. *The Psychic Life of Power: Theories in Subjection.* Stanford, CA: Stanford University Press.

———. 2004. *Precarious Life: The Powers of Mourning and Violence.* London: Verso.

Calabresi, Guido, and Bobbitt, Philip. 1978. *Tragic Choices.* New York: Norton.

Caruth, Cathy (ed.). 1995. *Trauma: Explorations in Memory.* Baltimore: Johns Hopkins University Press.

Castel, Robert. 1981. *La gestion des risques: De l'anti-psychiatrie à l'après-psychanalyse.* Paris: Éditions de Minuit.

———. 1995. *Les métamorphoses de la question sociale: Une chronique du salariat.* Paris: Fayard.

Césaire, Aimé. 1980. *Une tempête. D'après La Tempête de Shakespeare: Adaptation pour un théâtre nègre.* Paris: Le Seuil [1st French edition, 1969].

Cette France-là. 2009. Volume 1: 06/05/2007–30/06/2008. Paris: Association Cette France-là.

———. 2010. Volume 2: 01/07/2008–30/06/2009. Paris: Association Cette France-là.

Chaumont, Jean-Michel. 1997. *La concurrence des victimes: Génocide, identité, reconnaissance.* Paris: La Découverte.

Clastres, Pierre. 1977. *Society against the State.* Oxford: Mole Editions [1st French edition, 1974].

Clochard, Olivier, Decourcelle, Antoine, and Intrand, Chloé. 2003. "Zones d'attente et demande d'asile à la frontière: Le renforcement des contrôles migratoires?" *Revue européenne des migrations internationales* 19 (2): 157–189.

Clochard, Olivier, Gastaut, Yvan, and Schor, Ralph. 2004. "Les camps d'étrangers depuis 1938: Continuité et adaptations." *Revue européenne des migrations internationales* 20 (2): 57–87.

Collins, John. 2004. *Occupied by Memory: The Intifada Generation and the Palestinian State of Emergency.* New York: New York University Press.

Collovald, Annie. 2001. "De la défense des 'pauvres nécessiteux' à l'humanitaire expert: Reconversion et métamorphoses d'une cause politique." *Politix* 14 (56): 135–161.

Coronil, Fernando. 1997. *The Magical State: Nature, Money, and Modernity in Venezuela.* Chicago: University of Chicago Press.

Dalgalarrondo, Sébastien, and Urfalino, Philippe. 2000. "Choix tragique, controverse et décision publique: Le cas du tirage au sort des malades du sida." *Revue française de sociologie* 41 (1): 119–157.

Daniel, Valentine E., and Knudsen, John Chr. (eds.). 1995. *Mistrusting Refugees.* Berkeley: University of California Press.

Das, Veena. 1997. "Language and Body: Transactions in the Construction of Pain." In *Social Suffering,* ed. Arthur Kleinman, Veena Das, and Margaret Lock, 67–91. Berkeley: University of California Press.

———. 2007. *Life and Words: Violence and the Descent into the Ordinary.* Berkeley: University of California Press.

Das, Veena, and Kleinman, Arthur. 2001. "Introduction." In *Remaking a World: Violence, Social Suffering, and Recovery,* ed. Veena Das, Arthur Kleinman, Margaret Lock, Mamphela Ramphele, and Pamela Reynolds, 1–30. Berkeley: University of California Press.

Das, Veena, Kleinman, Arthur, Lock, Margaret, Ramphele, Mamphela, and Reynolds, Pamela (eds.). 2001. *Remaking a World: Violence, Social Suffering, and Recovery.* Berkeley: University of California Press.

Das, Veena, Kleinman, Arthur, Ramphele, Mamphela, and Reynolds, Pamela (eds.). 2000. *Violence and Subjectivity.* Berkeley: University of California Press.

Dauvin, Pascal, and Siméant, Johanna (eds.). 2002. *Le travail humanitaire: Les acteurs des ONG, du siège au terrain.* Paris: Presses de la Fondation de Sciences politiques.

Dejours, Christophe. 1998. *Souffrance en France: La banalisation de l'injustice sociale.* Paris: Le Seuil.

Deleuze, Gilles. 2003. *Nietzsche and Philosophy.* London: Athlone [1st French edition, 1962].

Demazière, Didier, and Pignoni, Maria-Teresa. 1999. *Chômeurs. Du silence à la révolte: Sociologie d'une vie collective.* Paris: Hachette littératures.

Derrida, Jacques. 2000. *Of Hospitality: Anne Dufourmantelle Invites Jacques Derrida to Respond.* Stanford, CA: Stanford University Press [1st French edition, 1997].

Descombes, Vincent. 2008. "Quand la mauvaise critique chasse la bonne . . ." *Tracés: Revue de Sciences humaines,* Special Issue 8: "Présent et futurs de la critique": 45–69.

De Waal, Alex. 2005. *Famine That Kills: Darfur, Sudan.* Oxford: Oxford University Press [1st English edition, 1989].

Didier, Élisabeth. 1992. "Torture et mythe de la preuve." *Plein droit: La revue du GISTI,* nos. 18–19 (October): 64–69.

Dodier, Nicolas. 2003. *Leçons politiques de l'épidémie de sida.* Paris: Éditions de l'École des Hautes Études en Sciences Sociales.

Donzelot, Jacques, and Roman, Joël. 1991. "Le déplacement de la question sociale." In *Face à l'exclusion: Le modèle français,* ed. Jacques Donzelot. Paris, Éditions Esprit.

Dorlin, Elsa. 2006. *La matrice de la race: Généalogie sexuelle et coloniale de la nation française.* Paris: La Découverte.

Dozon, Jean-Pierre, and Fassin, Didier. 1989. "Raison épidémiologique et raisons d'Etat: Les enjeux socio-politiques du sida en Afrique." *Sciences Sociales et Santé* 7 (1): 21–36.

Drescher, Seymour. 2009. *Abolition: A History of Slavery and Antislavery.* Cambridge: Cambridge University Press.

Duffield, Mark. 2001. *Global Governance and the New Wars: The Merging of Development and Security.* London: Zed Books.

Duprat, Catherine. 1993. *"Pour l'amour de l'humanité": Le temps des philanthropes. Volume 1: La philanthropie parisienne des Lumières à la monarchie de Juillet.* Paris: Éditions du CTHS.

Durkheim, Émile. 1974 *Sociology and Philosophy.* New York: Free Press.

Ehrenberg, Alain. 1998. *La fatigue d'être soi: Dépression et société,* Paris: Odile Jacob.

———. 2004. "Les changements de la relation normal-pathologique: À propos de la souffrance psychique et de la santé mentale." *Esprit* (May): 133–156.

Eliacheff, Caroline, and Soulez-Larivière, Daniel. 2006. *Le temps des victimes.* Paris: Albin Michel.

Elias, Norbert. 1987. *Involvement and Detachment.* Oxford: Blackwell [1st German edition, 1956].

Elster, Jon. 1992. *Local Justice: How Institutions Allocate Scarce Goods and Necessary Burdens.* New York: Russell Sage Foundation.

Elster, Jon, and Herpin, Nicolas (eds.). 1992. *Éthique des choix médicaux.* Arles: Actes sud.

Erner, Guillaume. 2006. *La société des victimes.* Paris: La Découverte.

Farmer, Paul. 1992. *AIDS and Accusation: Haiti and the Geography of Blame.* Berkeley: University of California Press.

Fassin, Didier. 1996. "Exclusion, *underclass, marginalidad:* Figures contemporaines de la pauvreté urbaine en France, aux États-Unis et en Amérique latine." *Revue française de sociologie* 37 (1): 37–75.

———. 1999. "L'ethnopsychiatrie et ses réseaux: Une influence qui grandit." *Genèses: Sciences sociales et histoire* 35: 146–171.

———. 2000. "La supplique: Stratégies rhétoriques et constructions identitaires dans les demandes d'aide d'urgence." *Annales: Histoire, Sciences sociales* 55 (5): 955–981.

———. 2001. "Une double peine: La condition sociale des immigrés malades du sida." *L'Homme* 160: 137–162.

———. 2004a. "La cause des victimes." *Les Temps modernes* 59 (627): 73–91.

———. 2004b. *Des maux indicibles: Sociologie des lieux d'écoute.* Paris: La Découverte.

———. 2004c. "Et la souffrance devint sociale: De l'anthropologie médicale à une anthropologie des afflictions." *Critique* 60 (680–681): 16–29.

———. 2005. "L'ordre moral du monde: Essai d'anthropologie de l'intolérable." In *Les constructions de l'intolérable: Études d'anthropologie et d'histoire sur les frontières de l'espace moral,* ed. Didier Fassin and Patrice Bourdelais, 17–50. Paris: La Découverte.

———. 2006. "La biopolitique n'est pas la politique de la vie." *Sociologie et sociétés* 38 (2): 35–48.

———. 2007a. "Humanitarianism, a Nongovernmental Government." In *Nongovernmental Politics,* ed. Michel Feher, 149–159. New York: Zone Books.

———. 2007b. *When Bodies Remember: Experience and Politics of AIDS in South Africa.* Berkeley: University of California Press [1st French edition, 2006].

———. 2009a. "Another Politics of Life Is Possible." *Theory, Culture and Society* 26 (5): 44–60.

———. 2009b. "Les économies morales revisitées." *Annales: Histoire, Sciences sociales* 64 (6): 1237–1266.

——— (ed.). 2010a. *Les nouvelles frontières de la société française.* Paris: La Découverte.

———. 2010b. "Ethics of Survival: A Democratic Approach to the Politics of Life." *Humanity: An International Journal of Human Rights, Humanitarianism, and Development* 1 (1): 81–95.

———. 2011a. "Ethnopsychiatry and the Postcolonial Encounter: A French Psychopolitics of Otherness." In *Unconscious Dominions: Psychoanalysis, Colonial Trauma and Global Sovereignties,* ed. Warwick Anderson, Deborah Jenson, and Richard Keller, 224–245. Durham, NC: Duke University Press.

———. 2011b. "*Noli Me Tangere:* The Moral Untouchability of Humanitarianism." In *Forces of Compassion: Humanitarianism between Ethics and Politics,* ed. Peter Redfield and Eric Bornstein, 35–52. Santa Fe: School of Advanced Research Press.

———. In press. "Adventures of South African Nevirapine: The Political Biography of a Magic Bullet." In *Changing States of Science: Ethnographic and Historical Perspectives on Government, Citizenship and Medical Research in Contemporary Africa,* ed. Paul Wenzel Geissler. Durham, NC: Duke University Press.

Fassin, Didier, and Bensa, Alban. 2008. *Les politiques de l'enquête: Épreuves ethnographiques*. Paris: La Découverte.

Fassin, Didier, and Defossez, Anne-Claire. 1992. "Une liaison dangereuse: Sciences sociales et santé publique dans les programmes de réduction de la mortalité maternelle en Équateur." *Cahiers des sciences humaines (Orstom)* 28 (1): 23–36.

Fassin, Didier, Le Marcis, Frédéric, and Lethata, Todd. 2008. "Life and Times of Magda A.: Telling a Story of Violence in South Africa." *Current Anthropology* 49 (2): 225–246.

Fassin, Didier, and Morice, Alain. 2001. "Les épreuves de l'irrégularité: Les sans-papiers, entre déni d'existence et reconquête d'un statut." *Exclusions au cœur de la cité*, ed. Dominique Schnapper, 260–309. Paris: Anthropos.

Fassin, Didier, Morice, Alain, and Quiminal, Catherine (eds.). 1997. *Les lois de l'inhospitalité: Les politiques de l'immigration à l'épreuve des sans-papiers*. Paris: La Découverte.

Fassin, Didier, and Pandolfi, Mariella (eds.). 2010. *Contemporary States of Emergency: The Politics of Military and Humanitarian Intervention*. New York: Zone Books.

Fassin, Didier, and Rechtman, Richard. 2009. *The Empire of Trauma: An Inquiry into the Condition of Victimhood*. Princeton, NJ: Princeton University Press [1st French edition, 2007].

Feldman, Allen. 1994. "On Cultural Anesthesia: From Desert Storm to Rodney King." *American Ethnologist* 21 (2): 404–418.

Felman, Shoshana. 1999. "Benjamin's Silence." *Critical Inquiry* 25 (2): 201–234.

Ferguson, James G. 2002. "Of Mimicry and Membership: Africans and the 'New World Society.'" *Cultural Anthropology* 17 (4): 551–569.

Fothergill, Alice. 2003. "The Stigma of Charity: Gender, Class, and Disaster Assistance." *Sociological Quarterly* 44 (4): 659–680.

Foucault, Michel. 1977. *Discipline and Punish: The Birth of the Prison*. London: Allen Lane [1st French edition, 1975].

———. 1979. *The History of Sexuality, Volume 1: The Will to Know*. London: Allen Lane [1st French edition, 1976].

———. 1989. *Résumé des Cours au Collège de France 1972–1980*. Paris: Julliard.

———. 1994. *Dits et écrits: 1954–1988, Volume IV*. Paris: Gallimard.

———. 2003. "What Is Enlightenment?" In *The Foucault Reader*, ed. Paul Rabinow and Nikolas Rose. New York: New Press.

———. 2007. *Security, Territory, Population: Lectures at the Collège de France 1977–1978*. New York: Picador [1st French edition, 2004].

Freyssinet, Jacques. 2004. *Le chômage*. Paris: La Découverte [1st French edition, 1984].

Fukuyama, Francis. 1992. *The End of History and the Last Man*. New York: Free Press.

Garfinkel, Harold. 1984. *Studies in Ethnomethodology*. Cambridge: Polity [1st American edition, 1967].

Gauchet, Marcel. 1999. *The Disenchantment of the World: A Political History of Religion*. Princeton, NJ: Princeton University Press [1st French edition, 1985].

Gauléjac, Vincent de. 1996. *Les sources de la honte*. Paris: Desclée de Brouwer.

Geremek, Bronislaw (ed.). 1980. *Inutiles au monde: Truands et misérables dans l'Europe moderne (1350–1600)*. Paris: Gallimard-Julliard.

Gilman, Sander L. 1985. *Difference and Pathology: Stereotypes of Sexuality, Race and Madness*. New York: Cornell University Press.

Godelier, Maurice. 1986. *The Making of Great Men: Male Domination and Power among the New Guinea Baruya*. Cambridge: Cambridge University Press [1st French edition, 1982].

Goffman, Erving. 1963. *Stigma: Notes on the Management of Spoiled Identity*. New York: Schuster.

Good, Anthony. 2007. *Anthropology and Expertise in the Asylum Courts*. Oxford: Routledge.

Graham, Mark. 2003. "Emotional Bureaucracies: Emotions, Civil Servants, and Immigrants in the Swedish Welfare State." *Ethos* 30 (3): 199–226.

Hacking, Ian. 1995. *Rewriting the Soul: Multiple Personality and the Sciences of Memory*. Princeton, NJ: Princeton University Press.

———. 1999. *Mad Travellers: Reflections on the Reality of Transient Mental Illnesses*. London: Free Association Books.

Halluin, Estelle d'. 2008. *Les épreuves du droit d'asile: De la politique du soupçon à la reconnaissance des réfugiés*. PhD diss., École des Hautes Études en Sciences Sociales, Paris.

Hartog, François. 2005. "Le témoin et l'historien." In *Évidence de l'histoire*, 191–214. Paris: Éditions de l'École des Hautes Études en Sciences Sociales.

Heyman, Josiah McC. 1998, *Finding a Moral Heart for U.S. Immigration Policy: An Anthropological Perspective*. American Ethnological Society Monograph Series, no 7.

Hoffman, Susanna M., and Oliver-Smith, Anthony (eds.). 2002. *Catastrophe and Culture: The Anthropology of Disaster*. Santa Fe: School of American Research Press.

Hoffmann, Stanley (ed.). 1996. *The Ethics and Politics of Humanitarian Intervention*. Notre Dame, IN: University of Notre Dame Press.

Horton, Richard. 1996. "Truth and Heresy about AIDS." *New York Review of Books* 43 (9).

Howell, Signe (ed.). 1997. *The Ethnography of Moralities*. London: Routledge.

Hyndman, Jennifer. 2000. *Managing Displacement: Refugees and the Politics of Humanitarianism*. Minneapolis: University of Minnesota Press.

Ignatieff, Michael. 2000. "The New American Way of War." *New York Review of Books* 47 (12).

James, Erica Caple. 2010. *Democratic Insecurities: Violence, Trauma, and Intervention in Haiti*. Berkeley: University of California Press.

Jewkes, Rachel, and Abrahams, Naeemah. 2002. "The Epidemiology of Rape and Sexual Coercion in South Africa: An Overview." *Social Science and Medicine* 55 (7): 1231–1244.

Jewkes, Rachel, Abrahams, Naeemah, and Mvo, Zodumo. 1998. "Why Do Nurses Abuse Patients? Reflections from South African Obstetric Services." *Social Science and Medicine* 47 (11): 1781–1795.

Joubert, Michel, Bertolotto, Fernando, and Bouhnik, Patricia (eds.). 1993. *Quartier, démocratie et santé: Mode de vie et santé des familles et des jeunes sur un quartier de banlieue, une recherche-action en santé communautaire.* Paris: L'Harmattan.

Kantorowicz, Ernst. 1957. *The King's Two Bodies: A Study in Medieval Political Theology.* Princeton, NJ: Princeton University Press.

Kleinman, Arthur. 1988. *The Illness Narratives: Suffering, Healing and the Human Condition.* New York: Basic Books.

Kleinman, Arthur, Das, Veena, and Lock, Margaret (eds.). 1997. *Social Suffering.* Berkeley: University of California Press.

Koselleck, Reinhart. 1985. *Futures Past: On the Semantics of Historical Time.* Cambridge, MA: MIT Press [1st German edition, 1979].

Laacher, Smaïn. 2002. *Après Sangatte: Nouvelles immigrations, nouveaux enjeux.* Paris: La Dispute.

Laé, Jean-François. 1996. *L'instance de la plainte: Une histoire politique et juridique de la souffrance.* Paris: Descartes et Cie.

Lalande, André. 1993. *Vocabulaire technique et critique de la philosophie.* 2 vols. Paris: Presses universitaires de France [1st French edition, 1926].

Lazarsfeld, Paul Felix. 1981. *Marienthal: The Sociography of an Unemployed Community,* with Marie Jahoda and Hans Zeisel [1st German edition, 1932].

Le Cour Grandmaison, Olivier. 2005. *Coloniser, exterminer: Sur la guerre et l'État colonial.* Paris: Fayard.

Lefort, Claude. 1986. *Essais sur le politique: XIXe–XXe siècles.* Paris: Le Seuil.

Lenoir, René. 1974. *Les exclus: Un Français sur dix.* Paris: Le Seuil.

Levi, Primo. 1960. *If This Is a Man.* New York: Orion [1st Italian edition, 1958].

Levinas, Emmanuel. 1969. *Totality and Infinity: An Essay on Exteriority.* The Hague: Martinus Nijhoff [1st French edition, 1961].

Leys, Ruth. 2000. *Trauma: A Genealogy.* Chicago: University of Chicago Press.

Lhuillier, Dominique. 2007. *Clinique du travail.* Paris: Erès.

Liagre, Romain, and Dumont, Frédéric. 2005. "Sangatte: Vie et mort d'un centre de 'réfugiés.'" *Annales de géographie* 641: 93–112.

Lock, Margaret. 1997. "Displacing Suffering: The Reconstruction of Death in North America and Japan." In *Social Suffering,* ed. Arthur Kleinman, Veena Das, and Margaret Lock, 207–244. Berkeley: University of California Press.

Lovell, Anne. 1998. "Sida-toxicomanie, un objet hybride de la nouvelle santé publique à Marseille." In *Les figures urbaines de la santé publique: Enquête sur des expériences locales,* ed. Didier Fassin, 203–238. Paris: La Découverte.

MacFarlane, S. Neil. 1999. "Humanitarian Action and Conflict." *International Journal* 54 (4): 537–561.

Maigret, Éric. 2002. "Pierre Bourdieu, la culture populaire et le long remords de la sociologie de la distinction culturelle." *Esprit* (March): 170–178.

Makaremi, Chowra. 2009. "Violence et refoulement dans la zone d'attente de Roissy-CDG." In *Enfermés dehors: Enquêtes sur le confinement des étrangers*, ed. Carolina Kobelinsky and Chowra Makaremi, 41–62. Bellecombe-en-Bauges: Éditions du Croquant.

Malkki, Liisa H. 1995. *Purity and Exile: Violence, Memory, and National Cosmology among Hutu Refugees in Tanzania*. Chicago: University of Chicago Press.

———. 1996. "Speechless Emissaries: Refugees, Humanitarianism, and Dehistoricization." *Cultural Anthropology* 11 (3): 377–404.

Marrus, Michael R. 1985. *The Unwanted: European Refugees in the Twentieth Century*. Oxford: Oxford University Press.

Messu, Michel. 1991. *Les assistés sociaux: Analyse identitaire d'un groupe social*. Toulouse: Privat.

Méténier, Isabelle. 2010. *Crise au travail et souffrance personnelle*. Paris: Albin Michel.

Mignolo, Walter D. 2000. *Local Histories/Global Designs: Coloniality, Subaltern Knowledges, and Border Thinking*. Princeton, NJ: Princeton University Press.

Minear, Larry, and Weiss, Thomas G. 1992. "Groping and Coping in the Gulf Crisis: Discerning the Shape of a New Humanitarian Order." *World Policy Journal* 9 (4): 755–777.

Morris, David B. 1991. *The Culture of Pain*. Berkeley: University of California Press.

Moyn, Samuel. 2010. *The Last Utopia: Human Rights in History*. Cambridge, MA: Belknap Press of Harvard University Press.

Nahoum-Grappe, Véronique. 1996. "L'usage politique de la cruauté: L'épuration ethnique (ex-Yougolsavie 1991–1995)." In *De la violence*, ed. Françoise Héritier, 273–323. Paris: Odile Jacob.

Nietzsche, Friedrich. 1986. *Human, All Too Human: A Book for Free Spirits*. Cambridge: Cambridge University Press [1st German edition, 1878].

Noiriel, Gérard. 1991. *La tyrannie du national: Le droit d'asile en Europe 1793–1993*. Paris: Calmann-Lévy.

Nussbaum, Martha C. 2001. *Upheavals of Thought: The Intelligence of Emotions*. Cambridge: Cambridge University Press.

Orford, Anne. 1999. "Muscular Humanitarianism: Reading the Narratives of the New Interventionism." *European Journal of International Law* 10 (4): 679–711.

Pandolfi, Mariella. 2008. "Laboratory of Intervention: The Humanitarian Governance of the Postcommunist Balkan Territories." In *Postcolonial Disor-*

ders, ed. Mary-Jo Del Vecchio Good, Sandra Teresa Hyde, Sarah Pinto, and Byron Good, 157–186. Berkeley: University of California Press.

———. 2010. "From Paradox to Paradigm: The Permanent State of Emergency in the Balkans." In *Contemporary States of Emergency: The Politics of Military and Humanitarian Intervention*, ed. Didier Fassin and Mariella Pandolfi, 153–172. New York: Zone Books.

Paugam, Serge. 1991. *La disqualification sociale: Essai sur la nouvelle pauvreté*. Paris: Presses universitaires de France.

———. 1993. *La société française et ses pauvres: L'expérience du revenu minimum d'insertion*. Paris: Presses universitaires de France.

Peschanski, Denis. 2002. *La France des camps: L'internement, 1938–1946*. Paris: Gallimard.

Peteet, Julie. 1994. "Male Gender and Rituals of Resistance in the Palestinian *Intifada*: A Cultural Politics of Violence." *American Ethnologist* 21 (1): 31–49.

Petryna, Adriana. 2002. *Life Exposed: Biological Citizens after Chernobyl*. Princeton, NJ: Princeton University Press.

Phillips, Alton. 2010. "The Life Course of Nevirapine and the Culture of Response to the Global HIV and AIDS Pandemic: Travelling in an Emergency." In *The Fourth Wave: Violence, Gender, Culture and HIV in the 21st Century*, ed. Jennifer Klot and Vinh-Kim Nguyen. New York: Social Science Research Council

Piven, Frances Fox, and Cloward, Richard A. 1993. *Regulating the Poor: The Functions of Public Welfare*. New York: Vintage Books [1st American edition, 1971].

Pollak, Michael. 1990. *L'expérience concentrationnaire: Essai sur le maintien de l'identité sociale*. Paris: Métailié.

Porras Ponceleón, Temir. 2000. "Venezuela: Les ambiguïtés de la 'révolution bolivarienne.'" *Problèmes d'Amérique latine* (39): 3–23.

Pugh, Michael. 1998. "Military Intervention and Humanitarian Action: Trends and Issues." *Disasters* 22 (4): 339–351.

Pupavac, Vanessa. 2001. "Therapeutic Governance: Psycho-social Intervention and Trauma Risk Management." *Disasters* 25 (4): 358–372.

Rancière, Jacques. 2006. *Hatred of Democracy*. London: Verso [1st French edition, 2005].

Rawls, John. 2000. *Lectures on the History of Moral Philosophy*. Cambridge, MA: Harvard University Press.

Razack, Sherene H. 2004. *Dark Threats and White Knights: The Somalia Affair, Peacekeeping, and the New Imperialism*. Toronto: University of Toronto Press.

Redfield, Peter. 2005. "Doctors, Borders and Life in Crisis." *Cultural Anthropology* 20 (3): 328–361.

———. 2010. "The Verge of Crisis: Doctors without Borders in Uganda." In *Contemporary States of Emergency: The Politics of Military and*

Humanitarian Intervention, ed. Didier Fassin and Mariella Pandolfi, 173–195. New York: Zone Books.

Renault, Emmanuel. 2008. *Souffrances sociales: Philosophie, psychologie et politique.* Paris: La Découverte.

Revault d'Allonnes, Myriam. 2008. *L'homme compassionnel.* Paris: Le Seuil.

Rey, Alain (ed.). 2006. *Dictionnaire historique de la langue française.* Paris: Le Robert [1st French edition, 1992].

Reynolds, Pamela. 2000. "The Ground of All Making: State Violence, the Family and Political Activists." In *Violence and Subjectivity,* ed. Veena Das, Arthur Kleinman, Mamphela Ramphele, and Pamela Reynolds, 141–170. Berkeley: University of California Press.

Ricoeur, Paul. 1986. *Lectures on Ideology and Utopia.* New York: Columbia University Press.

Robert, Philippe. 2002. *L'insécurité en France.* Paris: La Découverte.

Rodier, Claire, and Terray, Emmanuel (eds.). 2008. *Immigration: Fantasmes et réalités. Pour une alternative à la fermeture des frontières.* Paris: La Découverte.

Rosanvallon, Pierre. 1995. *La nouvelle question sociale: Repenser l'État-providence.* Paris: Le Seuil.

Rose, Nikolas. 1989. *Governing the Soul: The Shaping of the Private Self.* London: Free Association Books.

Royer, Solenn de. 2002. "L'épopée des Kurdes de l'East Sea: Drame en cinq actes." *Confluences Méditerranée* 42: 13–21.

Saint Augustine. 1991. *Confessions.* Oxford: Oxford World's Classics.

Sayad, Abdelmalek. 2004. *The Suffering of the Immigrant.* Cambridge: Polity [1st French edition, 1999].

Scheper-Hughes, Nancy. 1992. *Death without Weeping: The Violence of Everyday Life in Brazil.* Berkeley: University of California Press.

Scheper-Hughes, Nancy, and Bourgois, Philippe (eds.). 2004. *Violence in War and Peace: An Anthology.* Malden, MA: Blackwell.

Scheper-Hughes, Nancy, and Sargent, Carolyn (eds.). 1998. *Small Wars: The Cultural Politics of Childhood.* Berkeley: University of California Press.

Schneider, Joseph W. 1985. "Social Problems Theory: The Constructionist View." *Annual Review of Sociology* (11): 209–229.

Schmitt, Carl. 1985. *Political Theology: Four Chapters on the Concept of Sovereignty.* Chicago: University of Chicago Press [1st German edition, 1922].

Schwartz, Olivier. 1993. "L'empirisme irréductible" [postface]. In *Le hobo: Sociologie du sans-abri,* Nels Anderson, 266–308. Paris: Nathan.

Scott, James C. 1976. *The Moral Economy of the Peasant: Rebellion and Subsistence in Southeast Asia.* New Haven: Yale University Press.

Sennett, Richard. 1977. *The Fall of Public Man.* Cambridge: Cambridge University Press.

Simmel, Georg. 1998. *Les pauvres.* Paris: Presses universitaires de France [1st German edition, 1908].

Slim, Hugo. 2002. "Not Philanthropy but Rights: The Proper Politicisation of Humanitarian Philosophy." *International Journal of Human Rights* 6 (2): 1–22.

Smith, Adam. 1759. *The Theory of Moral Sentiments*. London: A. Millar, A. Kincaid and J. Bell.

Spencer, Jonathan. 2000. "On Not Becoming a 'Terrorist': Problems of Memory, Agency, and Community in the Sri Lankan Conflict." In *Violence and Subjectivity*, ed. Veena Das, Arthur Kleinman, Mamphela Ramphele, and Pamela Reynolds, 120–140. Berkeley: University of California Press.

Steinmetz, George. 2003. "The State of Emergency and the Revival of American Imperialism: Toward an Authoritarian Post-Fordism." *Public Culture* 15 (2): 323–345.

Stoléru, Lionel. 1977. *Vaincre la pauvreté dans les pays riches*. Paris: Flammarion.

Taussig, Michael. 1992. *The Nervous System*. London: Routledge.

Taylor, Charles. 1989. *Sources of the Self: The Making of the Modern Identity*. Cambridge, MA: Harvard University Press.

———. 2004. *Modern Social Imaginaries*. Durham, NC: Duke University Press.

Terry, Fiona. 2002. *Condemned to Repeat? The Paradox of Humanitarian Action*. Ithaca, NY: Cornell University Press.

Thénault, Sylvie. 2007. "L'état d'urgence (1955–2005): De l'Algérie coloniale à la France contemporaine: Destin d'une loi." *Le Mouvement Social* (218): 63–78.

Thomas, Hélène. 1997. *La production des exclus: Politiques sociales et processus de désocialisation socio-politique*. Paris: Presses universitaires de France.

Thompson, Edward Palmer. 1971. "The Moral Economy of the English Crowd in the Eighteenth Century." *Past and Present* 50 (1): 76–136.

Touraine, Alain. 1992. "Inégalités de la société industrielle, exclusion du marché." In *Justice sociale et inégalités*, ed. Joëlle Affichard and Jean-Baptiste de Foucauld, 163–174. Paris: Éditions Esprit.

Turner, Bryan S. 2002. "Sovereignty and Emergency: Political Theology, Islam and American Conservatism." *Theory, Culture and Society* 19 (4): 103–119.

Vallaeys, Anne. 2004. *Médecins Sans Frontières: La biographie*. Paris: Fayard.

Vásquez, Paula. 2010. *Poder y catástrofe: Venezuela bajo la Tragedia de 1999*. Caracas: Taurus, Santillana.

Veïsse, Arnaud. 2003. "Les lésions dangereuses." *Plein droit: La revue du GISTI* (56): 32–35.

Viet, Vincent. 1998. *La France immigrée: Construction d'une politique, 1914–1997*. Paris: Fayard.

Vogler, Candace, and Markell, Patchen. 2003. "Introduction: Violence, Redemption, and the Liberal Imagination." *Public Culture* 15 (1): 1–10.

Wahnich, Sophie. 1997. *L'impossible citoyen: L'étranger dans le discours de la Révolution française*. Paris: Albin Michel.

Walzer, Michael. 1988. *The Company of Critics: Social Criticism and Political Commitment in the Twentieth Century.* New York: Basic Books.

Weber, Max. 2008. *Complete Writings on Academic and Political Vocations.* New York: Algora.

Weber, Olivier. 1995. *French doctors: Les vingt-cinq ans d'épopée des hommes et des femmes qui ont inventé la médecine humanitaire.* Paris: Robert Laffont.

Weil, Patrick. 1991. *La France et ses étrangers: L'aventure d'une politique de l'immigration de 1938 à nos jours.* Paris: Gallimard.

Wheeler, Nicholas J. 2000. *Saving Strangers: Humanitarian Intervention in International Society.* Oxford: Oxford University Press.

Whiteside, Alan, and Sunter, Clem. 2000. *AIDS: The Challenge for South Africa.* Cape Town: Human and Rousseau-Tafelberg.

Wieviorka, Annette. 2006. *The Era of the Victim.* Ithaca, NY: Cornell University Press [1st French edition, 1998].

Wittgenstein, Ludwig. 1922. *Tractatus logico-philosophicus.* London: Routledge [1st German edition, 1921].

———. 2004. *Philosophical Investigations.* Oxford: Blackwell [1st German edition, 1953].

Woodward, Susan L. 2001. "Humanitarian War: A New Consensus?" *Disasters* 25 (4): 331–344.

Young, Allan. 1995. *The Harmony of Illusions: Inventing Post-Traumatic Stress Disorder.* Princeton, NJ: Princeton University Press.

Zago, Angela. 1998. *La rebelión de los ángeles: Reportaje. Los documentos del movimiento,* Caracas: Warp Ediciones.

Zemon Davis, Natalie. 1987. *Fiction in the Archives: Pardon Tales and Their Tellers in Sixteenth-Century France.* Stanford, CA: Stanford University Press.

Index

Note: Page numbers followed by *f* and *t* indicate figures and tables. Page numbers followed by n or nn indicate notes.

Text: 10/13 Aldus
Display: Aldus
Compositor: Westchester Book Group
Indexer: Judith Kip
Printer and Binder: Sheridan Books, Inc.